HEPATIC ENCEPHALOPATHY:

MANAGEMENT WITH LACTULOSE AND RELATED CARBOHYDRATES

Medi-Ed Press
Post Office Box 957, East Lansing, Michigan 48826-0957

Library of Congress Cataloging-in-Publication Data

Hepatic encephalopathy.

Includes bibliographies and index.
1. Hepatic encephalopathy--Treatment. 2. Lactulose--Therapeutic use. 3. Lactitol--Therapeutic use. 4. Lactose--Therapeutic use. I. Conn, Harold O., 1925- . II. Bircher, J. (Johannes) [DNLM: 1. Disaccharides--therapeutic use. 2. Hepatic Encephalopathy--drug therapy. WI 700 H5256]
RC848.H4H462 1988 616.3'62 88-9372
ISBN 0-936741-02-3

Third Printing

Manufactured in the United States of America

HEPATIC ENCEPHALOPATHY:

MANAGEMENT WITH LACTULOSE AND RELATED CARBOHYDRATES

Edited by

HAROLD O. CONN, M.D.
Professor of Medicine
Yale University School of Medicine
and the
West Haven Veterans Administration Medical Center
West Haven, Connecticut

JOHANNES BIRCHER, M.D.
Professor of Clinical Pharmacology
Georg-August-Universität Göttingen
Göttingen, Federal Republic of Germany

MEDI-ED PRESS
East Lansing, Michigan

CONTENTS

Acknowledgments ix
Contributors xi
Preface xvii

THE DISORDER

1 THE HEPATIC ENCEPHALOPATHIES 3
Harold O. Conn

2 PATHOGENESIS OF HEPATIC ENCEPHALOPATHY 15
Steven Schenker, Charles E. Brady, III

3 NITROGEN METABOLISM IN THE GUT 31
Peter B. Soeters, Paul A.M. van Leeuwen, Charles L.H. van Berlo

4 ENDOCRINE ASPECTS OF AMMONIA AND AMINO ACID METABOLISM 41
G. Marchesini, G.P. Bianchi, G.A. Checchia, M. Zoli

5 GABA IN HUMAN HEPATIC ENCEPHALOPATHY 53
Peter Ferenci

6 HEPATIC ENCEPHALOPATHY AND GABA-ERGIC NEUROTRANSMISSION 61
E. Anthony Jones

ITS THERAPY

7 THE THEORETIC THERAPY OF HEPATIC ENCEPHALOPATHY 83
Harold O. Conn

8 DIETARY MANAGEMENT OF PORTAL-SYSTEMIC ENCEPHALOPATHY 95
Misael Uribe

9 COLONIC METABOLISM OF LACTULOSE IN MAN 113
Ch. Florent

10 BRANCHED-CHAIN AMINO ACIDS IN THE TREATMENT OF HEPATIC ENCEPHALOPATHY 129
L. Siw Eriksson

LACTULOSE

11 THE PHARMACOLOGY OF LACTULOSE 145
Milton M. Lieberthal

12 CLINICAL PHARMACOLOGY OF LACTULOSE 177
Johannes Bircher, Dieter Ullrich

13 CLINICAL TRIALS OF LACTULOSE THERAPY IN HEPATIC ENCEPHALOPATHY 191
Francesco Orlandi, Eugenio Brunelli, Antonio Benedetti, Giampiero Macarri

14 ADVERSE REACTIONS AND SIDE EFFECTS OF LACTULOSE AND RELATED AGENTS 199
Harold O. Conn

15 COMBINATION THERAPY WITH LACTULOSE AND ANTIBIOTICS 207
Fredrick L. Weber, Jr.

SECOND GENERATION “LACTULOSES”

16 LACTITOL: CHEMICAL AND BIOLOGICAL PROPERTIES 221
John A. van Velthuijsen

17 LACTITOL FOR THE TREATMENT OF HEPATIC ENCEPHALOPATHY 245
Marsha Y. Morgan

18 LONG-TERM TREATMENT WITH CRYSTALLINE LACTULOSE 267
F. Rossi-Fanelli, C. Cangiano, F. Ceci, M. Familiari, M. Muscaritoli, O. Riggio, A. Cascino

19 EFFECT OF LACTULOSE AND LACTITOL ON HUMAN INTESTINAL FLORA 271
G. Lebek, M. Luginbühl

20 MANAGEMENT OF PORTAL-SYSTEMIC ENCEPHALOPATHY WITH LACTOSE 283
Misael Uribe

SUNDRY ASPECTS OF LACTULOSE

21 CATHARTIC PROPERTIES OF LACTULOSE 303
John Hamilton, Paul Bass

22 LACTULOSE IN PEDIATRICS 315
Dieter Ullrich, Johannes Bircher

23 EFFECTS OF LACTULOSE ON BILE AND CHOLESTEROL METABOLISM 333
Gianfranco Salvioli, Ruggero Lugli

24 LACTULOSE AND ANTIOXIDANT VITAMINS IN THE PREVENTION OF THE RECURRENCE OF ADENOMATOUS POLYPS 343
Maurizio Ponz de Leon, Paola di Donato, Luca Roncucci, Antonio Manenti, Gianpiero Rigo, Mario Perini, Alberto Ferrari, Aldo Antonioli, Marco Gandolfo, Guido Biasco and Luigi Barbara

25 HEPATIC ENCEPHALOPATHY IN THE 21ST CENTURY 351
Sheila Sherlock, Harold O. Conn

INDEX 359

ACKNOWLEDGMENTS

We are grateful to Dr. Herbert Falk for conceiving the need for a workshop on lactulose and for choosing us to design the program and to carry it out. We appreciate the freedom we had in selecting our coworkers and the topics to be discussed.

We acknowledge the prompt responses of our coauthors in our request for manuscripts and to our editorial changes, the latter of which were responded to with slightly less enthusiasm.

We thank Camille Rolfe Paglinco, Christa Kratz, Ursula Bircher and Marilyn Barr Conn for their technical assistance, which ranged from secretarial to redactorial to editorial, and for their continual encouragement.

We are grateful to Virginia Simon for her art and assistance.

We thank Dr. van Velthuijsen for allowing us to use his structural diagrams on the cover of the book.

Finally, we want to thank Sherlyn Martens for her swift and accurate translations of the typed manuscripts to finished pages and for never audibly complaining about the revisions, which never stopped until the cloth was on the binding.

The Editors

CONTRIBUTORS

Editors

HAROLD O. CONN, M.D.
Professor of Medicine, Yale University School of Medicine and the West Haven Veterans Administration Medical Center, West Haven, Connecticut 06516, U.S.A.

JOHANNES BIRCHER, M.D.
Professor of Clinical Pharmacology, University of Göttingen, Robert-Koch-Str. 40, D-3400 Göttingen, Federal Republic of Germany.

Chapter Authors

ALDO ANTONIOLI. M.D.
University of Modena, Cattedra di Gastroenterologia, Modena, Italy.

LUIGI BARBARA, M.D.
University of Bologna, Institute of Clinical Medicine, Bologna, Italy.

PAUL BASS, M.D.
Professor of Medicine, Department of Medicine, School of Medicine and School of Pharmacy, University of Wisconsin, Madison, Wisconsin 53706, U.S.A.

ANTONIO BENEDETTI, M.D.
Department of Gastroenterology, School of Medicine and General Hospital of Ancona, P.O.Box 538, I-60100 Ancona, Italy.

G.P. BIANCHI, M.D.
Universita di Bologna, Istituto di Patologia Medica I, Policlinico S. Orsola, Via Massarenti 9, I-40138 Bologna, Italy.

GUIDO BIASCO, M.D.
University of Bologna, Institute of Clinical Medicine, Bologna, Italy.

CHARLES E. BRADY, III, M.D.
Department of Medicine, Division of Gastroenterology and Nutrition, The University of Texas Health Science Center at San Antonio, San Antonio, Texas 78284, and Audie L. Murphy Memorial Veterans Hospital, San Antonio, Texas 78284, U.S.A.

EUGENIO BRUNELLI, M.D.
Department of Gastroenterology, School of Medicine and General Hospital of Ancona, P.O. Box 538, I-60100 Ancona, Italy.

A. CASCINO, M.D.
Laboratory of Clinical Nutrition, 3rd Department of Internal Medicine, University of Rome "La Sapienza," Viale dell'Universita 37, I-00185 Roma, Italy.

C. CANGIANO, M.D.
Laboratory of Clinical Nutrition, 3rd Department of Internal Medicine, University of Rome "La Sapienza," Viale dell'Universita 37, I-00185 Roma, Italy.

F. CECI, M.D.
Laboratory of Clinical Nutrition, 3rd Department of Internal Medicine, University of Rome "La Sapienza," Viale dell'Universita 37, I-00185 Roma, Italy.

G. A. CHECCHIA, M.D.
Universita di Bologna, Istituto di Patologia Medica I, Policlinico S. Orsola, Via Massarenti 9, I-40138 Bologna, Italy.

PAOLA DI DONATO, M.D.
University of Modena, Institute of Medical Pathology, Policlinico, Via del Pozzo 71, I-41100 Modena, Italy.

L. SIW ERIKSSON, M.D.
Associate Professor of Medicine, Department of Medicine, Section of Gastroenterology and Hepatology, Huddinge University Hospital, Karolinska Institute, S-14186 Huddinge, Sweden.

M. FAMILIARI, M.D.
Laboratory of Clinical Nutrition, 3rd Department of Internal Medicine, University of Rome "La Sapienza," Viale dell'Universita 37, I-00185 Roma, Italy.

PETER FERENCI, M.D.
Associate Professor of Medicine, 1st Department of Gastroenterology and Hepatology, University of Vienna, Lazarettgasse 14, A-1090 Vienna, Austria.

ALBERTO FERRARI, M.D.
University of Modena, Cattedra di Gastroenterologia, Modena, Italy.

CH. FLORENT, M.D.
Hôpital Saint Antoine, Service d'Hepatogastroenterologie, 184 Rue du Faubourg Saint Antoine, F-75571 Paris Cedex 12, France.

MARCO GANDOLFO, M.D.
University of Modena, Cattedra di Gastroenterologia, Modena, Italy.

JOHN HAMILTON, M.D.
Assistant Professor of Medicine, Section of Gastroenterology, Department of Medicine, School of Medicine and School of Pharmacy, University of Wisconsin, Madison, Wisconsin 53706, U.S.A.

E. ANTHONY JONES, M.D., F.R.C.P.
Chief, Liver Diseases Section, Digestive Diseases Branch, National Institute of Diabetes and Digestive and Kidney Diseases, National Institutes of Health, Bethesda, Maryland 20892, U.S.A.

G. LEBEK, M.D.
Emeritus Professor of Microbiology, University of Berne, Blinzernfeldweg 9, CH-3098 Köniz, Switzerland.

MILTON M. LIEBERTHAL, M.D.
Clinical Professor of Medicine, University of Cincinnati College of Medicine, Cincinnati, Ohio 45208, U.S.A.

M. LUGINBÜHL, M.D.
Mühleberg, Herbligen, CH-3526 Brenzikofen, Switzerland.

RUGGERO LUGLI, M.D.
University of Modena, Cattedra di Patologica Medica, Ospedale Estense, Viale Vittorio Veneto 9, I-41100 Modena, Italy.

GIAMPIERO MACARRI, M.D.
Department of Gastroenterology, School of Medicine and General Hospital of Ancona, P.O. Box 538, I-60100 Ancona, Italy.

ANTONIO MANENTI, M.D.
University of Modena, Istituto di Clinica Chirurgica, Modena, Italy.

G. MARCHESINI, M.D.
Associate Professor, Istituto di Clinica Medica Generale e Terapia, Universitá di Bologna, Policlinico S. Orsola, Via Massarenti 9, I-40138 Bologna, Italy.

MARSHA Y. MORGAN, M.B. CH.B. F.R.C.P.
Senior Research Fellow and Honorary Senior Lecturer, Academic Department of Medicine, The Royal Free Hospital and School of Medicine, Pond Street, Hampstead, London NW3 2QG, United Kingdom.

M. MUSCARITOLI, M.D.
Laboratory of Clinical Nutrition, 3rd Department of Internal Medicine, University of Rome "La Sapienza," Viale dell'Universita 37, I-00185 Roma, Italy.

FRANCESCO ORLANDI, M.D.
Professor of Gastroenterology, Department of Gastroenterology, School of Medicine and General Hospital of Ancona, P.O. Box 538, I-60100 Ancona, Italy.

MARIO PERINI, M.D.
University of Modena, Cattedra di Gastroenterologia, Modena, Italy.

MAURIZIO PONZ DE LEON, M.D.
Professor, University of Modena, Institute of Medical Pathology, Policlinico, Via del Pozzo 71, I-41100 Modena, Italy.

O. RIGGIO, M.D.
Laboratory of Clinical Nutrition, 3rd Department of Internal Medicine, University of Rome "La Sapienza," Viale dell'Universita 37, I-00185 Roma, Italy.

GIANPIERO RIGO, M.D.
University of Modena, Cattedra di Gastroenterologia, Modena, Italy.

LUCA RONCUCCI, M.D.
University of Modena, Institute of Medical Pathology, Policlinico, Via del Pozzo 71, I-41100 Modena, Italy.

F. ROSSI-FANELLI, M.D.
Professor of Medicine, Chief, Laboratory of Clinical Nutrition, 3rd Department of Internal Medicine, University of Rome "La Sapienza," Viale dell'Universita 37, I-00185 Roma, Italy.

GIANFRANCO SALVIOLI, M.D.
Professor, University of Modena, Cattedra di Patologica Medica, Ospedale Estense, Viale Vittorio Veneto 9, I-41100 Modena, Italy.

STEVEN SCHENKER, M.D.
Professor and Chairman, Department of Medicine, Division of Gastroenterology and Nutrition, The University of Texas Health Science Center at San Antonio, San Antonio, Texas 78284, and Audie L. Murphy Memorial Veterans Hospital, San Antonio, Texas 78284, U.S.A.

DAME SHEILA SHERLOCK, M.D.
Professor of Medicine, Emeritus, Professor of Surgery, The Royal Free Hospital and School of Medicine, Pond Street, Hampstead, London NW3 2QG, United Kingdom.

PETER B. SOETERS, M.D.
Professor of Surgery, University Hospital Maastricht, Department of Surgery, Rijksuniversiteit Limburg, St. Annadal Ziekenhuis, P.O. Box 616, NL-6200 Maastricht, The Netherlands.

DIETER ULLRICH, M.D.
Division of Clinical Pharmacology, University of Göttingen, Robert-Koch-Str. 40, D-3400 Göttingen, FRG.

MISAEL URIBE, M.D.
Professor of Medicine and Medical Sciences, Instituto Nacional de la Nutricion, "Salvador Zubiran," Calle Vasco de Quiroga 15, Delegacion Tlalpan, 14000 Mexico, D.F.

CHARLES L. H. VAN BERLO, M.D.
University Hospital Maastricht, Department of Surgery, Rijksuniversiteit Limburg, St. Annadal Ziekenhuis, P.O. Box 616, NL-6200 Maastricht, The Netherlands.

PAUL A.M. VAN LEEUWEN, M.D.
University Hospital Maastricht, Department of Surgery, Rijksuniversiteit Limburg, St. Annadal Ziekenhuis, P.O. Box 616, NL-6200 Maastricht, The Netherlands.

JOHN A. VAN VELTHUIJSEN, PH.D.
CCA biochem b.v., Research & Development, Arkelsedijk 46, P.O. Box 21, NL-4200 AA Gorinchem, The Netherlands.

FREDRICK L. WEBER, JR., M.D.
Associate Professor of Medicine, Department of Medicine, Division of Gastroenterology and Nutrition, VA Medical Center and Case Western Reserve University, School of Medicine, 2074 Abington Road, Cleveland, Ohio 44106, U.S.A.

M. ZOLI, M.D.
Istituto di Clinica Generale e Terapia, Universitá di Bologna, Policlinico S. Orsola, Via Massarenti 9, I-40138 Bologna, Italy.

PREFACE

The field of hepatic encephalopathy (HE), which includes a number of syndromes (1), is in the midst of an investigational revolution. To those on the periphery of this field, it often looks quiet and benign like a large cloud drifting serenely across the sky (Figure 1). Its shape appears to be constant; nothing is

FIGURE 1. A cloud passes peacefully above the sea.

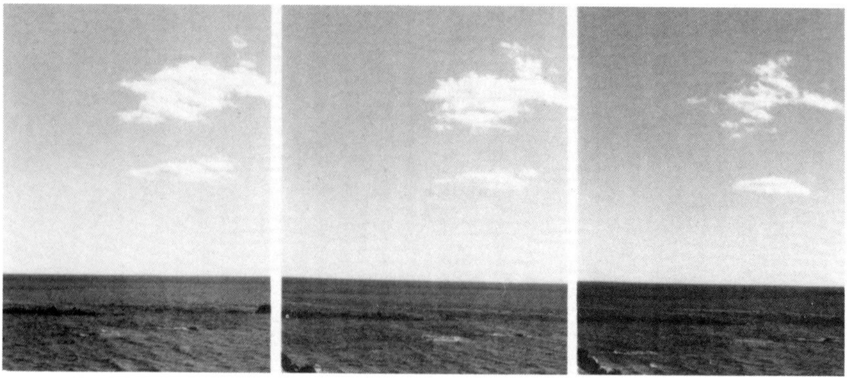

FIGURE 2. The cloud seen in Figure 1 is in the upper left. As the cloud moves to

changing. Or is it? If one focuses on the leading edge of the cloud, one realizes that its shape is continuously changing. Sometimes, a cloud will pass from an area of high humidity into a mass of dry air and the cloud will disappear (Figure 2). At other times, one can see clouds appear *de novo*, almost by magic. When one flies into a cloud, one quickly learns that clouds are not peaceful places, but rather centers of energy and activity. Like such a cloud, hepatic encephalopathy may appear to be floating peacefully across the horizon of medicine looking much as it did when we entered the field, but it too is very active and energetic and is continuously changing. Some advances like the gamma-aminobutyric acid (GABA) hypothesis appear (2), change their shape dramatically (3) and take their place in our understanding of these disorders. (GABA is the subject of several chapters in this volume.) Others like alpha-ketoglutaramate in the pathogenesis of HE (4) fade soon after they are introduced and are rarely heard of again. (This substance is not mentioned again in this volume.)

A major therapeutic breakthrough in this field was made largely as the consequence of the synthesis of ideas by one of the editors of this volume (JB). In approved scientific fashion, this contribution was made standing on the shoulders of giants. To oversimplify the story, one might say that the first recognition of hepatic encephalopathy was the result of Eck's creation in 1877 of the Eck fistula, an end-to-side portacaval shunt. Without the shunt, the HE it precipitated would not have been identified so early or so clearly. Almost 90 years later Franz Ingelfinger, on learning of the lactobacillophilic effects of lactulose, suggested that this synthetic disaccharide might be of use in the management of HE (5). Bircher read Ingelfinger's informal suggestion and subsequently demonstrated the clinical value of this nonabsorbable carbohydrate in patients with portal-systemic encephalopathy (PSE) (6). The introduction of this new therapeutic agent provided a great stimulus to the investigation of the pathogenesis of these syndromes. This historical sequence prompted the other editor (HOC) to dedicate his book coauthored with

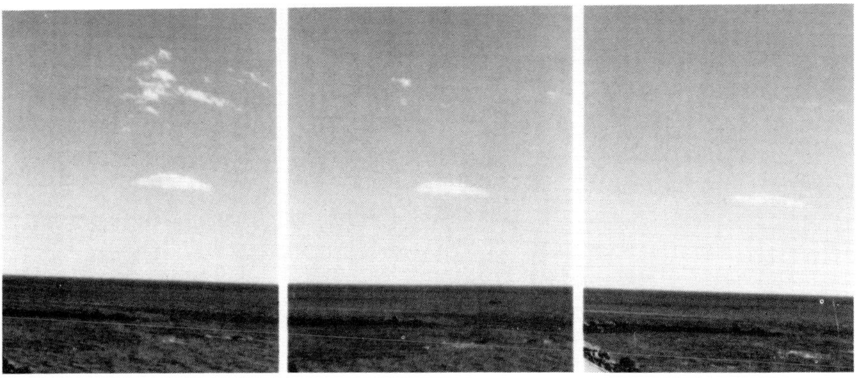

the left it rapidly dwindles and disappears.

Milton Lieberthal on this subject, "To Nickolai Eck, who exposed the darkness, to Franz Ingelfinger, who saw the light, and to Hannes Bircher, who turned it on."

Bacteriologists had suggested the concept that the administration of lactulose was useful in the induction of a lactobacillus flora in the colon (7, 8). In addition, the suggestion had been made that lactobacilli do not degrade urea to ammonia and that lactulose may, therefore, be beneficial in the treatment of PSE (5). Although this hypothesis was later shown to be wrong, lactulose proved to be effective in improving PSE, and now, 22 years after its introduction (6), the oral administration of lactulose is the treatment of choice for most patients. Thus, the lactulose story is another example of an incorrect hypothesis leading to a major advance.

The editors have identified a dozen major advances in the history of lactulose (5-18) which have been listed chronologically in Table 1. These 12 publications begin with the synthesis of lactulose which was a hitherto unknown carbohydrate, early insights into its bacterial activity and mechanism of action, and the introduction of a variety of clinical applications. They include the purposeful creation of lactitol, an advantageous analogue that is second generation lactulose, and new, broad-reaching application of the biologic activities of these substances. On reviewing the events summarized in Table 1, it becomes clear that although individual scientists contribute to progress, it is the complex interaction of human minds that really advances science.

The reader may ask how this book came about. The answer is simple: almost by accident.

The contributors to this volume were all participants in a Workshop on Lactulose that was directed by the editors of this book and sponsored by Herbert Falk. It had been decided that the contents of the workshop would not be published because the value of publishing "Proceedings" does not usually justify the effort involved. This workshop, however, was a very special event. Each of the participants had presented his or her view of one portion of the collage from a unique vantage point. Each reviewed the status of the area and presented new information and/or innovative aspects of current controversies. Furthermore, the presentations were clear, brief and relevant. Immediately afterward in a moment of weakness and enthusiasm the participants agreed that it would probably be worthwhile to explore the possibility of publishing it.

The late start was a blessing in disguise. In the search for a publisher, MEDI-ED Press, a young, state-of-the-art medical publishing firm with a refreshing, optimistic attitude and confident enthusiasm for this project was discovered. Several additional authors who had been unable to participate in the workshop were invited to prepare chapters on important, relevant aspects of topics that had not been included in the workshop.

It should be emphasized that this volume is not the "proceedings" of a workshop. It represents a coordinated attempt to have experts in the field summarize and synthesize the state of the art in a series of selected aspects of hepatic encephalopathy. The workshop was the stimulus, not the template. The workshop occurred almost two years before this book was published, but each chapter was

TABLE 1. Major Events in the History of Lactulose

1929 Description of lactulose by Montgomery and Hudson, who named it lactoketose (9).

1957 Identification of lactulose as a "bifidus factor" by F. Petuely (7, 10).

1965 Suggestion by F. Ingelfinger that the establishment of a lactobacillus flora in the gut with the aid of lactulose might be beneficial in patients with cirrhosis and encephalopathy (5).

1966 Initial report of successful treatment of portal-systemic encephalopathy with lactulose (6).

1971 Evaluation of nonionic diffusion of ammonia in the colon as mechanism of action of lactulose in PSE (11).

1974 Assessment of small intestinal transit time with lactulose and measurement of molecular hydrogen in exhaled air (12).

1975 Successful treatment of the salmonella carrier state with lactulose (13).

1977 Confirmation of equivalent efficacy of lactulose and neomycin in the treatment of PSE in a randomized clinical trial (14).

1977 Successful use of lactose in the treatment of portal-systemic encephalopathy in patients with lactase deficiency (15).

1978 Discovery of the bacterial utilization of ammonia as a source of nitrogen in the presence of lactulose as an additional mechanism of action in PSE (16).

1983 Initial description of lactitol in the treatment of PSE (17).

1987 Evaluation of lactulose as potential protective agent in colonic carcinogenesis (18).

reviewed, revised and updated within a few months of the date of publication.

The editors, who first met over lactulose almost 20 years ago, have each devoted considerable portions of their professional lives to the study of hepatic encephalopathy and its treatment with lactulose. One was the first to use lactulose in the management of HE and introduced it into clinical medicine; the other had helped establish its efficacy in a series of randomized clinical trials. Both were impressed with the rapidity with which the field has progressed, although it seemed to be moving at a snail's pace while it was happening. Both thought that a volume to mark the first two decades in the evolution of lactulose was in order.

As editors of journals, both were aware of the almost inherent deficiencies of books derived from symposia, i.e., various medical and investigational philosophies, different styles of writing and the Scylla and Charybdis of such anthologies, repetition and omission. The knowledge of these potential pitfalls was intensified by the multinational, multilingual backgrounds of the participants. With faith that quality will win out, however, it was decided to proceed and to focus on clarity, brevity, importance and relevance. Brevity, however, turned out not to be one of the virtues of the editors, as illustrated by this eight-page preface.

In preparing this Workshop the speakers, almost without exception, protested that the time allotted for their presentations was insufficient by a factor of at least two. Nevertheless, they managed to say what they wanted to say, and more, within the prescribed time limits. It is intriguing that in preparing the written version, almost without exception, these same authors had overestimated the numbers of pages they would need by a factor of two. This paradox suggests that the editors and authors of this volume are long-winded and short-handed. Other explanations are, of course, plausible.

This volume is concerned primarily with the current status of our knowledge of hepatic encephalopathy and its management, especially by carbohydrates, and to some of the other applications of lactulose administration.

We are fortunate to have as contributors to this volume many of the investigators from around the world who are currently creating lightning in the nonserene, ever-changing encephalopathy cloud.

One of the most fascinating aspects of editing this volume was the realization that its chapters were written by 21 authors or groups of authors from nine countries where seven different languages are used. Six were from the United States, five from Italy, two from Great Britain, two from the Netherlands, and one each from Austria, Federal Republic of Germany, France, Mexico, Sweden and Switzerland. It is impressive how well these chapters are written considering that two-thirds of the authors were writing in a second language. Medical investigation is a great English teacher.

It is hoped that the readers find this volume to be as useful and enjoyable as the authors and editors did in preparing it.

Harold O. Conn, New Haven, CT
Johannes Bircher, Göttingen, FRG

REFERENCES

1. Conn HO, Lieberthal MM. The syndrome of portal-systemic encephalopathy. In: The Hepatic Coma Syndromes and Lactulose. Baltimore, MD: Williams & Wilkins, 1978: 1-46.

2. Schafer DR, Jones EA. Hepatic encephalopathy and the gamma-aminobutyric acid neurotransmitter system. Lancet 1982; 1:18-20.

3. Hoyumpa AM. The unfolding GABA story. Hepatology 1986; 6:1042-1044.

4. Vergara F, Plum F, Duffy TE. Alpha-ketoglutaramate: increased concentrations in the cerebrospinal fluid of patients in hepatic coma. Science 1974; 183:81-83.

5. Ingelfinger F. Editorial comments. Beeson PB, et al., eds. Year Book of Medicine (1964-1965 Series). Chicago: Year Book Medical Publishers, 1964-1965: 591-592.

6. Bircher J, Müller J, Guggenheim P, et al. Treatment of chronic portal-systemic encephalopathy with lactulose. Lancet 1966; 1:890-893.

7. Petuely F, Lindner G. Untersuchungen über die Regulations - Mechanismen für die Darmflora und ihre Beeinflussung durch Terramycin: Bedeutung des Bakteriellen Umgebungsmilieus für die Darmflora. Zentralbl Bakteriol (Orig A) 1957; 169:178-195.

8. Hoffmann K, Mossel DA, Korus W, et al. Untersuchungen über die Wirkungsweise der Lactulose (ß-galactosido-fructose) im Darm. Klin Wochenschr 1964: 42:126-130.

9. Montgomery E, Hudson CS. Transformation of lactose to a new disaccharide, lactoketose. Science 1929; 69:556-557.

10. Petuely F. Der Bifidusfaktor. Dtsch Med Wochenschr 1957; 82:1957-1960.

11. Bircher J, Haemmerli UP, Trabert E, et al. The mechanism of action of lactulose in portal-systemic encephalopathy. Non-ionic diffusion of ammonia in the canine colon. Rev Europ Etudes Clin Biol 1971; 16:352-357.

12. Bond Jr, JH, Levitt MD. Use of pulmonary hydrogen (H_2) measurements to quantitative carbohydrate absorption. Study of partially gastrectomized patients. J Clin Invest 1974; 51:1219-1225.

13. Hoffmann K. Treatment of healthy salmonella carriers with lactulose (ß-galactosido-fructose). Dtsch Med Wochenschr 1975; 100:1429-1431.

14. Conn HO, Leevy CM, Vlahcevic ZR, et al. A comparison of lactulose and neomycin in the treatment of portal-systemic encephalopathy: a double-blind controlled trial. Gastroenterology 1977; 72:573-583.

15. Uribe M, Marquez MA, Garcia-Ramos G, et al. Treatment of chronic portal systemic encephalopathy with lactose in lactase deficient patients. Dig Dis Sci

1980; 25:924-928.
16. Vince A, Killingley M., Wrong OM. Effect of lactulose on ammonia production in a fecal incubation system. Gastroenterology 1978; 74:544-549.
17. Bircher J, Bührer M, Franz K, et al. Erstmalige Anwendung von Lactitol in der Behandlung der Porto-systemischen Enzephalopathie. Schweiz Med Wochenschr 1982; 112:1306-1307.
18. Van Berge Henegouwen GP, van der Werf SDJ, Ruben AT. Effect of long term lactulose ingestion on secondary bile salt metabolism in man: potential protective effect of lactulose in colonic carcinogenesis. Gut 1987; 28:675-680.

THE DISORDER

1

THE HEPATIC ENCEPHALOPATHIES

HAROLD O. CONN, M.D.

The hepatic encephalopathies are a diverse group of disorders that have two things in common: first, encephalopathy and second, a disorder of the liver that causes or predisposes to the encephalopathy. The encephalopathy *per se* is indistinguishable from the dementia that may occur in other disorders such as azotemia, carbon dioxide narcosis or barbiturate intoxication, although other aspects of these disorders may differ (Table 1). In other words, coma is coma, whether hepatic or nonhepatic. This statement is true for the various degrees of encephalopathy which range from minimal abnormalities of intellectual function to deep, unresponsive coma.

The prototype of HE is *portal-systemic encephalopathy,* hereafter referred to as PSE. It is seen almost exclusively in patients with advanced cirrhosis and portal hypertension. Its pathogenesis is determined by the presence and degree of portal-systemic shunting. These collateral veins carry blood from the portal vein into the systemic circulation, thus bypassing the liver. Potentially toxic substances, such as ammonia or mercaptans that arise in the lumen of the intestinal tract by bacterial action on alimentary substances that are usually removed or detoxified as the portal blood passes through the liver, are diverted around or through the liver and into the systemic circulation. Such comagenic substances are carried by the systemic blood flow to the brain where they cause coma.

PSE is characterized by several nonspecific components. First, the *encephalopathy* ranges from trivial impairment of orientation to full-blown coma (Figure 1). Various, similar, semiquantitative grading systems, usually on a 0 (normal) to IV (deep coma) scale have been devised (1-7). Second, *asterixis*, a nonspecific neurologic sign of impaired descending reticular system function, is seen in almost all types of encephalopathy of hepatic and nonhepatic origin (Figure 2). Third, *abnormal electroencephalograms* (EEGs) are characterized by

TABLE 1. Encephalopathies That May Be Indistinguishable in Patients with Chronic Liver Disease

I. Hepatic
    A. Portal-systemic encephalopathy
    B. Fulminant hepatic failure
    C. Urea cycle enzyme deficiencies
    D. Reye's syndrome
II. Metabolic
    A. Carbon dioxide narcosis
    B. Azotemia
    C. Diabetic coma
    D. Hypoglycemia
    E. Acid-base disturbances
        1. Metabolic alkalosis
        2. Metabolic acidosis
    F. Serum electrolyte abnormalities
        1. Hypokalemia
        2. Hypomagnesemia
III. Toxic
    A. Alcohol
    B. Drugs
        1. Hypnotic/sedative
        2. Analgesic
        3. Tranquilizer
        4. Beta adrenergic blocker
        5. Bromides
IV. Miscellaneous
    A. Constipation
    B. Multiple origin

slow waves of increased amplitude (Figure 3). The fewer the number of waves per second, the more severe the grade of encephalopathy. Elevated blood levels of a toxic substance that has induced the encephalopathy provide some specificity for the syndrome. In PSE the weight of evidence indicates that *ammonia* is that substance (8), and that the degree of elevation of the blood ammonia concentration parallels the severity of the encephalopathy (Figure 4). Other substances including methanethiol (9) and short-chain fatty acids have been implicated (10), and it has been suggested that ammonia, methanethiol and short-chain fatty acids in various combinations are responsible for PSE (11). Blood ammonia levels provide specificity for the PSE syndrome and help exclude non-nitrogenous, comagenic syndromes.

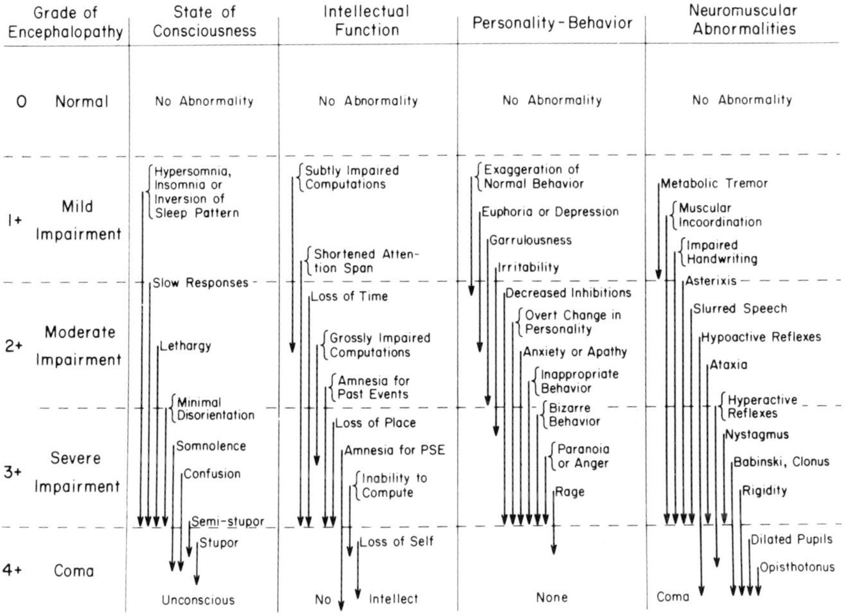

FIGURE 1. Spectrum of disordered mental state in PSE. The grade of PSE is indicated on the left. Each of the three components of mental state (state of consciousness, intellectual function, and personality-behavior) plus neuromuscular abnormalities are shown in the four columns. Within each column the grade at which specific abnormalities usually appear is shown by the tail of the arrow. The length of the arrow indicates the range of grades through which each abnormality may be observed. Many features of PSE are not detectable or measurable since testing may require a degree of cooperation not possible in comatose patients. Reproduced with permission of authors and publisher (8).

PSE is almost always seen in patients with advanced cirrhosis and portal hypertension who have developed portal-systemic collaterals. It is seen especially frequently in cirrhotic patients with portal-systemic shunts, and most commonly in those with *portacaval anastomoses* (PCA), the most frequently performed type of shunt. PSE has been claimed to occur less commonly after distal splenorenal shunts (DSRS) than after PCA (12), but several controlled comparisons show no difference in the frequency, severity or time of onset of PSE after DSRS or PCA (13, 14) (Figure 5).

In PSE, portal-systemic shunting is the primary abnormality, not hepatic function *per se*. Portacaval shunts performed during the resection of pancreatic

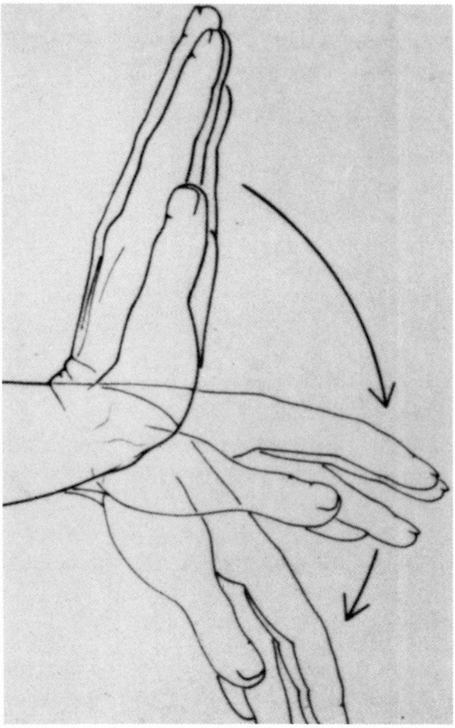

FIGURE 2. Asterixis. With the hand maintained in the dorsiflexed position, asterixis is characterized by the hand falling forward as shown by the arrows. The dorsiflexed position is instantaneously resumed, causing, in effect, a "flapping" motion. (Reprinted by permission of Conn HO: Current diagnosis and treatment of hepatic coma. Hosp Prac 1973; 8:65-72.)

neoplasms in noncirrhotic patients with normal livers and normal liver function are frequently followed by PSE. Moreover, spontaneous portal-systemic collaterals in otherwise normal patients or animals can induce severe encephalopathy (15).

A second type of hepatic encephalopathy is caused by deficiencies of any one of the five *urea cycle enzymes* (16). The most common and best studied enzyme deficiency, ornithine transcarbamylase deficiency, hereafter called OTC (Figure 6), is an autosomal recessive disorder that is transmitted by the heterozygous mother. In homozygous male infants in whom it is almost always lethal, it presents as severe encephalopathy that is precipitated by milk, other proteins or ammonia-liberating substances. The clinical picture consists of irritability, vomiting, coma, opisthotonos and, invariably, death. Blood ammonia levels are grossly elevated and the EEG shows the infantile equivalent of the EEG abnormalities seen in adults with PSE.

In the heterozygous state, the mothers of these infants are well unless they eat excessive amounts of dietary protein, which may induce a syndrome identical to PSE except that these patients do not have cirrhosis (16, 17). It is also seen rarely in adult men with an acquired OTC deficiency (18).

Similar syndromes exist for each of the other urea cycle enzymes, including carbamylphosphate synthetase (CPS), the other intramitochondrial en-

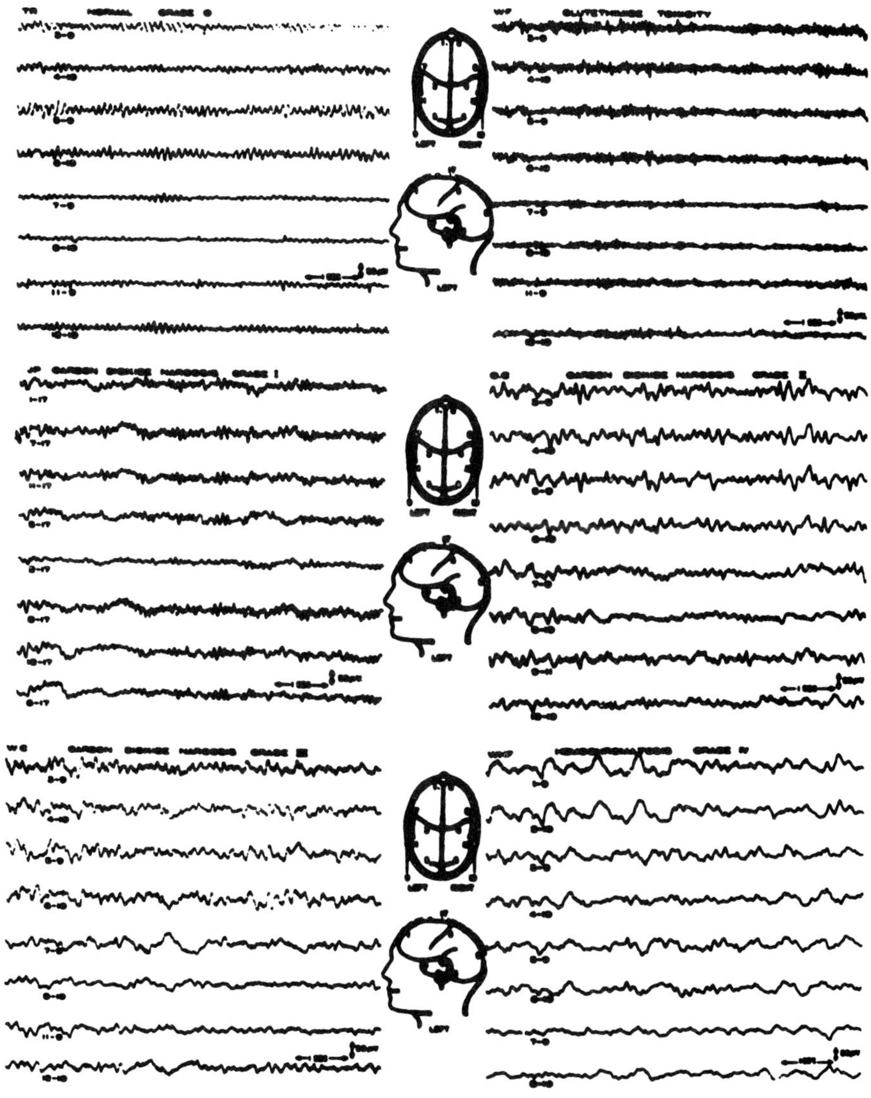

FIGURE 3. Electroencephalographic patterns in various types of encephalopathy. Upper left: Normal EEG. Regular 9-12 cps rhythm. Upper right: glutethimide encephalopathy is characterized by fast, irregular 18-20 cps activity. The next four EEGs are progressively more abnormal, characterized by waves of decreasing frequency and increasing amplitude. Lower right: grade IV PSE is characterized by 1 to 3 large, slow cps. (Reprinted by permission from Conn HO: Asterixis in nonhepatic disorders. Am J Med 1960; 29:647-661.)

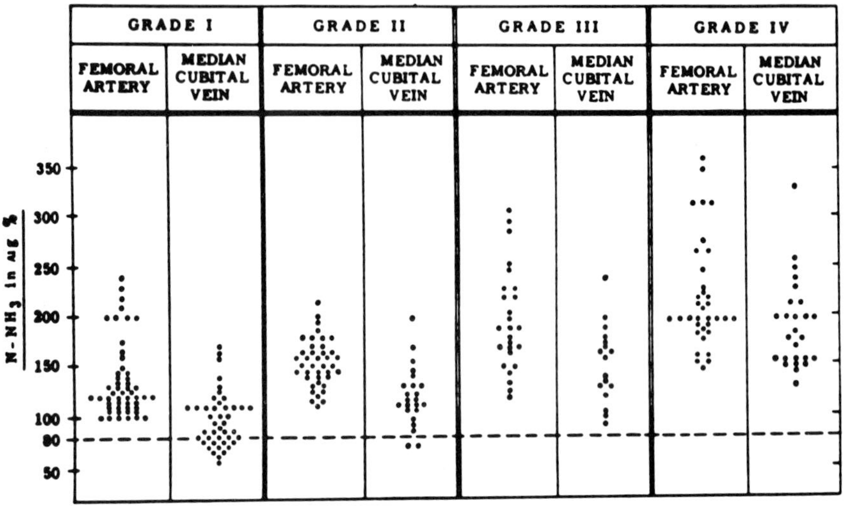

FIGURE 4. Association of blood ammonia concentration and the severity of PSE in untreated cirrhotic patients. There is a step-wise progression between the mean arterial ammonia levels and the degree of PSE. There is, however, much overlap in ammonia concentrations between adjacent grades of PSE. (Reprinted by permission from Stahl J: Studies of the blood ammonia in liver disease. Its diagnostic, prognostic and therapeutic significance. Ann Intern Med 1963; 58:1-24.)

zyme of this cycle, and the rate-limiting step in this pathway. In general, the earlier in the urea cycle the defect, the worse the encephalopathy and the higher the blood ammonia concentration (16).

The third syndrome is *Reye's syndrome*. It is a disorder of children which usually follows a viral infection such as influenza or chicken pox and is characterized by microvesicular fatty infiltration of the viscera and many other clinical and metabolic abnormalities (19). The encephalopathy appears to be a result of intense hyperammonemia (20). The decreased activity of OTC and/or CPS, the two intramitochondrial urea cycle enzymes, appears to be a transient acquired urea cycle enzyme deficiency caused by selective injury to the mitochondria (21) and appears to be a self-limited disorder; i.e., a transient metabolic insult occurs before the patient becomes encephalopathic, and if the patient doesn't die during the acute stage, the prognosis is excellent. In fact, the enzyme activity and blood ammonia concentration revert toward normal whether or not the patient recovers (22). The precise pathogenesis of the disorder is not known. Ammonia and salicylates have both been incriminated (23) and a combination of these effects may be responsible.

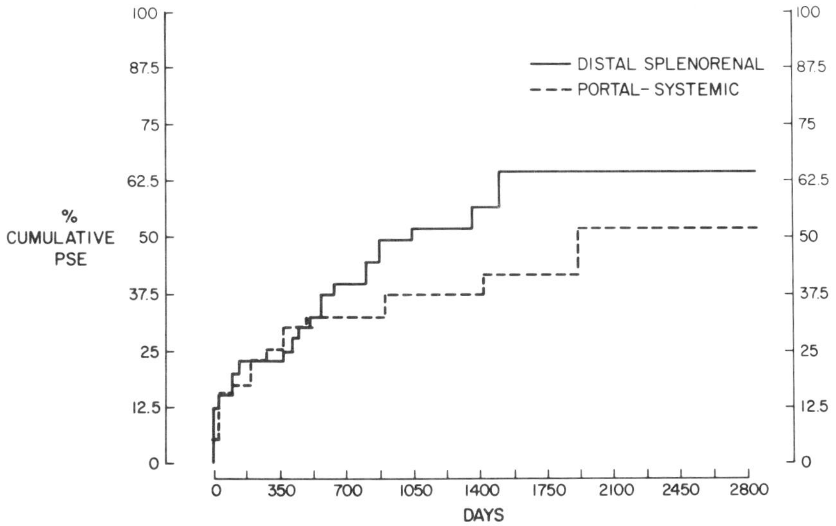

FIGURE 5. Cumulative prevalence of portal-systemic encephalopathy (PSE) after distal splenorenal shunts and after portal-systemic anastomoses, predominantly portacaval shunts. There were no significant differences in prevalence, mean time of onset after anastomosis or severity in the two groups of randomly selected patients. (Grace ND, et al., Hepatology, in press.)

The fourth encephalopathic syndrome is *fulminant hepatic failure* (FHF). This syndrome may be caused by viral hepatitis, usually due to hepatitis B virus, by alcohol or by drugs such as halothane. The drug toxicity may be due either to overdosage (acetaminophen), direct hepatotoxicity (carbon tetrachloride) or hypersensitivity (halothane). In this syndrome there is no underlying chronic liver disease or portal-systemic shunting, but severe hepatic injury results in an encephalopathy due to the failure of multiple hepatic systems resulting in hyperammonemia, hypoglycemia, and innumerable other abnormalities. The syndrome is recognized by its severe, frequently fatal hepatic dysfunction.

A number of clinical models such as carbon tetrachloride or acetaminophen toxicity exist, as do animal models such as galactosamine-induced liver injury. This later model has been the stimulus for the GABA hypothesis (24) and, subsequently, the endogenous phenodiazepine receptor-blocker hypothesis (25).

A basic fallacy of the FHF syndrome is that it is defined as acute or subacute hepatic injury of any etiology or severity, *in the presence of encephalopathy*. Technically, the superimposition of any degree of mental impairment on acute hepatic injury of any etiology or severity defines the term *fulminant* hepatic failure. Thus, one sometimes sees clinical inconsistencies. A patient with viral hepatitis may develop constipation, which under normal circumstances would be only a local, mechanical problem. In the presence of acute liver disease, constipation could

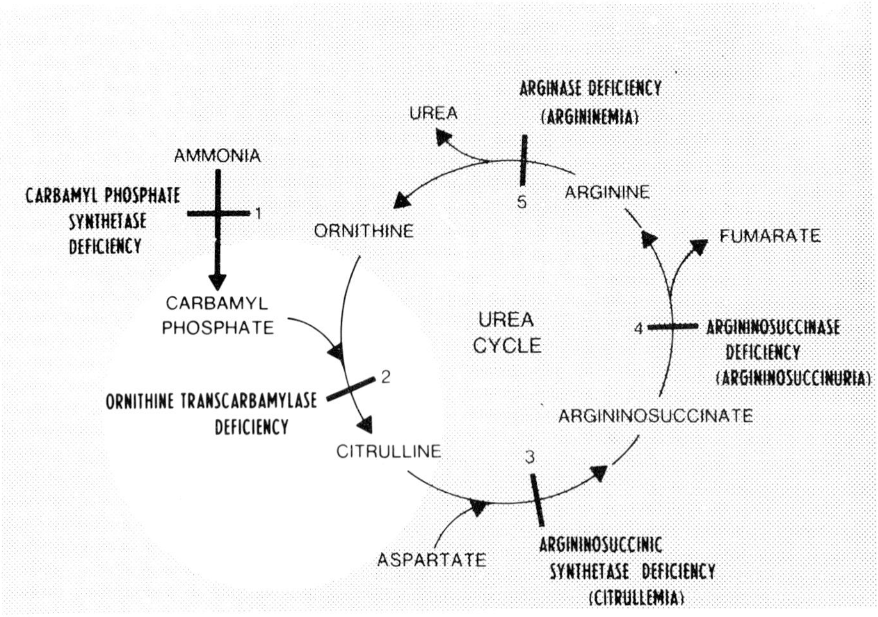

FIGURE 6. Ornithine transcarbamylase deficiency. The urea cycle is shown and the position of OTC in the cycle illuminated. (Reproduced with the permission of the authors and publisher (8).

cause encephalopathy which technically "creates" FHF. Happily, an enema or two may cure this highly lethal problem.

The fifth type of encephalopathy is *pseudo-PSE*. This is most frequently seen in patients with underlying liver disease, usually cirrhosis. It may be caused by a large number of drugs—particularly hypnotics, sedatives, analgesics or tranquilizers. It can probably also be precipitated in cirrhotic patients by metabolic abnormalities such as hypoglycemia, hypokalemia, alkalosis, hypoxemia or hypercarbia, which themselves are not comagenic. In principle, this syndrome looks like PSE, but is precipitated by nonammoniacal, comagenic substances in patients with an increased susceptibility for developing hepatic coma. Hyperammonemia is not present in these patients because the precipitant is non-nitrogenous. Whatever the toxic substance responsible, it can often be shown to be increased in the blood, the spinal fluid and/or in brain cells.

A number of Reye's-like syndromes with encephalopathy occur, some with hyperammonemia, some without. One of them, *Jamaica vomiting sickness*, is caused by hypoglycin, which appears to have metabolic activities similar to those of short-chain fatty acids, which may, under certain circumstances, be able to induce

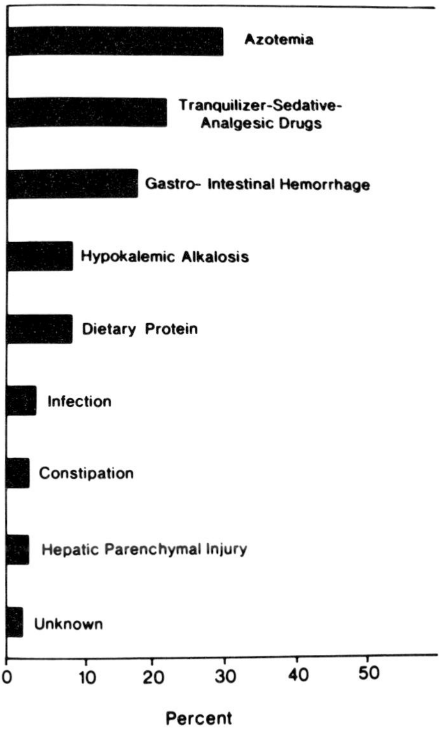

FIGURE 7. Distribution of causes of hepatic encephalopathy. This histogram shows the causes of encephalopathy in 100 patients with liver disease.

a Reye's-like encephalopathy (26, 27). A similar syndrome can be induced in experimental animals by 4-pentenoic acid (28). Note the structural similarity between these substances. Valproate is a drug that can sometimes give rise to a similar disorder, perhaps due to encephalopathy induced by some of its metabolites that resemble short-chain fatty acid analogues (29). These agents may be able to precipitate Reye's syndrome *de novo* or might, in susceptible patients, be able to precipitate pseudo-PSE, depending on their individual modes of action.

The distribution of the causes of 100 consecutive cases of hepatic encephalopathy helps put these diverse syndromes into clinical perspective (30) (Figure 7). Approximately 30% were associated with *azotemia* that developed spontaneously in half (15%) and after diuretic drugs in half (15%). Twenty percent were precipitated by *gastrointestinal hemorrhage.* The deepest coma occurred in the patients with GI bleeding. Another 10% were associated with excessive protein ingestion. Thus, 60% occurred in cirrhotic patients in whom a nitrogenous substance induced the disorder; these are classified as PSE. All exhibited an increased blood ammonia concentration. Central nervous system suppressant drugs, such as analgesic, sedative or tranquilizing drugs, accounted for another 20%. These cases and others, such as hypoglycemia, are not associated with elevated blood ammonia levels and are considered *pseudo-PSE. Fulminant hepatic failure* was only seen in 2% caused either by viral hepatitis or fulminant alcoholic hepatitis. We observed no *urea cycle enzyme deficiencies* or *Reye's syndrome* in our hospital which cares for war veterans and admits no children and few women. Each hospital differs in its patient mix, and the epidemiology of hepatic encephalopathy is therefore different for each different type of hospital.

The lumping of all these syndromes under a single rubric, HE, has impaired our understanding of these disorders. Many series of patients, even in randomized clinical trials, have included a) patients with spontaneous PSE induced by dietary protein, b) patients with secondary PSE precipitated by GI bleeding or azotemia, c) patients with fulminant hepatic failure and, certainly, d) patients with unrecognized pseudo-PSE. It behooves clinicians to differentiate these syndromes by determination of blood ammonia levels and to treat accordingly. It behooves investigators to study homogeneous groups of patients or, at least, to stratify such cases by their etiologic agents so that the effects of therapy can be judged rationally. Conceivably, a single substance or reaction may be, in the final biophysical analysis, common to all these disorders, but if so, it must be very close to the meaning of life and to the seat of the soul.

REFERENCES

1. Adams RD, Foley JM. The neurological disorder associated with liver disease. Res Publ Assoc Res Nerv Ment Dis 1953; 32:198-237.

2. Denis J, Opolon P, Nusinovici V. Treatment of encephalopathy during fulminant hepatic failure by hemodialysis with high permeability membranes. Gut 1978; 19:787-793.

3. Benhamou JP, Lenne C, Fauvert R. L'encephalopathic hépatique. Rev Int Hepatol 1986; 11:207-224.

4. Conn HO, Leevy CM, Vlahcevic ZR, et al. Comparison of lactulose and neomycin in the treatment of chronic portal-systemic encephalopathy—a double-blind controlled trial. Gastroenterology 1977; 72:573-583.

5. Leevy CM, Popper H, Sherlock S, eds. Diseases of the Liver and Biliary Tract. Fogarty International Center Proceedings No. 22, DHEW Publication No. (NIH) 77-725.

6. Teasdale G, Jennett B. Assessment of coma and impaired consciousness: a practical scale. Lancet 1974; 2:81-84.

7. Parsons-Smith BG, Summerskill WHJ, Dawson AM, et al. The electroencephalogram in liver disease. Lancet 1957; 2:867-871.

8. Conn HO, Lieberthal MM. Pathogenesis of portal-systemic encephalopathy. In: The Hepatic Coma Syndromes and Lactulose. Baltimore: Williams & Wilkins, 1978: 46-84.

9. Chen S, Zieve L, Mahadevan V. Mercaptans and dimethylsulfide in the

breath of patients with cirrhosis of the liver. J Lab Clin Med 1970; 75:628-635.

10. Zieve L, Nicoloff DM, Mahadevan V. Effect of hepatectomy on volatile free fatty acids of the blood (Abstract). Gastroenterology 1968; 54:1285.

11. Zieve L, Doizaki WM, Zieve FJ. Synergism between mercaptans and ammonia or fatty acids in the production of coma: a possible role for mercaptans in the pathogenesis of hepatic coma. J Lab Clin Med 1974; 83:16-28.

12. Rikkers LF, Rudman D, Galambos JT, et al. A randomized controlled trial of the distal splenorenal shunt. Ann Surg 1978; 188:271-282.

13. Harley HAJ, Morgan T, Redeker AG, et al. Results of a randomized trial of end-to side portacaval shunt and distal splenorenal shunt in alcoholic liver disease and variceal bleeding. Gastroenterology 1986; 91:802-809.

14. Grace ND, Conn HO, Resnick RH, et al. Distal splenorenal vs portal-systemic shunts after hemorrhage from varices: a randomized controlled trial (Submitted for publication).

15. Ohnishi K, Saito M, Sato S, et al. Direction of splenic venous flow assessed by pulsed doppler flowmetry in patients with a large splenorenal shunt. Relation to spontaneous hepatic encephalopathy. Gastroenterology 1985; 89:180-185.

16. Hsia YE. Inherited hyperammonemic syndromes. Gastroenterology 1974; 67:347-374.

17. Flannery DB, Hsia YE, Wolf B. Current status of hyperammonemic syndromes. Hepatology 1982; 2:495-506.

18. Meythaler JM, Varma RR. Reye's syndrome in adults. Arch Intern Med 1987; 147:61-64.

19. Reye RDK, Morgan B, Baral J. Encephalopathy and fatty degeneration of the viscera: a disease entity in childhood. Lancet 1963; 2:749-752.

20. Snodgrass PJ, DeLong GR. Urea-cycle enzyme deficiencies and an increased nitrogen load producing hyperammonemia in Reye's syndrome. N Engl J Med 1976; 294:855-860.

21. Partin JC, Shubert WK, Partin JS. Mitochondrial ultrastructure in Reye's syndrome: encephalopathy and fatty degeneration of the viscera. N Engl J Med 1971; 258:1339-1343.

22. Lovejoy FH Jr, Smith AL, Bresnan MJ, et al. Clinical staging in Reye's syndrome. Am J Dis Child 1974; 128:36-41.

23. Hurwitz E, Barrett MJ, Bregman DS, et al. Public Health Service study on Reye's syndrome and medications. Report of the pilot phase. N Engl J Med 1985; 313:849-857.

24. Jones EA, Schafer DF, Ferenci P, et al. The neurobiology of hepatic encephalopathy. Hepatology 1984; 4:1235-1242.

25. Scollo-Lavizzari G, Steinmann E. Reversal of hepatic coma by benzodiazepine antagonist (Ro 15-1788) (Correspondence). Lancet 1985; 1:1324-1325.

26. Tanaka K, Isselbacher KJ, Shih V. Isovaleric and alphamethylbutyric acidemias induced by hypoglycin. A mechanism of Jamaican vomiting sickness. Science 1972; 175:69-72.

27. Tanaka K, Kean EA, Johnson B. Jamaican vomiting sickness: biochemical investigation of two cases. N Engl J Med 1976; 295:461-463.

28. Glasgow AM, Chase HP. Production of the features of Reye's syndrome in rats with 4-pentenoic acid. Pediatr Res 1975; 9:133-138.

29. Zimmerman HJ, Ishak KG. Valproate-induced hepatic injury: analyses of 23 fatal cases. Hepatology 1982; 2:591-597.

30. Fessel JM, Conn HO. An analysis of the causes and prevention of hepatic coma (Abstract). Gastroenterology 1972; 62:191.

2

PATHOGENESIS OF HEPATIC ENCEPHALOPATHY

STEVEN SCHENKER, M.D., AND CHARLES E. BRADY, III, M.D.

Although the symptoms and signs of hepatic encephalopathy* seem to have been described in antiquity and much research in this area has been done, the exact pathogenesis of this disorder remains unknown (1-3). Some of the reasons for the uncertainty and controversy as to pathogenesis of this disorder are a) gaps in knowledge about the neurochemical/neurophysiological basis of normal consciousness (awareness) which make it difficult to search for and identify deviations from normal; b) the heterogeneity of the brain, both functional and biochemical, which extends to different cells (i.e., astroglial cells) in the brain (4) and compartmentation of neurochemical processes (i.e., gamma-aminobutyric acid, alpha-ketoglutarate) within them (5); c) problems in developing animal models as typical counterparts of the various forms of human hepatic encephalopathy and establishing that depression in mental/neurological status in such models is truly due to liver disease and not the physiological alterations accompanying the experimental procedure (6); and d) uncertainty when associated events (i.e., mental changes and biochemical findings) are causally related.

Hepatic encephalopathy is most easily defined as an alteration of mental state which accompanies and is due to impaired liver function and/or abnormal shunting of blood (spontaneous or postsurgical) from the portal to the systemic circulations. In the past, such encephalopathy has been characterized by abnormal mental status examination (i.e., lack of orientation, deficits in normal cerebration)

* As used here, the term *encephalopathy* embraces the wide spectrum of mental changes seen in patients with liver disease and due to it. It includes portal-systemic encephalopathy (PSE) seen with chronic liver disease and coma accompanying acute liver failure.

and by evidence of constructional apraxia and an impaired semiquantitative Numbers Connection (Trailmaking) Test. These features are often accompanied by evidence of liver disease and/or shunting of blood, by an abnormal EEG, elevated blood ammonia or spinal fluid glutamine levels, and, most importantly, by the absence of other cause(s) of encephalopathy. At times, a therapeutic trial is helpful in establishing the diagnosis (1).

More recently, there has been emphasis on the presence and diagnosis of minimal or subclinical hepatic encephalopathy. Such minimal disease may be first suspected through subtle intellectual changes noted by family members, and may be substantiated by the use of psychometric tests (7, 8), or perhaps by the use of specialized procedures such as analysis of changes in visual evoked potentials (9, 10), or by cerebral abnormalities seen with computerized tomography (11). The use of visual evoked potentials and computerized tomography requires further validation as to specificity and comparison to an accepted standard of hepatic encephalopathy, or perhaps by documenting reversibility in these parameters with therapy. Such an approach, however, presupposes that all aspects of hepatic encephalopathy, even the minimal ones, are reversible. This concept, generally held for hepatic encephalopathy other than hepatolenticular degeneration (Pseudo-Wilsonian hepatic encephalopathy) and spastic paraparesis, has been recently questioned (11) and may need to be reassessed.

There is a surprising absence of correlative studies of techniques for detection of early hepatic encephalopathy. Combined assessments utilizing psychometrics, visual evoked potentials, computerized tomography and the trailmaking test carried out longitudinally in the same patient prior to and after therapy for hepatic encephalopathy and comparison of such data with other encephalopathies would be helpful. Until the true sensitivity and specificity of visual evoked potentials are established and their neurophysiological basis is agreed upon, it appears premature to use these for categorization of animal models and mechanisms of coma.

Another important issue in considering the mechanism(s) of hepatic encephalopathy is the wide clinical spectrum of this disorder. Are the mechanisms of coma in patients with fulminant liver failure and portal-systemic encephalopathy (PSE) in cirrhotic patients the same? What about the largely irreversible and progressive neurological syndromes of hepatocerebral degeneration and spastic paraparesis? In the latter two situations, cerebral and spinal cord abnormalities, respectively, are found. Do studies in animal models with acute injury apply to patients with chronic liver failure? Again, it is our belief that until the issue is clarified, the findings in each experimental model should not be extrapolated to the others.

With these concerns expressed, what are the data with regard to the pathogenesis of hepatic encephalopathy? First, based on animal experimentation and studies in patients with localized brain lesions and neurosurgical procedures, it appears that consciousness is dependent on normal function of certain key brain areas. These are the reticular activating substance (RAS) in the brainstem, which is responsible for the "off" and "on" aspects of consciousness, and the cortex, which modulates the content (12, 13). Clearly such a restricted definition does not do justice to the various interacting circuits and cellular/subcellular pools in the brain, but it sets forth the minimum known gross cerebral areas likely to be affected in hepatic encephalopathy. Indeed, there is evidence that the brain responds in a heterogeneous manner to a variety of factors which accompany hepatic encephalopathy as evidenced by the variable distribution of hyperplastic astrocytes (Alzheimer type II astrocytes) in brains of patients with hepatic encephalopathy (14), the differential cerebral regional increase in glucose and ammonia consumption in hyperammonemia of animals with portacaval shunts (15, 16) and from selective depression of energy stores in the brainstem reticular activating system after hyperammonemia (17).

Second, patients with hepatic encephalopathy (both with acute and chronic liver disease), the disorder is largely reversible, which implies a metabolic (neurochemical/neurophysiological) rather than a structural disorder. The corollary of this aspect is that the astroglial changes and cerebral edema seen in many such patients are epiphenomena and not determinants of altered mental state. As indicated earlier, the exact role of hepatocerebral dysfunction and paraparesis in the spectrum of hepatic encephalopathy as regards central nervous system morphology and the issue of reversibility is uncertain. Also, should it turn out that bouts of more conventional hepatic encephalopathy leave subtle residua after treatment, as suggested by recent studies with computed tomography (11), the concept of potential reversibility may need to be rethought.

Third, although a deficiency of some key protective substance(s), more specific than albumin or glucose, has been postulated from time to time, the bulk of current evidence favors increased accumulation of "toxins" or an imbalance of false or true (excitatory vs. inhibitory) neurotransmitters as mechanisms for hepatic encephalopathy. Recently it has been suggested that accumulation of endogenous soporific ligands for cerebral benzodiazepine receptors may be found in patients with liver disease, and especially those with PSE (18, 19). If verified as to pathogenetic significance, this might serve as one explanation for the alleged benefit of inhibitors of benzodiazepine binding (20, 21). These reports are conceptually fascinating in pointing toward a novel site for therapy of hepatic encephalopathy (22), but as discussed later, they are currently conflicting or uncontrolled and anecdotal (20, 21, 23-28).

Within this general framework, there are three major, more specific hypotheses of the cause of hepatic encephalopathy. These are a) the toxin concept, b) the false neurotransmitter theory and c) the abnormal excitatory/inhibitory true neurotransmitter view, of which the gamma-aminobutyric acid (GABA) concept is a key component. Moreover, as will become evident later, some have formulated a combined (overlapping) view of the problem as the most logical explanation of the available data.

TOXIN CONCEPT

It is felt by many that excess ammonia is a candidate for the key toxin in hepatic encephalopathy. This is based on a) the frequent increase in blood (especially arterial) ammonia and spinal fluid glutamine (cerebral end product of ammonia detoxication) in patients with hepatic encephalopathy; b) good correlation of sequential ammonia levels and mental state in the same individual; c) abnormal mental status in children with urea cycle abnormalities and elevated ammonia; d) neurotoxicity in animals given ammonia or substances which generate ammonia; and e) improvement in mental status with treatment generally directed at ammonia production (3, 14).

On the other hand, blood ammonia is certainly not invariably increased in patients with hepatic encephalopathy, single values don't correlate well with the mental state, the acute EEG after ammonia administration may not resemble the pattern seen in patients with PSE and animal models with acute ammonia intoxication manifest a more convulsive picture than seen in most patients with this syndrome (22). These differences may, in part, be explained by the brief time frame of the acute studies and by lack of equivalence between blood and brain ammonia, with spinal fluid glutamine serving as a better index of encephalopathy.

However, a more intriguing proposal incorporates ammonia into a multifactorial toxin hypothesis for the pathogenesis of hepatic encephalopathy. Indeed, experimental studies have suggested a synergism between ammonia, mercaptans and short-chain fatty acids (3), with other, as yet undefined, endogenous or exogenous nitrogenous substances also a possibility.

In this multifactorial toxin hypothesis, the individual agents may impair cerebral function in different ways. For example, ammonia *in vitro* alters chloride flux across the neuronal membrane and may reversibly interfere with the nerve action potential (29). Ammonia, in the process of its detoxification to glutamic acid and then glutamine, may also result in a depletion of excitatory amino acid transmitters, aspartate and glutamate (Figure 1) (30, 31, 64). In this way, ammonia toxicity may relate very meaningfully to the true neurotransmitter imbalance concept. Aspartate and glutamate also help to shuttle hydrogen equivalents across the mitochondrial membrane, replenishing intramitochondrial NADH, a key component of the electron chain (30). Decreased availability of these key amino acids may thus impair shuttle of hydrogen equivalents from cytoplasm into mitochondria with a resultant decrease in intramitochondrial NADH/NAD ratio and impaired energy generation (30).

Indeed, phosphocreatine and ATP levels have been shown to be selectively decreased in the reticular activating system of rats given ammonia acutely (17) and in astrocytes exposed to ammonia in tissue culture, in the absence of cyclic

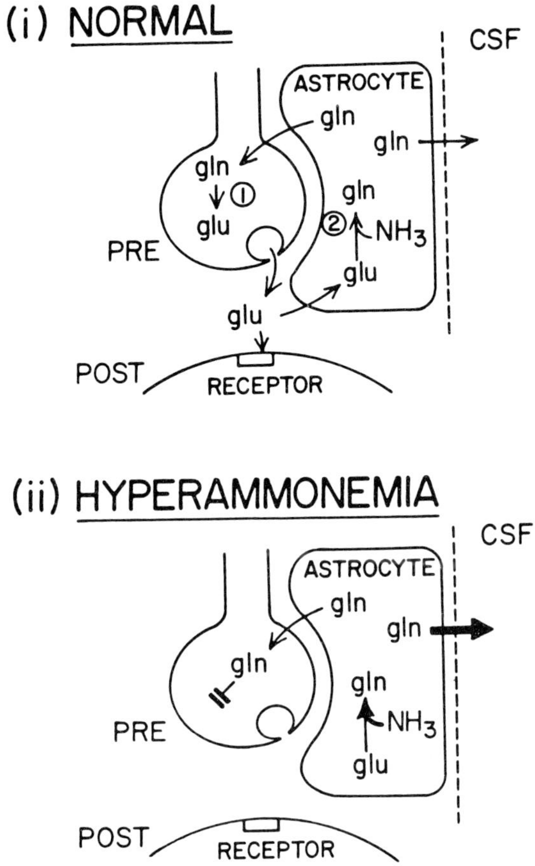

FIGURE 1. Simplified schematic representation of glutamate-glutamine cycle involved in regulation at the glutamatergic synapse: (1) glutaminase; (2) glutamine synthetase. Used with permission from Humana Press, Inc., *Neurochemical Pathology* 1987; 6:140, Butterworth, et al.

AMP (4). However, in the *in vivo* studies, it appears that changes in energy level were delayed until after the onset of coma and hence may be a secondary rather than a causal phenomenon (17, 30). Microregional turnover data, however, are not available, and relatively few studies (4, 31) have assessed the effects of ammonia on the metabolism of astrocytes, although these are the cells that primarily detoxify ammonia in brain, line the blood-brain barrier and show morphologic changes in patients with hepatic encephalopathy (1). Furthermore, the excess glutamine generated in brain from ammonia detoxication has been postulated to exchange with aromatic amino acids, the latter entering the brain in greater quantity and generating false (weak) neurotransmitters at the expense of norepinephrine and serotonin (32). While this last concept has been questioned on kinetic grounds, it shows how interactive the various hypotheses may be mechanistically.

To these multiple potential mechanisms of ammonia toxicity, one would add in the multifactorial toxin hypothesis the effect of mercaptans and short-chain fatty acids (3). These may interact with membranes, inhibit Na^+-K^+ ATPase, alter ammonia detoxication and have other detrimental effects. It is evident, therefore, that excess ammonia continues to qualify as *an* important likely toxin, that its toxic effects may be mediated by various mechanisms and may be potentiated by effects of other putative toxins. Furthermore, the toxic effects of ammonia may well relate to its detoxication and consequent disruption of normal cell metabolism (14, 33) and may especially affect cells (i.e., astroglia) which metabolize ammonia preferentially and in regions of the brain sensitive to ammonia (13, 15, 17, 31). Thus, studies of the whole brain may not be helpful, rendering animal models and cells in tissue culture, with all their caveats, necessary for further delineation of the pathogenesis of this disorder.

FALSE NEUROTRANSMITTER CONCEPT

The false neurotransmitter hypothesis stipulates that there is increased uptake of certain aromatic amino acids (phenylalanine, tyrosine) by the encephalopathic brain due to lower competitive uptake of branched-chain amino acids or, as stated earlier, in exchange for glutamine, which is present in high concentrations (1, 3, 33, 34). Such influx of phenylalanine in turn may interfere with normal generation of true excitatory neurotransmitters (norepinephrine and dopamine) from tyrosine. In addition, excess of tryptophan could result in increased serotonin. Moreover, tyrosine may then be metabolized to weak (false) neurotransmitters (i.e., octopamine). The net effect of such imbalance would be failure of proper neurosynaptic transmission. This interesting mechanism has likewise been questioned. While it is true that the branched-chain/aromatic amino acid ratio is decreased in many patients with PSE and that increased concentrations of false neurotransmitters and lower levels of norepinephrine are found in serum of such patients and in the brain of animals with experimentally induced hepatic coma (35), other data are much less supportive. For instance, the ratio of branched-chain/aromatic amino acids does not correlate well with encephalopathy and the value of providing branched-chain amino acids for the treatment of PSE is not established (3, 36, 37).

More importantly, administration of large quantities of false neurotransmitters intraventricularly to animals failed to produce coma and very low concentrations of norepinephrine and dopamine also were not associated with coma (38). Finally, in patients with PSE, no decrease in norepinephrine or dopamine has been detected in postmortem brains, and controlled trials of L-dopa have not shown benefit (39). Thus, while the above concept is far from proven, it has generated much exciting research into the neurotransmitter field and thus has opened new vistas. In addition, because of the functional heterogeneity of the brain and problems with animal models of PSE, it is possible that a critical imbalance of neurotransmitters in vital sites, perhaps augmented by accumulation of false neurotransmitters, may still be of importance in human PSE.

ABNORMAL EXCITATORY/INHIBITORY NEUROTRANSMITTER BALANCE

As regards the abnormal excitatory/inhibitory true neurotransmitter concept, one key aspect of this approach is the stipulation of imbalance of *various* neurotransmitters at critical brain sites. It is thus, in a sense, multifactorial and accommodates a multitude of findings. As alluded to earlier, such a concept would conform with decreased concentrations of the excitatory amino acids aspartate and glutamate demonstrated in the brains of animals exposed to ammonia and in patients with PSE. It would also fit with the proposed accumulation of various neuroinhibitory substances, some known (2) and others perhaps not yet identified.

Gamma-aminobutyric Acid Concept. A more restricted version of this true neurotransmitter imbalance concept is the so-called gamma-aminobutyric acid (GABA) hypothesis (2). GABA is one of the most prevalent inhibitory amino acids in the brain. Briefly, the GABA concept stipulates that excess GABA is generated in the gut by bacteria and that this substance bypasses the diseased/shunted liver, which normally metabolizes it. The excess GABA then may pass through a disrupted blood-brain barrier to cause inhibition of consciousness at the cerebral postsynaptic level (2, 40, 41). Another form of this concept postulates no increase in blood GABA and its enhanced passage into brain, but rather increased binding of GABA to GABA receptors in the brain of patients with hepatic encephalopathy (42-44). The cause of such increased binding is uncertain, but may be due to a decrease in endogenous ligands, "denervation" or other mechanisms for up-regulation of the GABA receptor.

As alluded to earlier, linked to the GABA concept is the finding of increased cerebral sensitivity of the brain of patients with chronic liver disease to various sedatives. The mechanisms of such increased sensitivity are unknown but may include decreased plasma binding of certain drugs, increased blood-brain permeability to such agents, increased cerebral receptor response (phenobarbital, benzodiazepine and GABA receptors are part of the same receptor cluster) (2, 45), displacement of normally present endogenous ligand or simply the summation of various subliminal toxic effects.

The initial evidence in favor of the GABA concept derives from an impressive array of studies showing increased GABA-like material in blood of animals with experimentally-induced hepatic coma (46) and in patients with PSE (47), formation of GABA by colonic bacteria (48), demonstration of uptake of GABA by liver (49), decreased GABA extraction by damaged liver (50), increased permeability of the blood-brain barrier to an analogue of GABA in animals with liver damage (51) and increased binding of GABA to synaptic GABA receptors in brain of animals with hepatic coma (2, 41, 52). This concept has been reinforced by suggestions that the proximity of benzodiazepine and phenobarbital receptors to the GABA receptor complex (2, 18, 45) may explain the apparent pharmacodynamic sensitivity of patients with PSE to these sedatives (53). Indeed, the visual evoked potential pattern recorded in animals with coma induced by liver damage and these sedatives was similar (54). In some studies, benzodiazepine antagonists were reported to reverse (at least in part) coma due to liver damage (20, 21, 25-28) and there appeared to be more cerebral benzodiazepine receptors in patients with PSE studied by positron emission tomography (55). This provocative hypothesis not only relates to the mechanism(s) of hepatic encephalopathy at the neurochemical/neurophysiological level, but also has implications for possible therapy of this disorder.

Unfortunately, there is also much evidence against the GABA hypothesis and the volume of this seems to be mounting. *First*, many recent studies in various model systems and using more specific analytical techniques have indicated that the GABA-like material originally analyzed by a radioreceptor assay, and felt to be GABA, represented other substances, possibly partly glutamine (43, 56-59). Thus, while some still find increased GABA in plasma of animals with liver damage or of patients with PSE (60, 61), most find no elevation, or only a small GABA increase (56, 58) which generally does not correlate with the degree of encephalopathy present. Furthermore, mass fragmentography has shown no increase of GABA in the cerebrospinal fluid of such patients (58).

Second, increased permeability of the blood-brain barrier to GABA analogues and various other substances in diverse models of liver injury has also not been uniformly reported (43, 62, 63). Certainly, increased transfer of larger molecules is increasingly felt to be an agonal (late) phenomenon and the cerebral edema seen in acute coma seems to be cytotoxic, not vasogenic, and may affect primarily astrocytes and the gray matter (4, 62, 63). Any enhanced permeability may be primarily for small molecules (63). The relevance of changes seen in acute experimental liver failure to human PSE can also be questioned. Permeability may differ with the model, the state of the disease and the marker used.

Third, animal models of human encephalopathy sometimes do not resemble the clinical state. For instance, the striking cerebellar signs noted in rabbits with galactosamine hepatotoxicity (18) are not usually seen in patients with either fulminant liver failure or PSE.

Fourth, many animal models of liver failure and brain tissue from patients with PSE have failed to show an alteration of the GABA system (GABA concentration or its metabolizing enzymes) or binding of GABA to its receptors (56, 59, 64-73). This lack of uniformity (Table 1) in animals and the negative data in humans require careful consideration. If there is an excess of GABA in key brain sites, one would expect down-regulation of binding as a compensatory phenomenon. Possi-

TABLE 1. Cerebral Gamma-aminobutyric Acid Binding in Various Studies of Experimental and Human Hepatic Encephalopathy

Model system	Binding	Reference (see list below)
1. Galactosamine toxicity in rabbits	Increased, low and high affinity site*	(13)
2. Galactosamine toxicity in rats	Increased initially*, lost for low affinity site with progression of failure	(1)
3. Portacaval shunting and dimethylnitrosamine in dogs	Increased for both sites initially, reduced or lost with progression of coma	(2)
4. Portacaval shunting in dogs	Unaltered	(14)
5. Alcoholics with and without HE	Unaltered	(6)
6. Patients with HE	Variable	(4) (Abstract)
7. Carbon tretrachloride-induced cirrhosis in rats	Increased	(11) (Abstract)
8. Thioacetamide toxicity in rats	Unaltered**	(9)
9. Viral liver failure in rats	Decreased	(11) (Abstract)
10. Portacaval shunting plus ligation of common bile duct	Unaltered**	(9)
11. Portacaval shunting and hepatic artery ligation in rats	Unaltered	(5)
12. Combined NH_4Cl, octanoic acid and dimethylsulfide administration in rats	Increased	(2)
13. Galactosamine toxicity in guinea pigs	Unaltered	(10) (Abstract)
14. Ethanolamine oleate injection via bile duct in guinea pigs	Unaltered	(10) (Abstract)
15. Portacaval shunting in dogs	Unaltered	(12) (Abstract)
16. Secondary biliary cirrhosis in dogs	Unaltered	(12) (Abstract)
17. Cirrhotic patients	Unaltered**	(7) (Abstract)

* Benzodiazepine binding increased; ** Benzodiazepine binding unaltered.

1. Baraldi M, et al. Science 1982; 216:427.
2. Baraldi M, et al. Arch Toxicol Suppl 1984; 7:103.
3. Baraldi M, et al. In: Kleinberger G, Ferenci P, Riederer P, et al., eds. Advances in Hepatic Encephalopathy and Urea Cycle Diseases. Basel: Karger, 1984: 353.
4. Ferenci P, et al. Gastroenterology 1983; 84:1371.
5. Ferenci P, et al. Metab Brain Dis 1987; 2:195.
6. Tran VH, et al. Ann Neurol 1981; 9:289.
7. Lavoie J, et al. J Neurochem 1987; 49:692.
8. Maddison JE, et al. Gastroenterology 1987; 93:1062.
9. Maddison JE, et al. Hepatology 1987; 7:621.
10. Nakatsukasa H, et al. Hepatology 1987; 7:1033.
11. Pappas SC, et al. Hepatology 1986; 6:1106.
12. Roy S, et al. Hepatology 1987; 7:1033.
13. Schafer DF, et al. J Lab Clin Med 1983; 102:870.
14. Thompson JS, et al. J Surg Res 1985; 38:143.

bly key brain sites, as yet unstudied, are important. Also, more consideration should be given to different affinity sites, with the low affinity site likely more important (56). On the other hand, a denervation phenomenon does not readily explain the usual reversibility of the encephalopathy.

Finally, and most interesting, are the studies with agonists and antagonists of GABA. These provocative reports, unfortunately, are conflicting in animals and uncontrolled so far in man (20, 21, 23-28). It may be that administration of various forms of benzodiazepine "antagonists" (22) in different animal models, at various stages of coma and with varying methods and end points for assessing recovery, explain the diversity of results. These possible reasons, however, do not apply to human PSE and do not explain a lack of controlled trials in this patient population. As regards the positron emission data (55), increased penetration of the benzodiazepine antagonist in patients with PSE could also explain the observations. Hence, in the future, nonspecific permeability markers should be included as part of such investigations and data obtained at various stages of liver disease with and without encephalopathy and after reversal of PSE. Moreover, data on endogenous benzodiazepine-like ligands so far have not been clearly related to hepatic encephalopathy, but rather to liver disease (18). Could the beneficial effects of benzodiazepine antagonists be exerted on the effects of such endogenous substances? In many ways, the concept of altered balance of various true neurotransmitters is more attractive than the GABA concept, as it is less restrictive and ties in to ammonia metabolism. More data in this area are eagerly awaited. The possible relationship of altered neurotransmitters to changes in the composition and structure of the neuronal membrane also need to be elucidated.

It is evident from this brief overview that the pathophysiology of hepatic encephalopathy is complex, controversial and certainly not fully elucidated. The comments, expressed above, are necessarily personal and thus may be somewhat biased. In brief, our view is that hepatic encephalopathy is primarily a metabolic and potentially reversible disorder of multifactorial, multimechanistic origin. Many of these factors and their mechanism(s) of action on the brain remain to be worked out. At present it appears that an imbalance of true excitatory vs. inhibitory neurotransmitters at key brain sites, possibly with secondary impairment of energy metabolism, seems likely. It also seems reasonable to postulate that ammonia and other amines contribute importantly to this neurotransmitter disequilibrium. The demonstration of an altered glutamate/aspartate neurotransmitter system in the brain of animals with experimental hepatic coma and some patients (66) is particularly provocative in this regard. This has been shown by numerous authors (Table 2) and clearly deserves further study. This overall view refers primarily to PSE and may not apply to coma of acute liver failure.

Further research in this area is necessary and should include a) better validated and diverse animal models, especially of the chronic liver damage/ shunting type, b) more emphasis on brain microheterogeneity, c) more studies of

TABLE 2. Cerebral Glutamatergic Function in Hepatic Encephalopathy: A Review of the Literature*

Reported finding(s)	Reference (see list below)
Glutamate concentration	
Reduced in portacaval shunted rats:	
(a) whole brain (by 10%)	(3)
(b) forebrain (by 20%)	(9)
(c) cerebral cortex (by 50%)	(6)
Reduced by 37% in cerebral cortex of patients with fulminant hepatic failure	(11)
Reduced by 20% in cerebral cortex of cirrhotic patients dying in hepatic coma	(2, 14)
Increased in hippocampus of galactosamine model of fulminant hepatic failure	(7)
Glutamate release	
Decreased by ammonia perfusion of hippocampal slices	(8)
Glutamate binding	
Increased in brain in acute hyperammonemia	(4)
Increased in cerebral cortex of shunted rats	(1, 2)
Normal in thioacetamide-induced liver failure in rats	(5)
Glutamate neurotransmission	
Decreased in hippocampal slice preparation following ammonia perfusion	(13)
Ammonia-induced decrease in hippocampus	(12)
Ammonia-induced decrease in spinal cord	(10)

* Adapted with permission from Humana Press, Inc., *Neurochemical Pathology* 1987; 6:142, Table 7, Butterworth, et al.

1. Butterworth RF, et al. Trans Am Soc Neurochem 1986; 17:242.
2. Butterworth RF, et al. Neurochem Path 1987; 6:131.
3. Cremer JE, et al. Neuropath Appl Neurobiol 1975; 3:292.
4. Ferenci P, et al. Hepatology 1984; 4:25.
5. Ferenci R, et al. Hepatology 1987; 7:1033.
6. Giguere JF, et al. Neurochem Res 1984; 9:1309.
7. Hamberger A, et al. Neurochem Res 1984; 9:1181.
8. Hamberger A, et al. J Neurochem 1979; 33:1295.
9. Hindfelt B, et al. J Clin Invest 1977; 59:386.
10. Raabe W. Neurochem Path 1987; 6:145.
11. Record CO, et al. Eur J Clin Invest 1976; 6:387.
12. Theoret Y, et al. Neuroscience 1985; 14:807.
13. Theoret Y, et al. Neuroscience 1985; 14:798.
14. Lavoie J, et al. J Neurochem 1987; 49:692.

astroglial cells which metabolize ammonia in brain, d) more correlative studies of neurochemistry and neurophysiology, e) further definition of the blood-brain barrier in the experimental models of liver failure in the hope of improving our understanding of liver damage-induced cerebral edema and f) *in vivo* studies of potential agonists and antagonists of coma in such animal models of liver failure with correlative assessments of dose given, receptor binding and functional impairment and recovery. In patients there is a need for a better definition of minimal encephalopathy with agreement on *practical* diagnostic tools, assessment of the potential for *full* recovery and the use of newer techniques (Nucleomagnetic Resonance [NMR], Positron Emission Spectrometry [PET], etc.) for defining brain metabolism. Above all, in this complex field, with many established, even fixed, opinions, there is a need for an open, but critical, mind to new data. What is clearly important is not who is right, but what is right.

REFERENCES

1. Schenker S, Hoyumpa AM Jr. Pathophysiology of hepatic encephalopathy. Hosp Pract 1984; 19:99-121.

2. Schafer DF, Jones EA. Potential neural mechanisms in the pathogenesis of hepatic encephalopathy. In: Popper H, Schaffner F, eds. Progress in Liver Diseases, Vol 7. New York: Grune & Stratton, 1982: 615-627.

3. Zieve L. Pathogenesis of hepatic encephalopathy. Metab Brain Dis 1987; 2:147-165.

4. Norenberg MD. The role of astrocytes in hepatic encephalopathy. Neurochem Pathol 1987; 6:13-33.

5. Cooper AJL, Lai JCK. Cerebral ammonia metabolism in normal and hyperammonemic rats. Neurochem Pathol 1987; 6:67-95.

6. Mullen KD, Gammal S, Geller D, et al. Correspondence. Hepatology 1987; 7:617-618.

7. Gilberstadt S, Gilberstadt H, Zieve L, et al. Psychometric performance defects in cirrhotic patients without overt encephalopathy. Arch Intern Med 1980; 140:519-521.

8. Rikkers L, Lenko P, Rudman D, et al. Subclinical hepatic encephalopathy: detection, prevalence and relationship to nitrogen metabolism. Gastroenterology 1978; 75:462-469.

9. Zeneroli ML, Pinelli G, Gollini G, et al. Visual evoked potential: a diagnostic trial for the assessment of hepatic encephalopathy. Gut 1984; 25:291-299.

10. Caselles F, Sagales T, Calzada MD, et al. Visual evoked potentials in hepatic encephalopathy. Lancet 1985; 1:394-395.

11. Bernthal P, Hays A, Tarter RE, et al. Cerebral CT scan abnormalities in cholestatic and hepatocellular disease and their relationship to neuropsychologic

test performance. Hepatology 1987; 7:107-114.

12. Plum F, Posner JB. The Diagnosis of Stupor and Coma. Contemporary Neurology Series, Vol 1. Philadelphia: Davis Publishing Company, 1980.

13. French JD, Magoun HW. Effects of chronic lesions in central cephalic brainstem of monkeys. Arch Neurol Psychiat 1952; 68:591-604.

14. Butterworth RF, Giguere JF, Michand J, et al. Ammonia: key factor in the pathogenesis of hepatic encephalopathy. Neurochem Pathol 1987; 6:1-12.

15. Lockwood AH, Ginsberg MD, Rhoades HM, et al. Cerebral glucose metabolism after portacaval shunting in the rat. J Clin Invest 1986; 78:86-95.

16. Girard GL, Giguere JF, Butterworth RF. The capacity for removal of excess ammonia in brain is reduced following portocaval anastomosis (Abstract). Hepatology 1987; 7:1033.

17. McCandless DW, Schenker S. Effect of acute ammonia intoxication on energy stores in the cerebral reticular activating system. Exp Brain Res 1981; 44:325-330.

18. Mullen KD, Szanter KM, Galloway PG, et al. CSF of patients with hepatic encephalopathy (HE) contains significant benzodiazepine (BZ) binding activity. Correlation with postmortem cortical BZ binding studies (Abstract). Hepatology 1987; 7:1103.

19. Basile AE, Gammal SH, Mullen KD, et al. Hepatic encephalopathy: evidence for the involvement of an endogenous benzodiazepine receptor ligand (Abstract). Hepatology 1987; 7:1103.

20. Baraldi M, Zeneroli ML, Ventura E, et al. Supersensitivity of benzodiazepine receptors in hepatic encephalopathy due to fulminant hepatic failure in the rat: reversal by a benzodiazepine antagonist. Clin Sci 1984; 67:167-175.

21. Bassett ML, Mullen KD, Skolnick P, et al. Amelioration of hepatic encephalopathy by pharmacologic antagonism of the $GABA_a$-benzodiazepine receptor complex in a rabbit model of fulminant hepatic failure. Gastroenterology 1987; 93:1069-1077.

22. Schafer D. Hepatic coma: studies on the target organ. Gastroenterology 1987; 93:1131-1134.

23. Rzepczynski D, Zieve L, Lindblad S, et al. In vivo studies of GABA-ergic effects in experimental hepatic encephalopathy. Hepatology 1986; 6:902-905.

24. Zieve L, Ferenci P, Rzepczynski D, et al. A benzodiazepine antagonist does not alter the course of hepatic encephalopathy or neural gamma-aminobutyric acid (GABA) binding. Metab Brain Dis 1987; 2:201-206.

25. Scollo-Lavizzari C, Steinmann E. Reversal of hepatic coma by benzodiazepine antagonist (Ro 15-1788) (Correspondence). Lancet 1985; 1:1324.

26. Bansky G, Meier PJ, Ziegler WH, et al. Reversal of hepatic coma by benzodiazepine antagonist (Ro 15-1788) (Correspondence). Lancet 1985; 1:1324-1325.

27. Ferenci P. Personal communication.

28. Bansky G, Meier PJ, Riederer E, et al. Effect of benzodiazepine antagonist in hepatic encephalopathy in man (Abstract). Hepatology 1987; 7:1103.

29. Raabe W. Synaptic transmission in ammonia intoxication. Neurochem Pathol 1987; 6:145-166.

30. Hindfelt B, Plum F, Duffy TE. Effect of acute ammonia intoxication or cerebral metabolism in rats with portacaval shunts. J Clin Invest 1977; 59:386-396.

31. Hertz L, Murphy Ch RK, Lai JCK, et al. Some metabolic effects of ammonia on astrocytes and neurons in primary culture. Neurochem Pathol 1987; 6:97-130.

32. James JH, Jeppson B, Ziparo V, et al. Hyperammonemia, plasma amino acid imbalance and blood/brain amino acid transport: a verified theory of portal systemic encephalopathy. Lancet 1979; 2:772-775.

33. Warner KS, Schenker S. Effect of an inhibitor of glutamine synthesis (methionine sulfoximine) ammonia toxicity and metabolism. J Lab Clin Med 1964; 64:442-449.

34. Fischer JE, Baldessarini RJ. Pathogenesis and therapy of hepatic coma. In: Popper H, Schaffner F, eds. Progress in Liver Disease, Vol 5. New York: Grune & Stratton, 1976: 363-397.

35. Dodsworth JM, James JH, Cummings MC, et al. Depletion of brain norepinephrine in acute hepatic coma. Surgery 1974; 75:811-820.

36. Weber FL, Reiser BJ. Relationship of plasma amino acids to nitrogen balance and portal systemic encephalopathy in alcoholic liver disease. Dig Dis Sci 1982; 27:103.

37. Zieve L, Onstad GR, Doizaki WM, et al. High brain concentrations of phenylalanine, tryptophan and methionine do not cause coma in rats or dogs (Abstract). Gastroenterology 1980; 79:1070.

38. Zieve L, Olsen RL. Can hepatic coma be caused by a reduction of brain noradrenaline or dopamine? Gut 1977; 18:688-691.

39. Michel H, Solere M, Grainer P, et al. Treatment of cirrhotic hepatic encephalopathy with L-dopa. A controlled trial. Gastroenterology 1980; 79:207-211.

40. Schafer DF, Jones EA. Hepatic encephalopathy and the gamma-aminobutyric acid neurotransmitter system. Lancet 1982; 1:18.

41. Jones EA, Schafer DR, Ferenci P, et al. The neurobiology of hepatic encephalopathy. Hepatology 1984; 4:1235-1242.

42. Baraldi M, Zeneroli ML. Experimental hepatic encephalopathy: changes in the binding of gamma-aminobutyric acid. Science 1982; 216:427.

43. Zeneroli ML, Iuliano E, Racogni G, et al. Metabolism and brain uptake of gamma-aminobutyric acid in galactosamine-induced hepatic encephalopathy in rats. J Neurochem 1982; 38:1219-1222.

44. Baraldi M, Zeneroli ML, Ventura E, et al. Portal systemic encephalopathy in dogs: changes in brain GABA receptors and neurochemical correlates. In: Kleinberger G, Ferenci P, Riederer P, et al., eds. Advances in Hepatic Encephalopathy and Urea Cycle Diseases. Basel: Karger, 1984: 353-359.

45. Tallman JF, Paul SM, Skolnich P, et al. Receptors for the age of anxiety: pharmacology of the benzodiazepines. Science 1980; 207:274-278.

46. Schafer DF, Waggoner JG, Jones EA. Sera from rabbits in acute hepatic coma inhibit the binding of (^{3}H)-gamma-aminobutyric acid to neural membranes. Gastroenterology 1980; 78:1320.

47. Ferenci P, Schafer DF, Kleinberger G, et al. Serum levels of gamma-aminobutyric acid-like activity in acute and chronic hepatocellular disease. Lancet 1983; 2:811-814.

48. Schafer DF, Fowler JM, Jones EA. Colonic bacteria: a source of gamma-aminobutyric acid in blood. Proc Soc Exp Biol Med 1981; 167:301-303.

49. Minuk GY, Vargula J, Ferenci P, et al. Identification of an acceptor system for gamma-aminobutyric acid on isolated rat hepatocytes. Hepatology 1984; 4:180-185.

50. Ferenci P, Schafer DF, Shrager R, et al. Metabolism of the inhibitory neurotransmitter gamma-aminobutyric acid in a rabbit model of acute hepatic failure. Hepatology 1983; 3:507-512.

51. Horowitz ME, Schafer DF, Molnar P, et al. Increased blood/brain transfer in a rabbit model of fulminant hepatic failure. Gastroenterology 1983; 84:1003-1011.

52. Schafer DF, Fowler VM, Munson PJ, et al. Gamma-aminobutyric acid and benzodiazepine receptors in an animal model of acute hepatic failure. J Lab Clin Med 1983; 102:870-880.

53. Bakti G, Fisch HV, Kazlganis G, et al. Mechanism of the excessive sedative response of cirrhotics to benzodiazepines: model experiments with triazolan. Hepatology 1987; 7:629-638.

54. Schafer DF, Pappas SC, Brody LE, et al. Visual evoked potentials in a rabbit model of hepatic encephalopathy. I. Sequential changes and comparisons with drug induced comas. Gastroenterology 1984; 86:540-545.

55. Samson Y, Bernau J, Pappata S, et al. Cerebral uptake of benzodiazepine measured by positron emission tomography in hepatic encephalopathy (Correspondence). N Engl J Med 1987; 316:414-415.

56. Maddison JE, Dodd PR, Morrison M, et al. Plasma GABA, GABA-like activity and the brain GABA-benzodiazepine receptor complex in rats with chronic hepatic encephalopathy. Hepatology 1987; 7:621-628.

57. Ferenci P, Ebner J, Zimmerman C, et al. Is blood GABA increased in hepatic encephalopathy? (Abstract). Hepatology 1986; 6:1157.

58. Moroni F, Riggio O, Carla V, et al. Hepatic encephalopathy: lack of changes of gamma-aminobutyric acid content in plasma and cerebrospinal fluid. Hepatology 1987; 7:816-820.

59. Maddison JE, Dodd PR, Johnston GAR, et al. Brain gamma-aminobutyric acid receptor binding is normal in rats with thioacetamide-induced hepatic encephalopathy despite elevated plasma gamma-aminobutyric acid-like activity. Gastroenterology 1987; 93:1062-1068.

60. Minule GY, Winder A, Burgess ED, et al. Serum gamma-aminobutyric acid (GABA) levels in patients with hepatic encephalopathy. Hepatogastroenterology 1985; 32:171-174.

61. Levy LJ, Leek J, Losowsky MS. Evidence for gamma-aminobutyric acid as the inhibitor of gamma-aminobutyric acid binding in the plasma of humans with liver disease and hepatic encephalopathy. Clin Sci 1987; 73:531-534.

62. Lo WD, Ennis SR, Goldstein GW, et al. The effects of galactosamine-induced hepatic failure upon blood-brain barrier permeability. Hepatology 1987; 7:452-456.

63. Trober PG, Canto MD, Granger DR, et al. Electron microscopic evaluation of brain edema in rabbits with galactosamine-induced fulminant hepatic failure: ultrastructure and integrity of the blood-brain barrier. Hepatology 1987; 7:1272-1277.

64. Butterworth RF, Lavoie J, Giguere JF, et al. Cerebral GABA-ergic and glutamatergic function in hepatic encephalopathy. Neurochem Pathol 1987; 6:131-144.

65. Ferenci P, Zieve L, Ebner J, et al. Postsynaptic gamma-aminobutyric acid receptor in hepatic coma following portacaval shunt and hepatic artery ligation in rat. Metab Brain Dis 1987; 2:195-200.

66. Lavoie J, Giguere JF, Layrargues GP, et al. Activities of neuronal and astrocytic marker enzymes in autopsied brain tissue from patients with hepatic encephalopathy. Metab Brain Dis 1987; 2:283-290.

67. Lavoie J, Giguere JF, Layrargues GP, et al. Amino acid neurotransmitters in autopsied brain tissue from cirrhotic patients with hepatic encephalopathy: no evidence for altered GABA function (Abstract). Hepatology 1987; 7:1103.

68. Ferenci P, Zimmermann Ch, Egner J. Gamma-aminobutyric acid (GABA)-ergic and glutamatergic neurotransmission in hepatic encephalopathy (HE) in thioacetamide (TAA) induced liver failure in rats (Abstract). Hepatology 1987; 7:1033.

69. Nakatsukasa H, Gordon VP, Martin P, et al. Brain gamma-aminobutyric acid (GABA) binding is unaltered in two guinea pig models of fulminant hepatic failure: further evidence conflicting with the GABA hypothesis (Abstract). Hepatology 1987; 7:1033.

70. Roy S, Pomier-Layrargues G, Bergeron M, et al. Lack of changes in GABA-ergic neurotransmission in cirrhotic and shunted dogs with hepatic encephalopathy (Abstract). Hepatology 1987; 7:1033.

71. Tran VH, Snyder SH, Major LF, et al. GABA receptors are increased in brains of alcoholics. Ann Neurol 1981; 9:289-292.

72. Thompson JS, Schafer DF, Schafer GJ, et al. Gamma-aminobutyric acid plasma levels and brain binding in Eck fistula dogs. J Surg Res 1985; 38:143-148.

73. Pappas SC, Levy CA, Gordon VP. Decreased brain GABA binding in a model of fulminant hepatic failure (FHF): evidence conflicting with the GABA hypothesis for hepatic encephalopathy (HE) (Abstract). Hepatology 1986; 6:1106.

74. Baraldi M, Zeneroli ML, Ventura E, et al. An increase in cerebral benzodiazepine receptors induced by a subacute administration of ammonia, mercaptans and short-chain fatty acids in rats. Clin Sci 1987; 73:669-671.

3

NITROGEN METABOLISM IN THE GUT

PETER B. SOETERS, M.D., PAUL A.M. VAN LEEUWEN, M.D.,
CHARLES L.H. VAN BERLO, M.D.

In the literature, the gut flora are still regularly indicated as the primary producers of ammonia (1-4). The predominant importance that is attached by clinicians to bacterial metabolism in the pathogenesis of hyperammonemia and hepatic encephalopathy, however, has resulted from two paramount factors:

First, Dame Sheila Sherlock emphasized the role of bacteria (5) and, second, the observation that antibiotics, notably chlortetracycline and, later, neomycin, lowered plasma levels of ammonia while ameliorating hepatic encephalopathy (5).

It is less well appreciated by clinicians that ammonia can also be generated by nonbacterial mechanisms. Nance and his associates reported that germfree dogs with Eck fistulae developed portal-systemic encephalopathy (PSE) with hyperammonemia (6). Several other reports also indicate that ammonia may be derived from intermediary metabolism in the gut. In 1973, Matsutaka and co-authors demonstrated that the small bowel of rats can take up glutamine *in vitro* and at the same time produce ammonia and glutamic acid (7).

In 1979, Weber reported that the small intestine of dogs liberates a large quantity of ammonia equal to that released by the uncleansed colon into the portal blood. In the small bowel, the amount of ammonia released by the small intestine is stoichiometrically related to the uptake of glutamine from arterial blood. Here glutamine was the most likely source of all the ammonia released. In the colon, half of the ammonia produced could be accounted for by deamidation of glutamine. Oxidation of the glutamine carbon provides an important source of energy for the epithelial cells of the intestinal mucosa where glutaminase is largely located (9). Arteriovenous (AV) glutamine across the nonhepatic organs of dogs (10, 11), sheep (12) and humans (13) furnished more direct clues. AV differences were larger across the small intestine than expected (14).

Watford et al. found that among added substrates glucose, glutamine and glutamate are the preferred fuels for mucosal respiration (15). Very important work was done by Windmueller, who reported in 1975 the use of an isolated, perfused preparation of rat intestine. He studied the fate of glutamine carbon and glutamine nitrogen (16). Isolated mucosa cells contain a group of enzymes that can account for the metabolism of glutamine (17). Fifty-seven percent of the glutamine carbon taken up appears in the portal blood as CO_2 (18). Nitrogen taken up by jejunum as glutamine could be accounted for by the release of ammonia (38%), citrulline (28%), alanine (24%), proline (7%), glutamate (2%) and ornithine (1%)(19, 20). About 75% of the glutamine amide nitrogen, released by glutaminase, could be accounted for as ammonia and the remainder as one of the two nitrogen atoms of citrulline.

It is therefore clear that in addition to ammonia generation by the bacterial flora, gut mucosa contains all the enzymes needed to produce NH_3 using glutamine as the main substrate.

INVESTIGATIONS

In order to establish the relative contributions of the bacterial flora and the gut mucosa, we conducted a series of experiments in germfree and conventional rats, employing techniques to manipulate the bacterial flora.

First, we repeated experiments done by Matsutaka (7) demonstrating that in tissue incubations the small bowel produces more NH_3 than the large bowel, and that this NH_3 production is glutamine-dependent (Table 1). Synchronously, glutamic acid and alanine are produced.

TABLE 1. Ammonia, Alanine, Glutamate and Glutamine Concentrations in Small and Large Intestine (Fasted State) of Conventional Rats after Incubations (90 min.). The values are the concentrations measured in the medium (n=7, mean±SEM). Glutamine in the incubation medium was 10mmol. Results are expressed in nmol/mg tissue w/w per 90 min.

	Ammonia	Alanine	Glutamine	Glutamate
	Small intestine (fasted state - glutamine)			
Medium	10.19±1.03	10.40±1.0	<2.5	5.19±0.84
	Small intestine (fasted state + glutamine 10mmol)			
Medium	35.40±3.76	24.70±1.25	448.30±19.9	12.56±2.53
	Large intestine (fasted state - glutamine)			
Medium	3.84±0.42	2.47±0.3	<2.5	1.47±0.14
	Large intestine (fasted state + glutamine 10mmol)			
Medium	15.20±1.07	6.94±0.5	448.3±19.2	6.26±1.07

In a second series of incubations employing crypt cells and villus cells of germfree and conventional rats, it was demonstrated after incubation in Krebs-Ringer buffer with glucose and after the addition of glutamine that both types of cells produce amounts of NH_3 that do not differ significantly in germfree and conventional rats (Table 2). Again, glutamic acid and alanine are simultaneously produced.

In a third series of experiments conventional rats were selectively "decontaminated" by administering antibiotics to eliminate either the anaerobic or the aerobic flora. Ammonia levels in portal venous blood decrease substantially only when the anaerobic flora are eradicated and may even approach the low portal venous ammonia levels seen in germfree animals (Table 3). When the aerobic flora were suppressed no significant decrements in ammonia levels were observed.

Another approach to this problem is to study germfree rats and to colonize them with either aerobic, anaerobic or conventional bacterial flora. Colonization with aerobic flora does not affect the portal venous ammonia concentration. Colonization with anaerobic flora results in a modest increase in NH_3 levels (Table 4), but does not reach the concentrations seen in conventional rats. These findings indicate that more organisms or longer periods are required for the gut and the gut flora to achieve normal levels.

In a fourth series of experiments we measured portal-arterial venous differences of amino acids and ammonia across the intestine in conventional and germfree rats (Figure 1).

The uptake of glutamine across the small bowel and the release of

TABLE 2. Ammonia, Alanine and Glutamic Acid Production in Conventional and Germfree Rats Incubated in Krebs-Ringer Buffer (glutamine 10 mmol) for 30 Minutes with and without Lactulose (2.5% - 10% W/V) and with Neomycin Added (81.4 µmol and 814 µmol). DNA content of each sample was 50 µg/ml. Results are the mean of the duplicate experiments and expressed in µmol/mg DNA/30 min. Intestinal cells harvested from four rats were pooled prior to each experiment.

	NH_3	NH_3	Alanine	Alanine	Glutamic acid	Glutamic acid
	-	+	-	+	-	+
Conventional						
Villus	0.77	8.83	0.25	5.12	0	3.39
Crypt	1.55	3.78	0.03	1.26	0	3.15
Germfree						
Villus	0.54	5.89	0.43	4.09	0	1.49
Crypt	0.95	7.63	0.42	2.84	0	5.49

TABLE 3. Mean Portal Ammonia Concentration of Small and Large Intestine in Controls, Selectively Decontaminated (without Enterobacteriaceae or without Anaerobic Flora) and Germfree Animals, in μmol/L(mean±SEM).

	Controls Plasma	Selectively decontaminated without entero-bacteriaceae Plasma	Selectively decontaminated with anaerobic flora Plasma	Germfree Plasma
	n=5	n=6	n=6	n=6
Small intestine	426±35.8	331±56	169.6±10.7	187±13
	n=5	n=6	n=6	n=5
Large intestine	548±57.4	545±49	262.5±24.8	186±10.2

ammonia are of the same order of magnitude in rats with conventional intestinal flora. In germfree animals, however, the uptake of glutamine and the release of ammonia across the small bowel are significantly lower than in conventional animals (Figure 2).

Windmueller has demonstrated that glutamine uptake from arterial blood in the gut is concentration-dependent (16). Consequently, both the uptake by the gut and the absolute levels of glutamine in arterial blood are important. Indeed, glutamine levels in the arterial blood of germfree rats are substantially lower than in conventional rats (Table 5). This difference may explain the lower uptake of glutamine in germfree animals and, subsequently, the smaller release of NH_3 from the intestine in the portal blood of germfree rats.

TABLE 4. Mean Portal Ammonia Concentration of Conventional, Gnotobiotic and Germfree Rats in μmol/L (mean±SEM)(n=5). Ammonia concentrations were determined in the combined portal effluent of small and large intestine.

	Conventional Plasma	Gnotobiotic aerobes Plasma	Gnotobiotic anaerobes Plasma	Gnotobiotic aerobes+anaerobes Plasma	Germfree Plasma
Portal vein	422±19.6	196±20.7	266±37	245.5±9.5	200±16.7

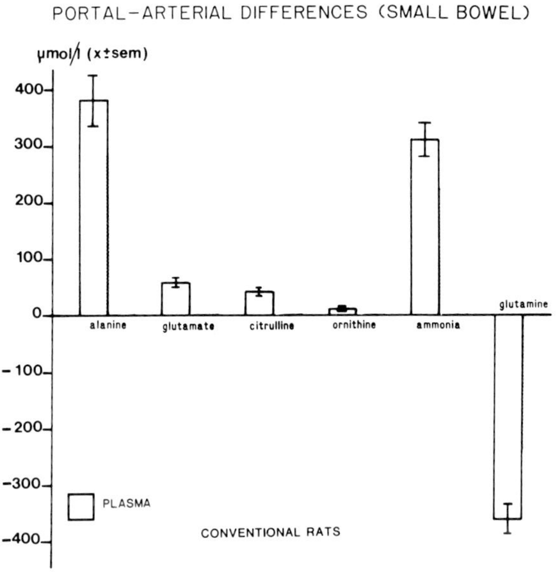

FIGURE 1. Portal-arterial differences of amino acids and ammonia in plasma of conventional male Wistar rats (fed state). Portal concentrations were selectively measured in the portal effluent of the small intestine. Positive and negative values represent output and uptake respectively in μmol/L (mean±SEM).

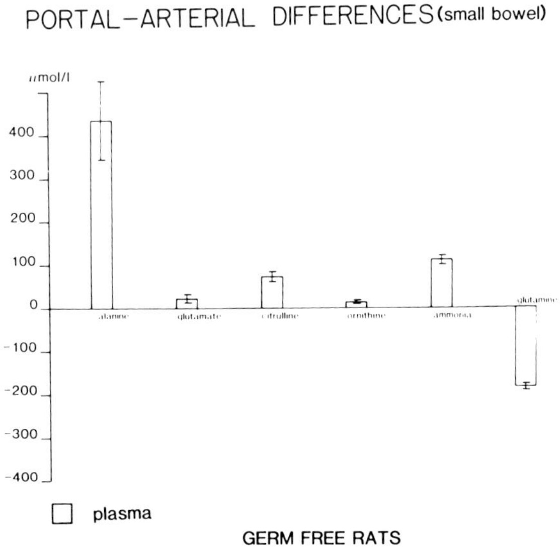

FIGURE 2. Portal-arterial differences of amino acids and ammonia in the plasma of germfree male Wistar rats (fed state). Portal concentrations were selectively measured in the portal effluent of the small intestine. Positive and negative values represent output and uptake respectively in μmol/L (mean±SEM).

TABLE 5. Arterial Ammonia and Amino Acid Concentrations in Plasma of Conventional and Germfree Rats (Fed State). Arterial blood was collected from the aorta of controls, lactulose- and neomycin-treated rats. Results are expressed in μmol/L (±SEM).

	Conventional controls Plasma n=6	Germfree controls Plasma n=6
Ammonia	114.0±13.6	85.0±3.7
Glutamic acid	48.0±3.0	89.1±13.7
Alanine	326.0±8.0	412.1±36.8
Citrulline	68.0±2.0	83.8±0.9
Ornithine	52.0±3.0	50.8±2.0
Glutamine	697.0±25.0	377.0±8.7

DISCUSSION

It is clear from data in the literature and from the results of our experiments that the presence of anaerobic bacteria in the gut increases ammonia generation by at least two mechanisms. First, anaerobic bacteria produce ammonia. Second, rats with normal gut flora exhibit arterial glutamine levels that are significantly higher than germfree rats. This difference leads to increased uptake of glutamine by the gut wall and, consequently, to increased production of ammonia in the intestinal wall.

It is not clear, however, why glutamine levels are higher in normal animals than in germfree animals. Glutamine concentrations and the glutamine/alanine ratio in the venous blood of the extremities have been shown to vary in different clinical states (19). In patients with cirrhosis, for instance, Imler has shown that the glutamine/alanine ratio is much greater than in healthy controls (19). The same phenomenon was demonstrated when experimental animals were infused with ammonium acetate.

In germfree rats the arterial glutamine/alanine ratio was much lower than in conventional rats (Table 5). The absolute level of glutamine in arterial plasma was also much lower. In accordance with the mechanisms postulated in patients with chronic liver disease or after ammonia infusions, the decreased glutamine/alanine ratio in germfree rats may be explained by the decrease in arterial ammonia levels that is present in germfree rats. Our data do not allow precise quantitation of bacterial and metabolic ammonia generation. We suggest, however, that the presence of bacteria in the gut increases the ammonia concentration in the portal vein, which is then largely taken up by the liver. However, a small portion escapes into the general circulation where ammonia affects the glutamine/alanine ratio and increases the glutamine concentration in the veins of the peripheral tissues and, consequently, in arterial blood. Potential differences in cardiac output, e.g., organ blood flow between normal and germfree animals, make interpretation of these data difficult. If, however, it is assumed that the blood flow is comparable, the modest increments in systemic ammonia levels in normal animals compared to germfree animals is insignificant in relation to the large increment in glutamine levels observed in normal rats (Table 5). Furthermore, the sum of glutamine and alanine is significantly higher in normal animals. It appears, therefore, that other factors may be active in animals with normal gut flora, thus increasing the systemic concentration of glutamine (and alanine). Windmueller has shown that the deamidation of glutamine in the small bowel is concentration-dependent (16). Our data confirm that an increase in systemic glutamine levels results in increased uptake and degradation of glutamine in the gut mucosa with enhanced production of ammonia.

These findings are relevant in terms of whole body nitrogen metabolism. More than 50% of all nitrogen released from peripheral proteolysis enters the systemic circulation as glutamine and alanine (20).

This phenomenon occurs in most organs, most notably skeletal muscle, heart muscle, adipose tissue and brain. To achieve homeostasis, the glutamine reduced is almost exclusively taken up by two organs: the gut and the kidney. In the kidney glutamine degradation is quantitatively less important than in the gut, but ammonia is also produced and released in the renal vein and in the urine depending upon its acidity. Therefore, it is likely that most glutamine is taken up by the gut mucosa. The first step in the degradation of glutamine is deamidation, which results in ammonia generation. Some 75% of this ammonia is released into the portal vein (18). It is evident that although exact quantities have not yet been measured, the flow through this pathway must be enormous. The chain of events described seems compatible with a scheme of evolutionary survival, i.e., it permits only small amounts of ammonia to gain access to the systemic circulation. Ammonia generated by the kidney is excreted into the urine when the urine is acid. Even when ammonium chloride or ammonium acetate is infused, glutamine is very quickly formed in most peripheral tissues including brain, muscle and fat. Glutamine then acts as a nontoxic nitrogen carrier, which is subsequently cleared by the gut and the kidneys. It should be appreciated, however, that almost all NH_3 taken up in the periphery and transformed into glutamine is later released into the portal vein, renal vein or urine as ammonia. Therefore, glutamine formation only temporarily utilizes ammonia. Most ammonia ultimately must be cleared by the liver. Only ammonia (NH_4^+) excreted in the urine escapes.

It can also be appreciated what happens in the presence of portal-systemic shunting. Ammonia produced in the gut gains free access to the systemic circulation and is cleared by the peripheral tissues. Glutamine produced in the periphery is taken up by the gut and the kidneys. In the gut, ammonia is released which again enters the systemic circulation, resulting in a vicious cycle.

These observations make it easy to understand how catabolism may precipitate hepatic encephalopathy. Increased breakdown of peripheral protein presents the organism with increased amounts of glutamine and alanine (21). Likewise, increased glutamine flux results in increased ammonia production in the gut, which gains access to the systemic circulation either because of diminished hepatic metabolic function or via the portal-systemic collateral circulation.

Some aspects of this discussion are speculative. More specifically, the flux through the pathways described has not been quantitated. We want to emphasize, however, that mucosal metabolism of glutamine in the gut and its interrelationships with intermediate metabolism elsewhere in the body are of greater importance in ammonia production than has previously been recognized in the literature.

REFERENCES

1. Walser M, Bodenloos LJ. Urea metabolism in man. J Clin Invest 1959; 38:1617-1626.

2. Wolpert E, Philips SF, Summerskill WHJ. Ammonia production in the human colon. N Engl J Med 1970; 283:159-164.

3. Phear EA, Ruebner B. The in vitro production of ammonium and amines by intestinal bacteria in relation to nitrogen toxicity as a factor in hepatic coma. Br J Exp Path 1956; 37:253-259.

4. Floch MH, Conn HO. Qualitative and quantitative relationships on fecal flora in cirrhotic patients with portal systemic encephalopathy and following portacaval anastomosis. Gastroenterology 1970; 59:70-79.

5. Phear EA, Ruebner B, Sherlock S, Summerskill WHJ. Methionine toxicity in liver disease and its prevention by chlortetracycline. Clin Sci 1956; 15:93.

6. Nance FC, Kline DG. Eck fistula encephalopathy in germ-free dogs. Ann Surg 1971: 174:856-861.

7. Matsutaka H, Aikawa T, Yamamoto H, et al. Gluconeogenesis and amino acid metabolism III. Uptake of glutamine and output of alanine and ammonia by nonhepatic splanchnic organs of fasted rats and their metabolic significance. J Biochem 1973; 74:1019-1029.

8. Weber FC, Veach G. The importance of the small intestine in gut ammonium production in the fasting dog. Gastroenterology 1979; 77:235-240.

9. Pinkus LM, Windmueller HG. Phosphate dependent glutaminase of small intestine. Localization and role in intestinal glutamine metabolism. Arch Biochem Biophys 1977; 182:506-517.

10. Addae SK, Lotspeich WB. Relation between glutamine utilization and production in metabolic acidosis. Am J Physiol 1968; 215:269-277.

11. Elwyn DH, Parikh HC, Shoemaker WC. Amino acid movements between gut, liver and periphery in unanesthetized dogs. Am J Physiol 1968; 215:1260-1275.

12. Wolf JE, Bergman EM, Williams HH. Net metabolism of plasma amino acids by liver and portal drained viscera of fed sheep. Am J Physiol 1972; 223:438-446.

13. Felig P, Wahren J, Karl I, et al. Glutamine and glutamate metabolism in normal and diabetic subjects. Diabetes 1973; 22:573-576.

14. Windmueller HG, Spaeth AE. Uptake and metabolism of plasma glutamine by the small intestine. J Biol Chem 1974; 249:5070-5079.

15. Watford M, Lund P, Krebs HA. Isolation and metabolic characteristics of rat and chicken enterocytes. J Biochem 1979; 178:589-596.

16. Windmueller HG, Spaeth AE. Intestinal metabolism of glutamine and glutamate from the lumen as compared to glutamine from blood. Arch Biochem Biophys 1975; 171:662-672.

17. Windmueller HG. Glutamine utilization by the small intestine. In: Meiser A, ed. Advances in Enzymology, Vol 53. New York: Wiley, 1982: 201-237.

18. Windmueller HG, Spaeth AE. Respiratory fuels and nitrogen metabolism in vivo in small intestine of fed rats. J Biol Chem 1980; 255:107-112.

19. Imler M, Schlienger JL, Frick A. Study of muscular glutamine and alanine release in cirrhotics with hyperammonaemia and in ammonium infused rats. In: Holm E, ed. Aminosguren und Ammoniak Stoffwechsel bei Leber Insuffizienz. Baden Baden: Verlag Gerard Witstrock, 1982: 33-39.

20. Rudermann NB. Muscle amino acid metabolism and gluconeogenesis. Ann Rev Med 1975; 26:245.

21. Souba WW, Smith RJ, Wilmore DW. Review: glutamine metabolism by the intestinal tract. JPEN 1985; 9:608-617.

4

ENDOCRINE ASPECTS OF AMMONIA AND AMINO ACID METABOLISM

G. MARCHESINI, M.D., G.P. BIANCHI, M.D.,
G.A. CHECCHIA, M.D., M. ZOLI, M.D.

The fine regulation of nitrogen metabolism depends on the counterbalancing action of anabolic and catabolic hormones, mainly insulin and glucagon, which, in turn, are regulated by substrate availability.

Ammonia is one of the principal end products of nitrogen metabolism. It is an unstable substrate, which may be utilized by several tissues during transamination processes. Therefore, ammonia metabolism is intimately connected to amino acid metabolism. Because its concentration in the portal vein exceeds peripheral levels by 5 to 10 times, the gastrointestinal tract is believed to be the main source of ammonia. From the splanchnic area, ammonia reaches the liver, where it is converted to urea by a series of enzymatic reactions. Part of the ammonia reaches the general circulation and becomes available to the peripheral muscle tissues and to the brain. This review will focus on the role of insulin and glucagon in ammonia and amino acid metabolism, on the site of the biologic action of these hormones and, conversely, on the stimulatory effects of amino acids and ammonia on insulin and glucagon secretion.

Particular emphasis will be given to the disturbed amino acid and ammonia metabolism in the course of chronic liver diseases.

SITE OF AMMONIA METABOLISM IN MAN

A direct evaluation of the site of ammonia metabolism in man, using total body scanning, was performed by Lockwood et al. (1), who injected ^{13}N-ammonium chloride into normal volunteers and into patients with cirrhosis (Table 1). After 20 minutes, approximately 6% of the injected dose of ammonia was retained in the

TABLE 1. The Distribution of Ammonia Metabolism in Man following ^{13}N-ammonia Injection

Organ	Controls (n=5) (%)	Severe liver diseases (n=12) (%)	Statistical signifigance
Brain	6.9±0.5	7.7±0.3	p<0.10, >0.05
Liver	7.1±0.7	10.6±0.5	Uptake dependent on size
Urine and bladder	6.4±1.1	2.8±0.6	p<0.01
Blood	6.4±0.3	6.4±0.6	NS
Thigh	1.7±0.1	1.2±0.1	p<0.025

From Lockwood et al. (1).

vascular bed, while 6% to 7% was in the brain, and another 7% was in the liver (Figure 1). The bladder (and the urine in it) of normal subjects contained another 6% to 7% of injected ammonia. The bladder radioactivity apparently represents the amount of ammonia converted to urea, and is reduced in patients with liver disease because of decreased urea synthesis. The decreased activity in urine was balanced by increased ^{13}N-activity in the diseased liver, unrelated to the size of the liver. Hepatic radioactivity increased from 7% in healthy subjects to 10% in cirrhotic patients. The activity in the thigh area, assumed to be a measure of ammonia metabolism in muscle, was only 1% to 2%, but a rough calculation of total muscle uptake gives values greater than 50% in healthy subjects, and less in patients with liver disease depending on the degree of muscle wasting.

These data stress the relevance of peripheral ammonia metabolism in ammonia detoxication. However, during resting, the arteriovenous difference of ammonia is close to zero (2), suggesting that there is no significant ammonia uptake or release. ^{13}N-activity in muscle is likely to result from the conversion of ammonia to other nitrogen compounds, among which alanine and mainly glutamine are the putative candidates, as pointed out by studies on interorgan amino acid exchange (3).

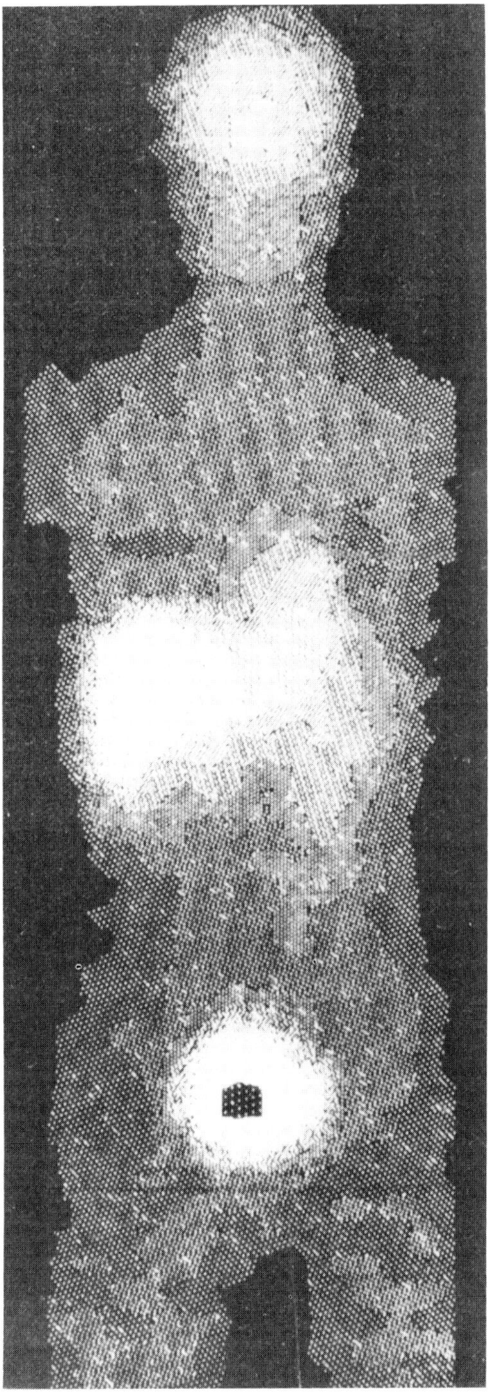

FIGURE 1. ^{13}N-ammonia total body High Energy Gamma rectilinear scan of a normal subject 20 minutes after the intravenous injection of $^{13}NH_4Cl$. Dot density is proportional to ^{13}N activity. The bladder, liver and brain are easily seen. Radioactivity can also be seen in the heart and in the left kidney. The torso is outlined by muscle activity. (Reproduced with permission of Dr. A.H. Lockwood and the American Society for Clinical Investigation.)

HORMONAL CONTROL OF PERIPHERAL AMMONIA AND AMINO ACID METABOLISM

The sole source of organic nitrogen for the body is dietary protein. The daily amount of protein turnover in the intact organism is approximately 300 g, which is roughly three times higher than the average protein intake. Therefore, most of the nitrogen released from protein degradation must be reused for protein synthesis. There is substantial evidence that an interorgan exchange of amino acids occurs to provide for the needs of the body under different conditions. In the postabsorptive state, amino acids are released from the periphery and reach the liver, while after a protein meal selected amino acids may escape hepatic uptake and replenish the peripheral tissues with the nitrogen lost during fasting. Only a small amount of nitrogen is completely degraded to ammonia and is eventually lost in the form of urea.

During this complex interorgan exchange, specific amino acids play a specific role; notably, alanine and glutamine are the major carriers of nitrogen from the periphery to the liver. In the postabsorptive state, the output of alanine and glutamine greatly exceeds that of all other amino acids, and accounts for approximately 50% of total nitrogen release (4). It should be noted that the output of alanine and glutamine also exceeds the alanine and glutamine content of muscle protein, thus suggesting a possible intraorgan exchange of nitrogen between different amino acids. Skeletal muscle, like liver tissue and brain, contains glutamine synthetase, which is the enzyme responsible for glutamine synthesis from glutamate and amino groups derived from amino acid degradation. There is also evidence that ammonia circulating in the blood can be used for glutamine synthesis (5).

The peripheral release of alanine and glutamine is matched by a remarkable uptake in the splanchnic area, as shown by hepatic vein catheterization (6). The liver itself is the main site of alanine disposal, while the gut probably accounts for most glutamine uptake. Studies performed during portal vein catheterization have demonstrated a gut uptake of glutamine and a release of alanine, which is transported to the liver in amounts that are in the same order of magnitude as the release of alanine from peripheral tissues (7). The net hepatic uptake of alanine is therefore nearly doubled through the contribution of the gut to alanine disposal. Only a part of glutamine reaches the kidney where it is transformed into alanine or degraded to ammonia and glutamate.

After a protein meal the amino acids absorbed in the gut after protein digestion are delivered to the liver, which regulates their entry into the peripheral circulation. A remarkable role of the gut itself has been demonstrated. It selectively releases alanine in amounts greater than had been expected on the basis of the amino acid content of dietary proteins. Glutamic acid and glutamine, as well as the glutamine reaching the gut through the mesenteric arteries, are probably transaminated within the mucosal cells to form alanine (8). Alanine is efficiently taken up by the liver, which also removes most of the other amino acids, so that the peripheral plasma levels of amino acids change little. Only the hepatic uptake of the branched-chain amino acids — valine, isoleucine and leucine — does not increase so that most of the branched-chain amino acids are delivered to the peripheral muscle tissue where their uptake can be demonstrated. Branched-chain amino acid uptake accounts for about half the nitrogen taken up by the muscle tissue during the first two hours after protein ingestion, while from two to three hours after the load almost all the amino nitrogen removed is derived from the branched-chain amino acids (9).

Within the muscle tissue, approximately 20% of the branched-chain amino acids are directly used for protein synthesis, but most of their amino nitrogen can be reused for the *de novo* synthesis of nonessential amino acids (10). This suggests that the branched-chain amino acids are nonspecific nitrogen carriers to the periphery, where their fate may be either protein synthesis or transamination.

All these complex metabolic reactions are regulated by insulin and/or glucagon (Table 2). According to Unger's theory of bihormonal modulation of the metabolic reactions, the molar ratio of insulin to glucagon has been suggested to regulate overall metabolism (11). However, evidence is accumulating that these hormones have different target organs.

The anabolic action of insulin on peripheral tissues has long been recognized. Insulin has been reported to stimulate protein synthesis, to facilitate amino

TABLE 2. Amino Acid Metabolism in Relation to the Hormonal Status in the Liver and in the Peripheral Muscle Tissue

State	Hormonal status	Hepatic metabolism	Peripheral metabolism #
Fasting	Low insulin	Amino acid uptake	High amino acid release
Oral glucose load	High insulin, low glucagon	Reduced amino acid uptake	Inhibition of amino acid release
Protein meal	High insulin, high glucagon	Increased amino acid uptake	Amino acid uptake *

While both insulin and glucagon produce remarkable effects on the liver, there is no evidence for an effect of glucagon on muscle tissue.

* Also dependent on increased substrate availability.

acid transport into the cells, and to inhibit protein degradation and amino acid efflux (12). In eviscerated animals, insulin infusions significantly reduce plasma amino acid levels (13), suggesting that the muscle tissue is the target organ. Furthermore, in humans exogenous insulin or glucose-induced hyperinsulinemia significantly reduces plasma amino acid levels, especially branched-chain amino acids (14). Pozefsky et al. (15) investigated the role of insulin on amino acid balance in peripheral muscle tissue. High physiologic levels of insulin, besides stimulating glucose uptake, significantly reduce alpha-amino nitrogen release and, notably, the release of branched-chain amino acids, but no net amino acid uptake is observed. After a protein meal, when insulin is increased and the periphery is flooded with branched-chain amino acids, a net uptake of branched-chain amino acids may be demonstrated, and it nearly equals the total amino acid uptake. These studies suggest that insulin acts primarily by decreasing amino acid efflux, while its anabolic action occurs only in the presence of large substrate availability.

Increasing glucagon to high physiologic levels does not significantly affect forearm amino acid metabolism (16). However, glucagon infusions stimulate insulin secretion, possibly masking the direct effects of glucagon. In patients with glucagonomas, hypoaminoacidemia is present (17), but it is more likely to result from increased amino acid utilization in the liver than from any peripheral effect.

HORMONAL CONTROL OF HEPATIC AMINO ACID AND AMMONIA METABOLISM

The amino acids transported to the liver during fasting, notably alanine, are used as glucogenic precursors via pyruvate, while the nitrogenous part of the molecule is used for urea synthesis. The role of pancreatic hormones is again crucial, as demonstrated by studies performed during glucagon infusion or after stimulation of endogenous insulin secretion by the administration of intravenous or oral glucose.

Following glucose administration, the splanchnic uptake of alanine is reduced, despite levels of arterial alanine being increased or unchanged (18). In the isolated, perfused liver model, insulin infusion decreases the incorporation of ^{14}C-alanine into glucose, suggesting a direct role of insulin in the regulation of gluconeogenesis (19).

Certainly, the liver is the main or the sole site of the regulatory action of glucagon. Glucagon levels are high in the fasting postabsorptive state, and decrease after oral glucose ingestion, which eliminates the need for hepatic gluconeogenesis. On the contrary, glucagon increases soon after a protein meal, as the amino acid supply to the liver increases and gluconeogenesis becomes necessary to compensate for insulin-induced hypoglycemia. Jennings et al. (20) have shown conclusively that glucagon infusions stimulate gluconeogenesis from alanine, while in glucagon deficiency, gluconeogenesis slows down.

Boden et al. (21) infused normal volunteers with somatostatin plus insulin or somatostatin plus insulin and glucagon in excess. In the second part of the experiment, insulin and glucagon levels were maintained within physiologic ranges after somatostatin infusion at appropriate infusion rates. In a few patients, glucose levels were maintained at nearly basal concentrations by Biostator-controlled glucose infusions. By doing so, they created a model of selective glucagon deficiency and glucagon excess, respectively, in the presence of normal insulin levels. Under these experimental but nearly physiologic conditions, hypoglucagonemia was accompanied by an increase in the plasma levels of most amino acids, while selective hyperglucagonemia caused a decrease of most plasma amino acids, most notably of alanine. In both studies no significant changes in branched-chain amino acid levels were observed. The effect of glucagon on amino acid concentrations became apparent after two to three hours and persisted until the end of the experiment after eight hours, suggesting a long-lasting regulatory effect of glucagon. A specific action of glucagon on the liver is supported by the finding that changes in glucagon concentration were paralleled by changes in urea nitrogen excretion.

Within the liver, the fate of amino acids is either their use for protein synthesis or deamidation, ammonia generation and urea synthesis. Urea synthesis is a specific hepatic function that has received considerable attention as a tool for a quantitative measurement of liver function. The urea nitrogen synthetic rate, however, depends on several conditions which were recently reviewed (22). When amino acid mixtures, or single ureagenic amino acids, are infused into normal subjects, urea nitrogen synthesis rates increase linearly with increased amino acid levels, in agreement with a dependence on substrate availability. However, the slope of the regression line varies according to the intrinsic ability of the liver to convert amino acid nitrogen into urea.

Urea nitrogen synthesis rates are linearly dependent upon glucagon concentrations, too (23), being reduced during the infusion of large amounts of glucose, which decreases gluconeogenesis and suppresses glucagon release. The effects of glucagon are independent of substrate availability.

The end product of amino acid catabolism is ammonia. A specific hepatic ammonia detoxication system prevents the rise of the blood ammonia concentration above those levels that may be toxic to other tissues. Häussinger et al. (24) have extensively studied this process in the isolated, perfused rat liver. Ammonia detoxication is due to a high-affinity system located in the perivenous area (zone III), where glutamine synthesis occurs, and to a low-affinity, high-capacity system in the periportal area (zone I), where the enzymes of the urea cycle are located and where glutaminase promotes glutamine degradation. The simultaneous activity of glutaminase and glutamine synthetase results in an intrahepatic, intercellular, glutamine cycle which improves ammonia removal. The flux through this cycle is under the control of ammonium ions and of glucagon in the physiologic range of portal ammonia concentrations. Glucagon stimulates glutaminase in the periportal area and inhibits glutamine synthetase in the perivenous hepatocytes, thus increasing ammonia availability for urea synthesis.

AMINO ACIDS AND AMMONIA AS SECRETAGOGUES

The interaction between amino acids or ammonia and pancreatic, glucoregulatory hormones includes the stimulatory action of these substrates on hormone secretion.

The effects of acute elevation of individual free amino acids on insulin and glucagon secretion has not been extensively studied in humans. A single study was reported in dogs (25). Although some problems may arise in applying these results to humans, they provide some clues which deserve consideration.

The glucagon response to supraphysiologic doses of amino acids varies with the metabolic type of the individual amino acids. Of twenty amino acids tested, only the three branched-chain amino acids—valine, isoleucine and leucine—which are metabolized in muscle, failed to stimulate glucagon secretion. The group of amino acids which enter the gluconeogenic pathway as pyruvate, the most important of which is alanine, are the most potent stimulators of glucagon secretion. Quite logically, amino acids seem able to stimulate the secretion of the substance which is responsible for their metabolism.

The insulin response to amino acids is also variable, but is usually less overt than that of glucagon. No relationship exists between the glucagon-stimulating and the insulin-stimulating activity of the individual amino acids.

In man, the glucagon-stimulating activity of alanine is well established (26), while the three branched-chain amino acids, even in large supraphysiologic doses, have little effect (27). Moreover, plasma insulin levels do not appreciably increase after the infusion of branched-chain amino acids (27). However, the fall in glucose levels induced by the branched-chain amino acids (26, 27) is likely to influence insulin and glucagon secretion.

As for the insulin- and glucagon-stimulating activity of ammonia, either after intravenous infusion or after ammonium chloride ingestion, the results are conflicting. In normal subjects (28) and in fed rats (29), no significant changes in pancreatic glucoregulatory hormones have been observed.

CHANGES IN AMMONIA AND AMINO ACID METABOLISM IN CHRONIC LIVER DISEASE

In patients with chronic liver diseases, several additional problems must be considered.

First, the amount of ammonia generated from the hydrolysis of urea in the gastrointestinal tract varies widely and tends to be greater than in control subjects

(30). In addition, because of spontaneous intra- and extra-hepatic portal-systemic shunting, ammonia and amino acids are not completely cleared by the liver before entering the systemic circulation, as they are in non-cirrhotic subjects. The liver uptake of alanine is reduced in strict correlation with the decreased liver cell mass (31), while urea synthesis is reduced and higher amino acid levels are necessary to maintain adequate ureagenesis (32).

However, the most remarkable changes occur in the periphery, where a reduced muscle mass may impair ammonia detoxication and amino acid metabolism. In the periphery, there is reduced release of branched-chain amino acids during fasting (27), while postprandial levels are greatly increased (33).

In spite of increased levels of insulin (34) and glucagon (35), the effects of these hormones on overall metabolism are reduced. In the periphery, altered sensitivity and responsiveness to insulin impair glucose and amino acid metabolism (36, 37), while the liver itself does not properly respond to the gluconeogenic activity of glucagon (38, 39). The finding that glucagon may increase ammonia levels in these patients is controversial (40). It has been suggested that in cirrhotic patients, because of glycogen depletion, fasting blood glucose is maintained within the normal range by increased gluconeogenesis, stimulated by glucagon. Under these conditions, the nitrogen part of the amino acids, oxidized to provide energy and glucose, might escape liver uptake and urea synthesis, thus contributing to hyperammonemia (41). However, increased amino acid catabolism in the liver should result in reduced plasma concentrations of glucogenic amino acids (mainly alanine and glutamine), which have never been demonstrated. The possibility that gluconeogenesis may occur in organs other than the liver is not supported by studies in normal human subjects, since no extrahepatic effects of glucagon have ever been reported (21).

The insulin and glucagon response to ammonia was tested in healthy control subjects and in patients with chronic liver disease in the course of an ammonia tolerance test (28). In control subjects, in which ammonia levels do not change following ammonium chloride ingestion, no changes in insulin and glucagon were observed. In patients with chronic liver disease, who exhibited a variable degree of hyperammonemia after the oral load, post-load ammonia levels were linearly related to post-load glucagon levels ($r=0.801$; $n=27$) and, in addition, the changes in ammonia concentrations paralleled the changes in glucagon ($r=0.707$; $n=17$).

CONCLUSIONS

In recent years, remarkable progress has been made in understanding protein metabolism, amino acid exchange, and ammonia detoxication. These advances are mainly due to greater availability of tracer techniques and developments in amino acid analysis. However, the problem is becoming more and more complex, since many variables must be considered for each experimental or physiologic state. Ammonia, which is a small and unstable molecule that turns over and exchanges rapidly, is a fundamental component of nitrogen metabolism.

The hormonal status is also important in changing the direction of metabolism. However, while hormonal levels can be easily measured in biological fluids, their concentration may have little correlation with their metabolic effects.

A lot of interest has been focused on receptor concentration and affinity, but receptor binding has little to do with the biologic activity of the hormones, due to postreceptor defects, demonstrated in several disease states (42-44).

Future research has to cope with all these problems, and only careful studies carried out by infusing hormones in *physiologic* concentrations are likely to provide further answers.

REFERENCES

1. Lockwood AH, McDonald JM, Reiman RE, et al. The dynamics of ammonia metabolism in man. Effects of liver disease and hyperammonemia. J Clin Invest 1979; 63:449-460.

2. Ganda OP, Ruderman NP. Muscle nitrogen metabolism in chronic hepatic insufficiency. Metabolism 1976; 25:427-435.

3. Felig P. Amino acid metabolism in man. Annu Rev Biochem 1975; 44:933-955.

4. Marliss EB, Aoki TT, Pozefsky T, et al. Muscle and splanchnic glutamine and glutamate metabolism in postabsorptive and prolonged starved man. J Clin Invest 1971; 50:814-817.

5. Garber AJ, Karl IE, Kipnis DM. Alanine and glutamine synthesis and release from skeletal muscle. II. The precursor role of amino acids in alanine and glutamine synthesis. J Biol Chem 1976; 251:836-843.

6. Felig P, Owen OE, Wahren J, et al. Amino acid metabolism during prolonged starvation. J Clin Invest 1969; 48:584-594.

7. Owen OE, Reichle RA, Mozzoli MA, et al. Hepatic gut, and renal substrate flux rates in patients with hepatic cirrhosis. J Clin Invest 1981; 68:240-252.

8. Windmueller HG, Spaeth AE. Intestinal metabolism of glutamine and glutamate from the lumen as compared to glutamine from blood. Arch Biochem Biophys 1975; 171:662-672.

9. De Fronzo RA, Felig P. Amino acid metabolism in uremia: insight gained from normal and diabetic man. Am J Clin Nutr 1980; 33:1378-1386.

10. Elia M, Livesey G. Branched-chain amino and oxo acid metabolism in human rat muscle. In: Walser M, Williamson JR, eds. Metabolism and Clinical Implications of Branched-chain Amino and Keto Acids. New York: Elsevier/North

Holland, 1981: 257-262.

11. Unger RH. Glucagon and the insulin:glucagon ratio in diabetes and other catabolic illnesses. Diabetes 1971; 20:834-838.

12. Fulks RM, Li JB, Goldberg AL. Effects of insulin, glucose, and amino acids on protein turnover in rat diaphragm. J Biol Chem 1975; 250:290-298.

13. Russel JA. Hormonal control of amino acid metabolism. Fed Proc 1955; 14:696-706.

14. Felig P, Marliss E, Cahill GF Jr. Plasma amino acid levels and insulin secretion in obesity. N Engl J Med 1969; 281:211-216.

15. Pozefsky T, Felig P, Tobin JD, et al. Amino acid balance across tissues of the forearm in postabsorptive man. Effects of insulin at two dose levels. J Clin Invest 1969; 48:2273-2282.

16. Pozefsky T, Tancredi RG, Moxley RT, et al. Metabolism of forearm tissues in man. Studies with glucagon. Diabetes 1976; 25:128-135.

17. Mallinson CN, Bloom SR, Warin AP. A glucagonoma syndrome. Lancet 1974; 2:1-5.

18. Felig P, Wahren J, Hendler R. Influence of oral glucose ingestion on splanchnic glucose and gluconeogenic substrate metabolism. Diabetes 1975; 24:468-475.

19. Rudorff KH, Albrecht G, Staib W. Effect of insulin and proinsulin on the metabolism of alanine in rat liver. Horm Metab Res 1970; 2:49-51.

20. Jennings AS, Cherrington AD, Liljenquist JE, et al. The roles of insulin and glucagon in the regulation of gluconeogenesis in the postabsorptive dog. Diabetes 1977; 26:847-856.

21. Boden G, Rezvani I, Owen OE. Effects of glucagon on plasma amino acids. J Clin Invest 1984; 73:785-793.

22. Vilstrup H. Urea synthesis in humans. Precondition of quantitation and relation to liver function. In: Kleinberger G, Ferenci P, Riederer H, Thaler H, eds. Advances in Hepatic Encephalopathy and Urea Cycle Diseases. Basel; Karger, 1984: 141-146.

23. Vilstrup H. Effects of glucose on alanine-derived urea synthesis. Clin Physiol 1984; 4:495-507.

24. Häussinger D, Sies H, Gerok W. Functional hepatocyte heterogeneity in ammonia metabolism. The intercellular glutamine cycle. J Hepatol 1984; 1:3-14.

25. Marreiro Rocha D, Faloona GR, Unger, H. Glucagon-stimulating activity of 20 amino acids in dogs. J Clin Invest 1972; 51:2346-2351.

26. Muller WA, Faloona GR, Unger H. The effects of alanine on glucagon secretion. J Clin Invest 1971; 50:2215-2221.

27. Marchesini G, Bianchi GP, Vilstrup H, et al. Plasma clearances of branched-chain amino acids in control subjects and in patients with cirrhosis. J Hepatol 1987; 3: (in press).

28. Marchesini G, Zoli M, Dondi C, et al. Ammonia-induced changes in pancreatic hormones and plasma amino acids in patients with liver cirrhosis. Dig

Dis Sci 1982; 27:406-412.

29. Mulloy AL, Visek WJ. Plasma insulin, glucagon, and gut glucagon-like immunoreactivity during experimentally induced hyperammonemia in rats. Proc Soc Exp Biol Med 1980; 163:137-140.

30. Hansen BA, Vilstrup H. Increased intestinal hydrolysis of urea in patients with alcoholic cirrhosis. Scand J Gastroenterol 1985; 20:346-350.

31. Bianchi GP, Zoli M, Checchia GA, et al. Plasma amino acid exchange in patients with liver cirrhosis. Ital J Gastroenterol 1987; 19:70-75.

32. Vilstrup H. Synthesis of urea after stimulation with amino acids: relation to liver function. Gut 1980; 21:990-995.

33. Marchesini G, Bianchi GP, Zoli M, et al. Plasma amino acid response to protein ingestion in patients with liver cirrhosis. Gastroenterology 1983; 85:283-290.

34. Megyesi C, Samols E, Marks V. Glucose tolerance and diabetes in chronic liver disease. Lancet 1967; 2:1051-1056.

35. Marco J, Diego J, Villaneuva ML, et al. Elevated plasma glucagon levels in cirrhosis of the liver. N Engl J Med 1973; 289:1107-1111.

36. Iversen J, Vilstrup H, Tygstrup N. Kinetics of glucose metabolism in relation to insulin concentrations in patients with alcoholic cirrhosis and in healthy persons. Gastroenterology 1984; 87:1138-1143.

37. Marchesini G, Forlani G, Zoli M, et al. Effect of euglycaemic insulin infusion on plasma levels of branched-chain amino acids in cirrhosis. Hepatology 1983; 3:184-187.

38. Sherwin RS, Fisher M, Bessoff J, et al. Hyperglucogonemia in cirrhosis: altered secretion and sensitivity to glucagon. Gastroenterology 1978; 74:1224-1228.

39. Marchesini G, Melli A, Checchia GA, et al. Pancreatic B-cell function in cirrhotic patients with and without overt diabetes. C-peptide response to glucagon and to meal. Metabolism 1985; 34:695-701.

40. Kabadi UM, Eisenstein AB, Konda J. Elevated plasma ammonia levels in hepatic cirrhosis: role of glucagon. Gastroenterology 1985; 88:750-756.

41. Kabadi UM. The association of hepatic glycogen depletion in cirrhosis with hyperammonemia. Hepatology 1987; 7:821-824.

42. Kolterman OG, Insel J, Saekow M, et al. Mechanism of insulin resistance in human obesity. Evidence for receptor and postreceptor defects. J Clin Invest 1980; 65:1272-1284.

43. Kolterman OG, Gray RS, Griffin J, et al. Receptor and postreceptor defects contribute to the insulin resistance in non-insulin dependent diabetes mellitus. J Clin Invest 1981; 68:957-969.

44. Iversen J, Vilstrup H, Tygstrup N. Kinetics of glucose metabolism in relation to insulin concentrations in patients with alcoholic cirrhosis and in healthy persons. Gastroenterology 1984; 87:1138-1143.

5

GABA IN HUMAN HEPATIC ENCEPHALOPATHY

PETER FERENCI, M.D.

Assessment of the actual role of impaired GABA-ergic neurotransmission in the pathogenesis of human hepatic encephalopathy (HE) is difficult. For obvious reasons, appropriate neurochemical or neuropharmacological studies are not feasible in these patients. In this overview, the available data on serum GABA concentrations and on brain GABA and benzodiazepine receptors in patients with HE will be reviewed and the preliminary experience with benzodiazepine antagonists in the treatment of HE will be discussed.

THE GABA HYPOTHESIS OF THE PATHOGENESIS OF HEPATIC ENCEPHALOPATHY

Findings in experimental models of HE indicate that an alteration of GABA-ergic neurotransmission may induce the neural inhibition of HE (1). In rabbits and rats with galactosamine-induced liver failure, the density of cortical postsynaptic GABA receptors is increased (2, 3). GABA catabolism in the brain (4) as well as in the liver (5) is impaired. Furthermore, sera of rabbits with HE inhibit the specific binding of ^{3}H-GABA to postsynaptic membranes (2) and this inhibitory activity was suggested to be mediated by GABA itself. An increase in serum GABA concentration may contribute to the development of HE since in fulminant hepatic failure the blood-brain barrier is permeable to GABA (6). GABA taken up by the brain may interact with "supersensitive" postsynaptic GABA receptors.

The neurochemical findings that suggest impairment of GABA-ergic neurotransmission in HE are well supported by electrophysiologic studies. Visual evoked potentials (VEP) observed in HE are almost identical to those induced by the administration of benzodiazepines or by barbiturates (7). As the action of both drugs is mediated by their interaction with GABA receptors, the similarities of VEPs support the concept that GABA-ergic neurotransmission is activated in HE. The postsynaptic GABA receptor is a supramolecular complex consisting of several proteins including the GABA receptor itself, a receptor for benzodiazepines and one for picrotoxin. These different proteins are functionally coupled. In rats and rabbits with galactosamine-induced liver failure and HE, the density of cortical benzodiazepine receptors is increased (2). The administration of various benzodiazepine or GABA antagonists can cause a complete but transient recovery from HE together with complete normalization of the abnormal VEPs (8, 9). Although some of the findings were not reproduced in other experimental models of HE, these findings support the concept that alterations of the GABA receptor complex are involved in HE pathogenesis.

BLOOD GABA CONCENTRATIONS IN PATIENTS WITH HEPATIC ENCEPHALOPATHY

Based on experiences in rabbits with galactosamine-induced liver failure, the radioreceptor assay was used to measure serum levels of "GABA-like" activity in 170 patients with various liver diseases with and without HE (10). They were found to be increased in all patients with overt HE due to acute or chronic hepatocellular failure. Particularly high levels were detected in patients with cirrhosis 12 to 16 hours after gastrointestinal hemorrhage. The "GABA-like"

TABLE 1. Serum GABA Concentrations in Patients with Hepatic Encephalopathy

Authors and references	Method	Underlying liver disease
Minuk et al. (14)	Ion exchange chromatography	Cirrhosis
Goetcheus et al. (13)	Enzymatic	Cirrhosis
Moroni et al. (12)	Gas-chromatography-mass spectroscopy	Cirrhosis
Ferenci et al. (15)	Radioreceptor assay	Fulminant hepatic failure and cirrhosis

activity was not further characterized and it was suggested that it may be GABA itself. In a further study aimed to test the validity of the GABA-radioreceptor assay for the measurement of serum GABA levels in HE, it was found that it lacks specificity and overestimates serum "true GABA" levels in HE. Among several amino acids tested, five inhibited specific GABA-binding within their physiological blood concentrations. The GABA binding inhibitory activity of a serum sample of a patient with HE was purified by gel-chromatography and was found to contain several amino acids at concentrations of about 0.1 mmol to 3.5 mmol glutamine, but no detectable GABA (11).

No major increase in serum GABA levels in HE was found by other analytical methods (Table 1). Serum GABA concentrations measured by gas-chromatography-mass-spectroscopy (12) or by the rather insensitive, enzymatic GABA assay (13) were not different in patients with HE and in controls, whereas they were increased in HE up to 3-fold when assayed by ion-exchange-chromatography (14). Based on the *in vivo* kinetics of the plasma clearance of ^{3}H-GABA in rabbits, a 60% to 100% increase in serum "true GABA" concentration can be expected to occur in liver failure (5). However, it should be stressed that no "gold standard" is available for the determination of serum concentration of "true GABA." For example, serum GABA concentrations in healthy subjects measured by high pressure liquid chromatography, ion-exchange-chromatography or the radioreceptor assay were substantially lower than those measured by gas-chromatography-mass-spectroscopy (Table 1). Thus, it is unknown whether serum GABA levels are increased in HE and, if so, how such levels may affect the functional status of the GABA-ergic neurotransmitter system in the brain.

GABA in controls (µmol)	GABA in patients with HE	
	% with increased level	Range (x upper limit of normal)
0.25 - 0.50	100	1.1 - 3.5
0.05 - 0.20	25	1.1 - 2
0.5 - 1.8	27	1.1 - 1.4
0.2 - 0.8	96	1.1 - 30

BRAIN GABA RECEPTORS IN PATIENTS WITH HEPATIC ENCEPHALOPATHY

Using a standard binding assay of GABA to neural membranes isolated from the brain, it has been estimated that the number of receptors for GABA on postsynaptic neurons increases significantly in animal models of fulminant hepatic failure (2, 3). Whereas this type of study is straightforward in experimental animals, caution is necessary in interpreting data derived from similar studies in humans. It is important to emphasize that the control patients in such a study cannot be classified as "healthy" controls and that the effects of the duration of HE, of the therapies used to treat HE and of the type and severity of the underlying liver disease on cerebral GABA receptors are not known. Furthermore, there are inherent difficulties in the interpretation of human postmortem receptor-binding studies. Nevertheless, measurement of specific GABA binding to synaptic membranes in the brains of patients who have died with HE may be useful to assess possible changes of GABA-ergic neurotransmission in human HE.

In a preliminary study, brains obtained at autopsy from 11 patients who had died of causes unrelated to liver disease and from 11 patients who had died of chronic liver disease were examined (15). Eight of the group with liver disease had overt HE at the time of death. Specific binding of GABA to synaptic membranes prepared from the frontal cortex was similar in the control subjects to those of cirrhotic patients with or without HE. However, when data were analyzed according to the severity of HE at the time of death, GABA binding in patients with mild HE (grade I-III) was substantially higher than that in control subjects or in patients with severe HE (grade IV) (Figure 1). This analysis, however, is based on very few patients. Furthermore, all of the patients in the hepatic disease group had chronic liver disease; the majority had alcoholic cirrhosis. No data are available from patients who died of fulminant hepatic failure.

From these preliminary data, it remains unclear whether human HE is associated with changes in brain GABA receptors or not. Clearly, more patients have to be studied including patients with acute and chronic HE of various types. In addition, GABA binding must be measured in different brain areas. No data are available on brain benzodiazepine receptors in human HE.

Positron emission tomography of the brain may be useful for receptor studies *in vivo*. ^{11}C-labeled compounds are administered intravenously and regional, cerebral ^{11}C-radioactivity can be measured sequentially by positron emission tomography. When ^{11}C-Ro 15-1788 was used as label for benzodiazepine receptors in patients with advanced cirrhosis and a history of HE, an increase of ^{11}C-Ro 15-1788 activity in their brains was observed as compared to those of control subjects (16). While these findings suggest changes of benzodiazepine receptors in patients with HE, several mechanisms other than increased affinity or density of benzodiazepine receptors may account for the increased cerebral uptake of the label. Further studies using this exciting new technology should help to document the occurrence and the nature of changes in neurotransmission in patients with HE.

EFFECTS OF BENZODIAZEPINE ANTAGONISTS IN PATIENTS WITH HEPATIC ENCEPHALOPATHY

In certain experimental models of HE, the density of postsynaptic benzodiazepine binding sites is increased (2) and an endogenous benzodiazepine antagonist is present in the brain (17). In rabbits and rats with galactosamine-induced liver failure, benzodiazepine antagonists work effectively to reverse HE (8, 9).

A few anecdotal reports on the effects of benzodiazepine antagonists in humans have been noted. In a patient with fulminant hepatitis B and grade IV HE, the intravenous injection of 0.5 mg of the benzodiazepine antagonist Ro 15-1788 (Flumazenil®, Hoffman-LaRoche) resulted in marked improvement both in clinical features and electroencephalographic findings of HE (Scollo-Lavizzari G, and Steinmann E, Lancet 1985; 1:1324, Correspondence). This improvement lasted for one hour and was reproduced with additional injections of Ro 15-1788.

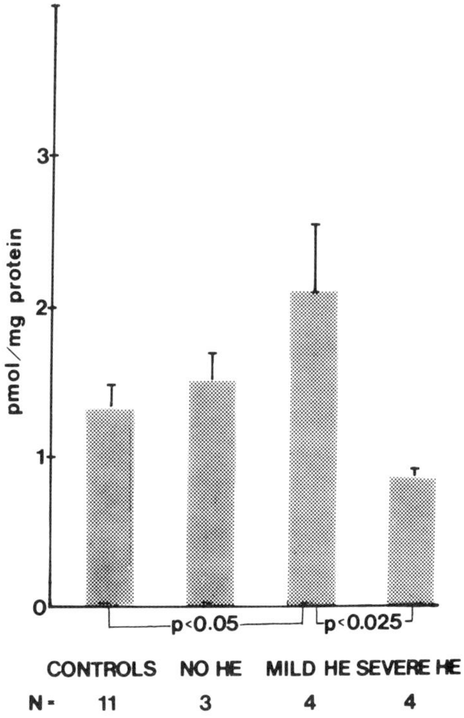

FIGURE 1. Mean specific binding of GABA to synaptic membranes isolated from the frontal cortex of brains obtained at autopsy from patients who died of causes unrelated to liver disease (controls) and from patients with chronic liver disease who died with and without overt features of hepatic encephalopathy. The concentration of the ligand was 16 mmol. Data are expressed as mean ± S.D.

A similar observation was reported in two patients with alcoholic cirrhosis and HE (grade IV) following gastrointestinal hemorrhage. In two other patients with alcoholic cirrhosis and HE (grade III), only slight clinical improvement was achieved, although much higher doses of Ro 15-1788 were used (Bansky et al., Lancet 1985; 1:1324-1325, Correspondence). Grimm et al. (18) reported their experience with Ro 15-1788 in five patients with fulminant liver failure and grade IV HE. Two of these five patients had a prompt arousal reaction and eventually recovered completely. Two patients had a slight transient improvement of HE but died later. In one of these patients, the clinical improvement was also documented by almost complete normalization of abnormal, long latency auditory and somatosensory evoked potentials. No effects were seen in the fifth patient who apparently had irreversible brain damage characterized by absence of clinical activity at the time of the administration of the drug.

In all patients who reacted to treatment with Ro 15-1788, improvement was observed within one to two minutes of the administration of the drug. Therefore, a randomized controlled study is feasible, and would permit more objective assessment of the effects of benzodiazepine antagonists in HE.

So far, only one patient with chronic portal-systemic encephalopathy who was treated with benzodiazepine antagonists has been reported (19). In February 1984, a 42-year-old woman without previous history of liver disease underwent two-thirds hepatectomy with construction of an end-to-side portacaval shunt because of an inflammatory gall bladder tumor. Six weeks after surgery, she developed hepatic coma and was successfully treated with lactulose enemas and infusions of branched-chain amino acids. However, on treatment with a 40 g protein diet and lactulose, she remained encephalopathic and had six further attacks of coma in the following year. Coma was always associated with marked hyperammonemia and highly abnormal EEGs. Oral antibiotics (neomycin, metronidazole, paromomycin) were tried without effect. One year after the shunt she improved markedly on treatment with amoxicillin and supplementation of diet with 30 g branched-chain amino acids (Travasorb® hepatic) per day. No further attacks of hepatic coma occurred until October 1985, but she was in a mild stage of HE most of the time. Over the next six months seven additional attacks of coma occurred. Thereafter, treatment with Ro 15-1788 (25 mg after breakfast and lunch orally) was started. Lactulose and amoxicillin were continued. The amount of dietary protein was gradually increased; after three months she tolerated an unrestricted protein diet. The patient was well, without evidence of recurrent HE until December 1986 when the Ro 15-1788 was stopped. Three days after stopping the medication the patient was in HE grade IV and had four further attacks until February 1987. Treatment with Ro 15-1788 was restarted in March 1987. Since then she has not experienced any attacks of HE and does not require a protein restriction. This remarkable clinical response indicates that benzodiazepine antagonists may be useful for treatment of some patients with chronic HE. However, a randomized controlled study should be performed to evaluate the effects of such therapy.

SUMMARY

The pathogenesis of HE is still not known at present. The "GABA hypothesis" of the pathogenesis of HE adds further information to the understanding of this syndrome. This attractive hypothesis has led to intensive investigations on the role of GABA-ergic neurotransmission in various experimental models of HE. The results of these studies are controversial. In human HE, the role of impairment of GABA-ergic neurotransmission is even less well studied and understood. The magnitude of the increase in serum GABA concentration in patients with HE has been overestimated by the radioreceptor assay. Apparently, HE is only associated with a minor increase in serum GABA concentrations. The role of such small increments in serum GABA in HE in influencing brain function is unknown. Data on brain GABA receptors in postmortem studies or on cerebral benzodiazepine uptake *in vivo* in patients with HE are preliminary and do not allow any conclusion on the status of the GABA-ergic neurotransmitter system in patients with HE. Based on a handful of anecdotal reports, treatment of HE with benzodiazepine antagonists appears to be promising, but these observations need validation by prospective, randomized, controlled studies.

REFERENCES

1. Schafer DF, Jones EA. Hepatic encephalopathy and the gamma-aminobutyric acid neurotransmitter system. Lancet 1982; 2:18-19.

2. Schafer DF, Fowler JM, Munson PJ, et al. Gamma-aminobutyric acid and benzodiazepine receptors in an animal model of fulminant hepatic failure. J Lab Clin Med 1983; 102:870-880.

3. Baraldi M, Zeneroli ML. Experimental hepatic encephalopathy—changes in gamma-aminobutyric acid. Science 1982; 216:427-431.

4. Ferenci P, Covell D, Schafer DF, et al. Metabolism of the inhibitory neurotransmitter gamma-aminobutyric acid in a rabbit model of fulminant hepatic failure. Hepatology 1983; 3:507-512.

5. Ferenci P, Jacobs R, Pappas SC, et al. Enzymes of cerebral GABA metabolism and synaptosomal GABA uptake in acute liver failure in the rabbit: evidence for decreased cerebral GABA-transaminase activity. J Neurochem 1984; 42:1487-1490.

6. Horowitz ME, Schafer DF, Molnar P, et al. Increased blood brain transfer in a rabbit model of acute liver failure. Gastroenterology 1983; 84:1003-1011.

7. Schafer DF, Pappas SC, Brady LE, et al. Visual evoked potentials in a rabbit model of hepatic encephalopathy. I: Sequential changes and comparisons with

drug induced comas. Gastroenterology 1984; 86:540-545.

8. Baraldi M, Zeneroli ML, Ventura E, et al. Supersensitivity of benzodiazepine receptors in hepatic encephalopathy due to fulminant hepatic failure in the rat: reversal by a benzodiazepine antagonist. Clin Sci 1984; 67:167-175.

9. Bassett ML, Mullen KD, Skolnick P, et al. GABA and benzodiazepine receptor antagonists ameliorate hepatic encephalopathy in a rabbit model of fulminant hepatic failure (Abstract). Hepatology 1985; 5:1032.

10. Ferenci P, Schafer DF, Kleinberger G, et al. Serum levels of gamma-aminobutyric acid-like activity in acute and chronic hepatocellular disease. Lancet 1983; 2:811-814.

11. Ferenci P, Ebner J, Zimmermann Ch, et al. Overestimation of serum concentration of gamma-aminobutyric acid by the GABA-radioreceptor assay. Hepatology 1988; 8:69-72.

12. Moroni F, Riggio O, Carla V, et al. Hepatic encephalopathy: lack of changes of gamma-amino-butyric acid content in plasma and cerebrospinal fluid. Hepatology 1987; (in press).

13. Goetcheus JS, Webster LT. Gamma-aminobutyrate and hepatic coma. J Lab Clin Med 1985; 65:257-267.

14. Minuk GY, Winder A, Gurgess ED, et al. Serum gamma-aminobutyric acid (GABA) levels in patients with hepatic encephalopathy. Hepatogastroenterology 1985; 32:171-174.

15. Ferenci P, Riederer P, Jellinger, et al. Changes in gamma-aminobutyric acid receptor in patients with hepatic encephalopathy (Abstract). Gastroenterology 1983; 84:1371.

16. Samson Y, Bernuau J, Pappata S, et al. Cerebral uptake of benzodiazepine measured by positron emission tomography in hepatic encephalopathy. N Engl J Med 1987; 316:414.

17. Mullen KD, Martin JV, Bassett ML, et al. Hepatic encephalopathy: a syndrome modulated by an endogenous benzodiazepine receptor ligand? (Abstract) Hepatology 1986; 6:1221.

18. Grimm G, Lenz K, Kleinberger G, et al. Ro 15-1788 improves coma in 4 out of 5 patients with fulminant hepatic failure; verification by long latency auditory and somatosensory evoked potentials (Abstract). J Hepatol 1987; Suppl. 1:S21.

19. Ferenci P, Grimm G, Gangl A. Successful longtime treatment of chronic hepatic encephalopathy (HE) with a benzodiazepine antagonist (Abstract). Hepatology 1987; 7:1064.

6

HEPATIC ENCEPHALOPATHY AND GABA-ERGIC NEUROTRANSMISSION

E. ANTHONY JONES, M.D., F.R.C.P.

Since the publication of the original hypothesis which suggested that the GABA (gamma-aminobutyric acid) neurotransmitter system may play a role in the pathogenesis of hepatic encephalopathy (HE) (1), this hypothesis has undergone a series of modifications and this process is continuing (2-5). An involvement of the GABA neurotransmitter system in HE would not exclude a role for substances implicated in other hypotheses that relate to the pathogenesis of this syndrome. As is the case for other hypotheses of the pathogenesis of HE, the one implicating the GABA system has neither been definitively confirmed nor refuted.

The results of a series of experiments in a single model of HE (galactosamine [GalN]-induced fulminant hepatic failure [FHF] in rabbits) led to the original hypothesis being proposed (1). As further relevant experimental data have become available, not only has the original hypothesis evolved, but it has become clear that the current hypothesis implicating the GABA system in HE is not dependent on all of the experimental findings that led to the original hypothesis. Failure to appreciate this basic point is likely to lead to a considerable amount of entirely unnecessary confusion.

A CURRENT SIMPLE HYPOTHESIS

The central postulate of the hypothesis implicating the GABA neurotransmitter system in the mediation of HE is that increased GABA-ergic tone contributes to the neural inhibition which is a prominent component of this syndrome. In other words, it is postulated that in HE there is increased inhibitory neurotransmission mediated by GABA-gated Cl^- conductance from synaptic clefts to the cytoplasm of postsynaptic neurons. Thus, according to this hypothesis the GABA/benzodiazepine receptor/chloride ionophore (supramolecular) complex in the brain is involved in HE (Figure 1A, 1B).

THEORETICAL CONSIDERATIONS

Increased GABA-ergic tone could arise in liver failure as a consequence of increased interaction between GABA and its receptors as was suggested in the original hypothesis (1). Such increased interaction could occur if more GABA is available in synaptic clefts and/or if the density or affinity of GABA receptors is increased. Increased amounts of GABA in synaptic clefts may occur if there is augmented release of GABA from presynaptic neurons or if there is increased transfer of plasma GABA (which would include gut-derived GABA) across the blood-brain barrier to synaptic clefts. Increased GABA-ergic tone could also arise in liver failure if events at benzodiazepine and/or barbiturate receptor sites on the supramolecular complex promote an increase in the frequency or open time of Cl^- channel openings (6). Such changes in Cl^- conductance could arise from the presence of an endogenous benzodiazepine or barbiturate receptor agonist in HE.

FACTORS ON WHICH THE HYPOTHESIS IS NOT DEPENDENT

It is most important to emphasize that the hypothesis is not dependent on the results of certain types of study which are widely quoted as either supporting or detracting from the hypothesis. For example, this point applies in particular to studies of GABA levels in peripheral blood serum (or cerebrospinal fluid [CSF]) and to studies of the densities and affinities of GABA and benzodiazepine receptors in the brain in models of HE.

Nevertheless, data generated in such studies are of considerable interest and have been most useful in stimulating additional research on the GABA system in relation to HE (4). Indeed, binding data compatible with an increase in the density of GABA receptors in HE in some studies has afforded one potential explanation for the occurrence of increased GABA-ergic tone in HE (7, 8). However, data on serum GABA levels and the status of GABA and benzodiazepine receptors in different models of HE are not consistent (4). Therefore, it would appear that the manifestations of HE are not dependent on any particular changes in serum GABA levels or in GABA or benzodiazepine receptors (9). Until more is known regarding the potential significance of the results of *in vitro* neurotransmitter receptor binding studies, it seems prudent to defer drawing any definitive conclusions from data on the status of other neurotransmitter receptors in models of HE, e.g., receptors for the excitatory amino acid neurotransmitters, glutamate and aspartate.

A

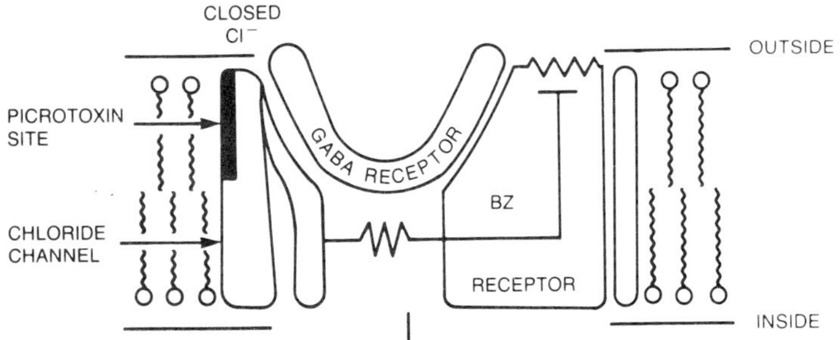

B

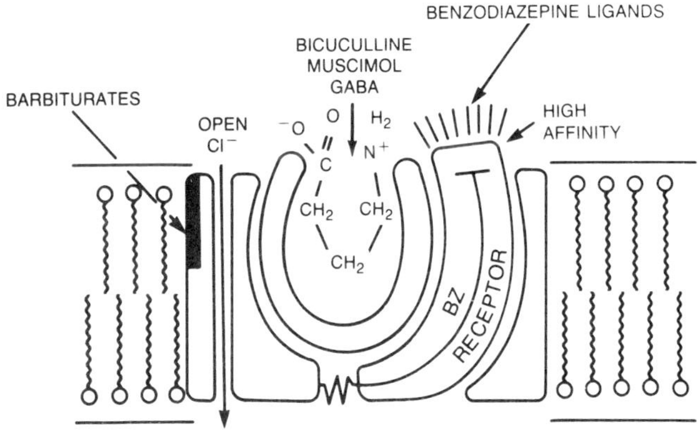

FIGURE 1. Diagramatic representation of the GABA benzodiazepine receptor/ chloride ionophore complex in the surface membrane of a postsynaptic neuron. Receptors are depicted for: (a) GABA, GABA receptor agonists (e.g., muscimol), and GABA receptor antagonists (e.g., bicuculline); (b) picrotoxin (the barbiturate binding site); and (c) benzodiazepine receptor agonists (e.g., diazepam), benzodiazepine receptor antagonists (e.g., CGS 8216, Ro 15-1788), and benzodiazepine receptor inverse agonists (e.g., beta-carbolines). A—The receptor complex in the unactivated state with the Cl^- channel closed. B—The receptor complex in the activated state with the Cl^- channel open. Activation is induced by GABA or GABA agonists binding to GABA receptors or barbiturates or benzodiazepine agonists interacting respectively with their specific receptors in the presence of GABA. Activation of the receptor complex is associated with conformational changes and opening of the Cl^- channel. These phenomena promote Cl^- conductance from synaptic cleft across the cell membrane to the cytoplasm and transformation of the cell membrane from a depolarized to a hyperpolarized state with resultant mediation of inhibitory neurotransmission. Reproduced with modifications from Biological Psychiatry (33).

SOURCES OF SUPPORT FOR THE HYPOTHESIS

The hypothesis is currently supported by the results of five types of investigation: a) in animals, drugs which induce encephalopathy by increasing GABA-ergic tone induce changes in visual evoked response (VER) recordings which closely resemble those in experimental HE (10, 11); b) drugs which antagonize the GABA/benzodiazepine receptor complex induce clinical and electrophysiologic remissions of HE in animal models (3, 12, 13); c) benzodiazepine receptor antagonists have been reported to induce clinical and electrophysiologic remissions of encephalopathy in humans with HE due to FHF (14, 15), HE associated with cirrhosis (16, 17) and chronic intractable portal-systemic encephalopathy (PSE) (18); d) benzodiazepine binding activity has been found in the CSF in an animal model of HE (19) and in humans with HE (20); e) neurons in brain slices from animals in HE exhibit increased sensitivity to depression by agonists of the GABA/benzodiazepine receptor complex (21) and, in contrast to control neurons, are excited by benzodiazepine receptor antagonists (22).

EVOLUTION OF SUPPORT FOR THE HYPOTHESIS

Studies of Visual Evoked Responses. To attempt to quantitate the abnormal electrophysiologic changes associated with HE in a way that was more useful than is possible from electroencephalograms (EEGs), even with computer analysis (23), VERs were recorded (10, 24). VERs are generated in response to repeated flashes of light emitted from a strobe (10) or light-emitting diode goggles (3). The VER is buried within the EEG trace and is derived from it by systematically averaging signals that are time-locked to the photic stimulus using a signal averager (computer of average transients). The result is a VER trace which is devoid of incoherent background EEG activity. The VER is plotted using an X-Y plotter. Conventionally, units of the X axis are milliseconds and units of the Y axis are microvolts—negative above a horizontal line and positive below it (10). The VER consists of a series of positive and negative peaks of electrical activity, each peak being characterized by its amplitude in relation to zero microvolts and its latency in relation to zero time (10). VERs are considered to represent summations of the electrical activity from volleys of excitatory and inhibitory postsynaptic potentials (25-27). With progression of HE, changes in the amplitudes and latencies of individual peaks of the VER become more pronounced. These changes in a given model of HE (10, 11) are highly reproducible. In rabbits with HE due to GalN-induced FHF, four clinical and VER stages of HE can be readily recognized (10).

The first clues that the GABA/benzodiazepine receptor complex may be involved in the mediation of HE were observations in rabbits that the abnormalities of the VER in HE (due to GalN-induced FHF) were almost identical to those associated with pentobarbital-induced coma, but were fundamentally different from those associated with ether-induced coma. These observations were first published as an abstract by Schafer et al. in 1980 (28) (Figure 2). The similarities between the abnormal VER induced by acute liver failure and by pentobarbital (10, 28) raised the possibility that the mechanisms involved in pentobarbital-induced coma may also be involved in the mediation of HE (10). Accordingly, the mechanisms by which pentobarbital induces neuronal inhibition became of interest.

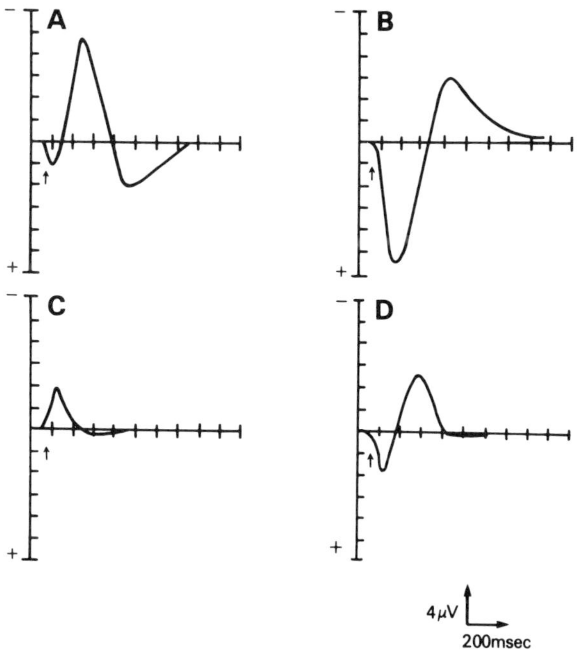

FIGURE 2. The first experimental observation that suggested that the GABA neurotransmitter system might be implicated in the mediation of hepatic encephalopathy (HE). To obtain an objective measurement of postsynaptic neural events in different encephalopathies, visual evoked responses (VERs) were recorded in rabbits. A—Normal; B—Galactosamine-induced hepatic coma or pentobarbital-induced coma; C—Ether-induced coma; D—Hyperammonemic encephalopathy. The VER associated with hepatic coma is not similar to that associated with either ether-induced coma, or hyperammonemic encephalopathy, but is similar to that associated with pentobarbital-induced coma. These observations raised the possibility that increased chloride ion conductance across postsynaptic neural membranes due to activation of the GABA neurotransmitter system may play a role in the mediation of the neural inhibition of HE. The VER waveforms depicted are reproduced with permission from Gastroenterology (10, 38).

Pentobarbital is known to stimulate GABA-ergic neurotransmission as a consequence of its interaction with specific binding sites for barbiturates on the GABA/benzodiazepine receptor/chloride ionophore complex on postsynaptic neurons (6, 29, 30). On this receptor complex there are binding sites, not only for barbiturates, but also for the inhibitory neurotransmitter, GABA, and for benzodiazepines (6, 29-34). When this receptor complex is in the inactive depolarized state, the chloride channel is closed (Figure 1A). With activation of the complex, initiated for example by the binding of GABA to its binding site, or the binding of a benzodiazepine or a barbiturate to its binding site in the presence of GABA, conformational changes take place in the receptor complex (Figure 1B). These changes result in opening of the chloride channel, chloride conductance across the membrane, the transformation of the membrane from a depolarized to a hyperpolarized state and the consequent promotion of GABA-ergic inhibitory postsynaptic neurotransmission (6, 29-34). Increased GABA-ergic tone is known to cause encephalopathy (3, 10, 13, 35).

Additional assessments of the potential involvement of the GABA/ benzodiazepine receptor complex in the mediation of HE included further studies of VERs. The abnormal pattern of the VER in HE was found to be almost identical, not only to that in pentobarbital-induced encephalopathy (10, 11), but also to that in encephalopathy induced by a GABA receptor agonist, muscimol (10), a GABA transaminase inhibitor, gamma-vinyl-GABA (3) or a benzodiazepine receptor agonist, diazepam (3, 10). In addition, recently the abnormal pattern of the VER in rats with HE due to thioacetamide-induced FHF has also been shown to be very similar to that in rats with pentobarbital-induced coma (11). In contrast, in several encephalopathies induced by agents which are not believed to mediate their neurobehavioral effects by promoting GABA-ergic neurotransmission, the associated abnormal VER patterns did not resemble those in HE (10, 11, 36-38). Thus, in models of HE, implication of the GABA/benzodiazepine receptor complex in the mediation of the encephalopathy was suggested by patterns of VERs consistent with increased GABA-ergic tone (10, 11, 39).

Studies Using Antagonists and Agonists of the GABA Receptor Complex in Animal Models. If the GABA/benzodiazepine receptor complex plays a role in the neurochemical mechanisms that mediate the syndrome of HE due to FHF, as suggested by VER studies, then agents that affect the components of this supramolecular complex should either mimic or reverse this syndrome (3). To test the validity of this hypothesis in rabbits, the effects of antagonists of the GABA/benzodiazepine receptor complex on HE were assessed and encephalopathies induced by agents which promote GABA-ergic neurotransmission were compared with HE. The antagonist drugs used were bicuculline (a GABA receptor antagonist) (30, 40, 41), Ro 15-1788 (a benzodiazepine receptor antagonist) (41) and isopropylbicyclophosphate (IPPO). IPPO is a chloride channel blocker which binds to a site near the chloride channel, which is distinct from both GABA or benzodiazepine binding sites (42-44). Ro 15-1788 counteracts the effects of benzodiazepine ligands by displacing them from benzodiazepine receptors; it mediates few behavioral effects alone in normal animals, but it abruptly reverses benzodiazepine-induced sedation (3, 41). The relationship of Ro 15-1788 to benzodiazepines is analogous to the relationship between naloxone (Narcan) and morphine (45).

Rabbits were studied in grade II to grade IV encephalopathy (3) induced by GalN, gamma-vinyl-GABA or diazepam. GalN induces HE due to FHF (46). Gamma-vinyl-GABA (a GABA transaminase inhibitor) induces encephalopathy as a consequence of the accumulation of uncatabolized GABA in the brain (47,48) and diazepam (a benzodiazepine receptor agonist) induces encephalopathy by potentiating GABA-ergic neurotransmission (6,30-34). Responses to receptor antagonists were assessed in terms of both clinical neurologic status and electrophysiologic status. Clinical improvement was expressed in terms of a composite neurologic response score which was based on clinical assessments of changes in alertness, responses to a standard painful stimulus, muscle tone and spontaneous movement. An unequivocal improvement in any of these assessments constituted one point in the response score. Electrophysiologic status was assessed from VER recordings (3).

No clinical improvement in HE occurred after the intravenous administration of the vehicles for the receptor antagonist drugs. In contrast, the intravenous administration of bicuculline or Ro 15-1788 consistently induced transient but unequivocal clinical ameliorations of HE. In addition, bicuculline (intravenous) also induced a transient clinical improvement in gamma-vinyl-GABA-induced encephalopathy, and Ro 15-1788 (intravenous) induced a rapid clinical reversal of diazepam-induced coma. Bicuculline and Ro 15-1788 together induced a similar degree of clinical amelioration of HE to that observed when each drug was given alone. Thus, there was no evidence that the two drugs acted synergistically. IPPO also induced a similar degree of clinical amelioration of HE as did the other two drugs (3).

In HE a pathologic increase in the amplitude of the first positive wave of the VER trace (P1) occurred. The intravenous injection of the vehicles for the receptor antagonist drugs alone had no effect on the amplitude of P1 in HE. In contrast, the intravenous injection of bicuculline, Ro 15-1788 or IPPO normalized the increased amplitude of Pl in HE (Figures 3 and 4). Abnormalities of the VER waveform in gamma-vinyl-GABA-induced encephalopathy and diazepam-induced coma were similar to those in HE (increased amplitude of Pl) and were corrected by the intravenous administration of bicuculline and Ro 15-1788 respectively (3).

In normal rabbits, small doses of bicuculline induced slow wave EEG complexes and larger doses induced convulsions. In animals with HE, bicuculline caused slow wave complexes and convulsions only after injection of doses that were significantly larger than the corresponding doses in controls (3). These observations indicate that there is increased resistance to the convulsive effects of bicuculline in HE due to FHF and consequently are compatible with this syndrome being associated with increased GABA-ergic tone.

In analogous studies in rats with GalN-induced encephalopathy, CGS 8216, a benzodiazepine receptor antagonist with a more prolonged pharmacologic action than Ro 15-1788, has been shown to induce both clinical and electrophysiologic (VER) ameliorations of the encephalopathy (12). Furthermore, in rats with thioacetamide-induced FHF, Ro 15-1788 induced unequivocal clinical and electrophysiologic (VER) ameliorations of HE (13). Thus, Ro 15-1788-induced ameliorations of HE are neither species- nor model-specific. A partial inverse agonist of the benzodiazepine receptor, Ro 15-4513, produced even more dramatic (clinical

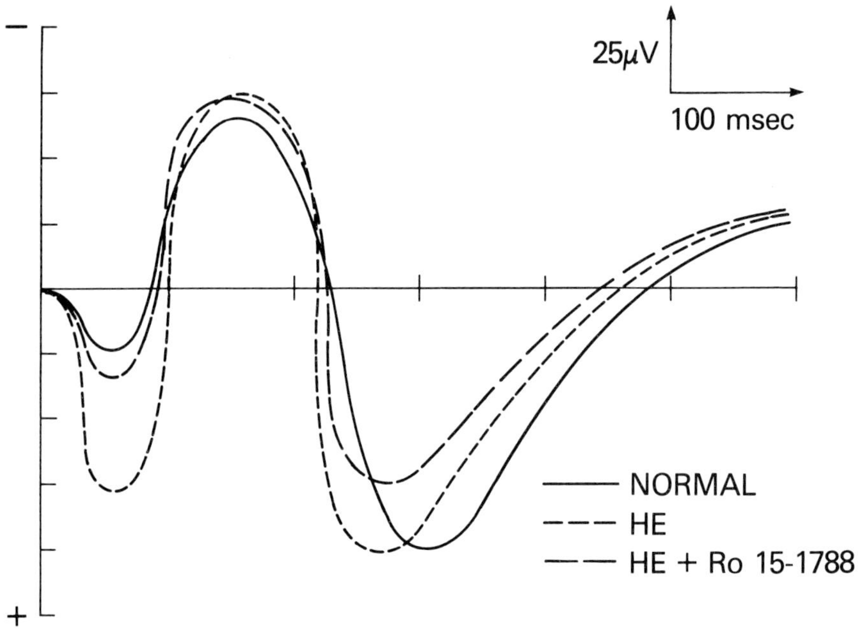

FIGURE 3. Electrophysiologic amelioration of hepatic encephalopathy (HE) in a rabbit model of fulminant hepatic failure induced by the intravenous administration of the benzodiazepine receptor antagonist, Ro 15-1788. Depicted are composite visual evoked responses in normal rabbits, rabbits in HE and rabbits in HE following the intravenous administration of Ro 15-1788. Ro 15-1788 corrected the pathological increase in the amplitude of the first positive wave (P1) which was associated with HE. Reproduced with permission from Gastroenterology (3).

and electrophysiologic) ameliorations of HE in thioacetamide-treated rats than did Ro 15-1788 (13). Inverse agonists of the benzodiazepine receptor not only compete with benzodiazepine agonists but also decrease the ability of GABA to promote chloride conductance (9). Thus, these neuropharmacologic findings provide further support for the hypothesis that the GABA/benzodiazepine receptor complex is implicated in the mediation of HE. The clinical and electrophysiologic amelioration of HE induced by benzodiazepine receptor antagonists cannot be explained by increased levels of GABA in synaptic clefts or by increased density or affinity of GABA receptors. Clearly another factor must be involved to account for these

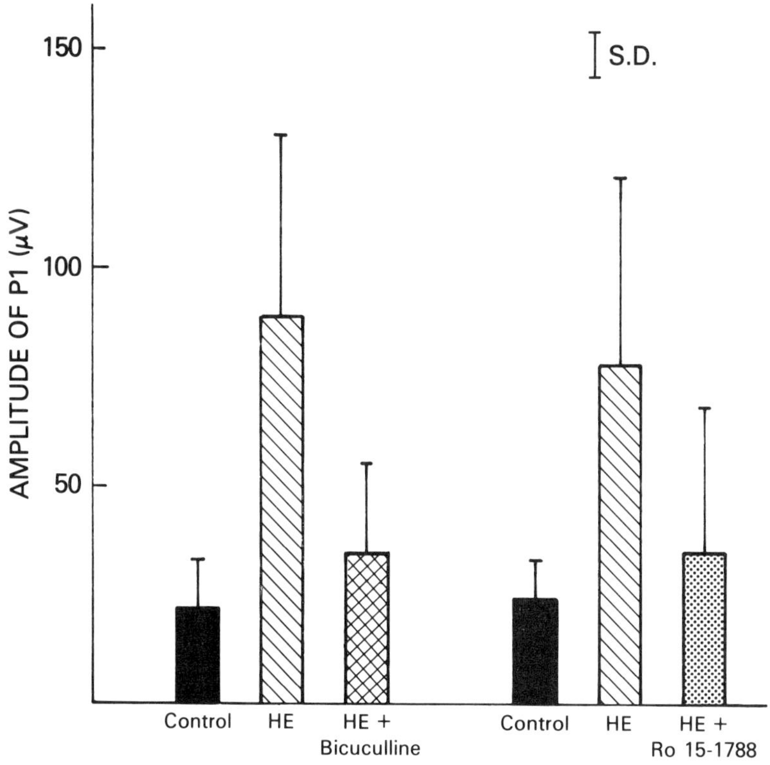

FIGURE 4. Electrophysiologic amelioration of fulminant hepatic encephalopathy (HE) in a rabbit model of hepatic failure induced by the intravenous administration of a GABA receptor antagonist, bicuculline, or a benzodiazepine receptor antagonist, Ro 15-1788. Amplitudes of the first positive wave (P1) of the visual evoked response are depicted as means ± SD for control rabbits, rabbits in HE and rabbits in HE following the intravenous administration of bicuculline or Ro 15-1788. Both bicuculline and Ro 15-1788 corrected the pathologic increase in the amplitude of P1 which was associated with HE. The data depicted were published in tabular form in Gastroenterology (3).

ameliorations, such as the presence of an endogenous benzodiazepine agonist ligand.

Benzodiazepine Receptor Antagonist-induced Ameliorations of HE in Man. The studies relating to the GABA/benzodiazepine receptor complex in animal models of HE provide a rationale for trials in humans with HE of drugs which modulate the function of this receptor complex by decreasing GABA-ergic neurotransmission. Such drugs would not include those acting at the GABA receptor site, such as bicuculline, or chloride channel blockers, such as IPPO, as such drugs have a low therapeutic index with a marked propensity to induce convulsions (3, 9, 42-44). However, certain drugs, such as benzodiazepine receptor antagonists, which act at the benzodiazepine receptor site, have the potential of modulating GABA-ergic neurotransmission with a high therapeutic index and without inducing convulsions (9, 41). Indeed, Ro 15-1788 is not only a benzodiazepine receptor antagonist, but has also recently been shown to have partial benzodiazepine receptor agonist properties (22, 49). Recently, there have been preliminary reports of unequivocal clinical and electrophysiologic (EEG or evoked response) ameliorations of HE in humans following the administration of Ro 15-1788. Such ameliorations have been observed in patients with FHF (14, 15), acute HE associated with cirrhosis (16, 17) (Figure 5) and chronic intractable PSE (18). These findings are compatible with HE due to FHF or chronic liver disease being associated with increased GABA-ergic tone mediated by an endogenous benzodiazepine ligand which can be displaced from benzodiazepine receptors by benzodiazepine receptor antagonists.

Evidence for Benzodiazepine Binding Activity in CSF. During the past decade evidence for the existence of an endogenous ligand for benzodiazepine receptors has been sought in normal animals without definitive success (50). The recent reports of benzodiazepine receptor antagonists inducing clinical and electrophysiologic ameliorations of HE in animal models and humans raises the possibility that in HE benzodiazepine receptor antagonists may be reducing augmented GABA-ergic tone by displacing an endogenous benzodiazepine agonist ligand from benzodiazepine receptors. The existence of such a ligand can be sought by examining the ability of a biological fluid to displace [^{3}H]-beta-carboline ethyl ester or [^{3}H]-Ro 15-1788 from fresh brain preparations. By the application of this approach, benzodiazepine receptor binding activity has been found in the CSF in an animal model of HE (19) and in humans with HE (20).

Responses of Neurons to Agonists and Antagonists of the GABA/Benzodiazepine Receptor Complex in Vitro. The studies in which clinical and electrophysiologic remissions of HE were induced in rabbits with GalN-induced FHF by antagonists of the GABA/benzodiazepine receptor complex, and particularly by Ro 15-1788 (3), directly led to experiments being undertaken in which recordings were made of changes in the electrical activity of single neurons in brain slices in response to pharmacologic agents specific for the supramolecular complex. These studies were prompted by the need to apply techniques which enabled a high resolution of neuronal function in order to ascribe with any degree of confidence the results of the studies which employed VERs to changes in the function of a specific neurotransmitter system. The spontaneous activity of Purkinje neurons in cerebellar slices maintained *in vitro* was recorded. Unlike studies of VERs, this technique precludes correlating electrophysiologic and behavioral changes. However, this experimental approach is particularly useful because it eliminates variables attributable to changes in the blood-brain barrier and peripheral drug metabolism.

Using this technique, the spontaneous activity of Purkinje neurons from rabbits in HE was found to be 3 to 5 times more sensitive to depression by muscimol (a GABA agonist) or flunitrazepam (a benzodiazepine agonist) than that of corresponding control neurons (21). This hypersensitivity to depression appeared to be specific to agents acting at the supramolecular complex as no difference in the sensitivity of these neurons was apparent in response to treatment with a depressant alpha-adrenergic receptor agonist (A.S. Basile, unpublished observations). Furthermore, pretreatment of these neurons with a benzodiazepine receptor antagonist (Ro 14-7437) eliminated the hypersensitivity of neurons from rabbits with HE to

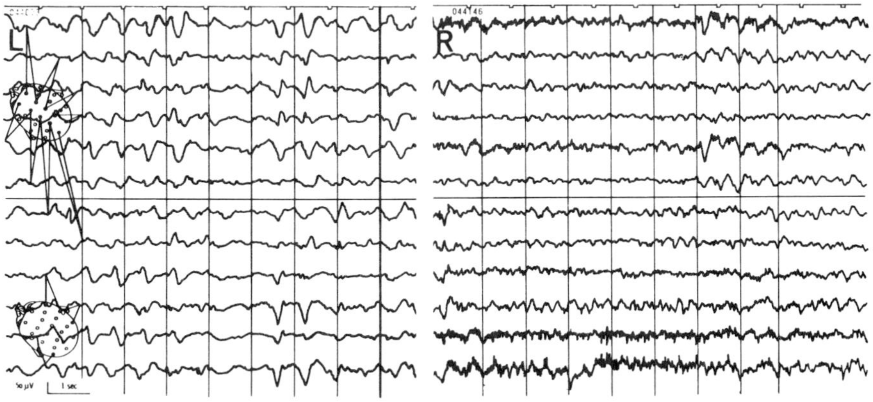

FIGURE 5. Electrophysiologic amelioration of hepatic encephalopathy in a 58-year-old woman with cirrhosis following the intravenous administration of the benzodiazepine receptor antagonist, Ro 15-1788. Left— Before treatment, when the patient was in grade IV HE, the EEG showed continuous 1- to 2- Hz triphasic wave activity. Right—40 sec after the administration of 0.3 mg of Ro 15-1788, the patient's degree of HE had improved: clinically the patient was in grade II HE and the EEG showed 4- to 5-Hz theta background activity. Reproduced with permission from The Lancet (16).

depression by muscimol (A.S. Basile, unpublished observations). Increases in the levels of GABA in synaptic clefts or increases in the densities or affinities of GABA receptors could potentially account for the increased sensitivity of neurons from animals in HE to muscimol and flunitrazepam. In addition, administration of benzodiazepine receptor antagonists (Ro 15-1788 or Ro 14-7437) significantly increased the spontaneous activity of Purkinje neurons from rabbits with HE at concentrations which had no effect or depressed the activity of control rabbit Purkinje neurons (22). These findings, together with the results of the VER studies (3, 10-13), provide strong evidence that GABA-ergic tone is increased in the models of HE studied. Increases in the levels of GABA in synaptic clefts or increases in the densities or affinities of GABA receptors cannot account for the increased spontaneous activity of Purkinje neurons from animals with HE induced by benzodiazepine receptor antagonists. Another factor must be involved to account for these effects, such as the presence of an endogenous benzodiazepine receptor agonist ligand.

THE ROLE OF THE GUT

So far, this chapter has concentrated on phenomena in the central nervous system (CNS) in relation to HE. This emphasis on the CNS reflects the fact that the brain is the end organ of the syndrome of HE. However, it is well recognized that gut factors are involved in the precipitation and amelioration of HE, at least in patients with chronic liver disease (51-54). Accordingly, it is pertinent to consider whether gut-derived GABA could contribute to HE, even though a role for gut-derived GABA is not a necessary prerequisite for the hypothesis that increased GABA-ergic tone is involved in HE.

The intestine (gut wall and enteric bacteria) is a major source of GABA outside the CNS (55, 56). However, GABA is only one of many neuroactive substances that arise in the intestine. Nevertheless, specific mechanisms for the uptake (57) and catabolism (58) of GABA by the liver have been shown to exist; hepatic clearance of GABA is reduced in an animal model of acute liver failure (59); GABA levels in peripheral blood plasma of humans in HE tend to be elevated (60, 61) (Figure 6); and increased permeability of the blood-brain barrier to GABA has been convincingly demonstrated using two entirely different methods in a model of acute liver failure (GalN-induced FHF in rabbits) (62, 63). Therefore, it is likely that liver failure, at least in one acute model, is associated with increased quantities of gut-derived GABA gaining access to brain extracellular fluid. However, whether such gut-derived GABA can reach GABA receptors in synaptic clefts and augment GABA-ergic tone is uncertain as efficient, neuronal, carrier-mediated transport systems exist which remove GABA from synaptic regions (64).

Whether the increased blood-brain barrier permeability to GABA found in rabbits with GalN-induced FHF also applies to other apparently satisfactory models of acute or chronic liver failure is uncertain, and whether blood-brain barrier permeability to GABA is increased in human HE is unknown. At the present time a role for gut-derived GABA in the mediation of HE has neither been confirmed nor refuted. Indeed, it is also true to say that none of the gut-derived neuroactive substances that have been implicated in HE has been proven to play a definitive role in the mediation of this syndrome. It is possible that gut-derived substances that play an important role in HE have yet to be identified. For example, if an endogenous substance with benzodiazepine agonist-like properties (or a precursor of such a substance) arose in the gut, such a substance might well contribute to the neural inhibition of HE (3, 9, 12-20, 22). The possibility that a normal diet may contain benzodiazepines has been raised (65).

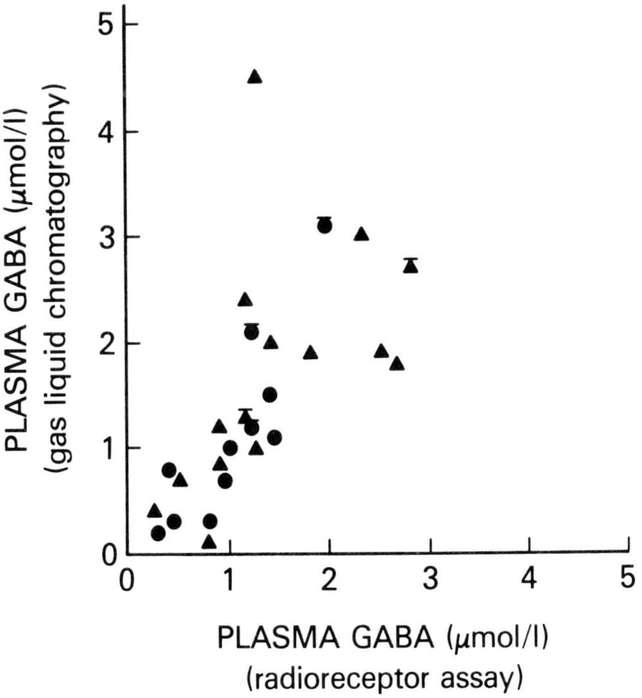

FIGURE 6. Correlation between values for plasma GABA concentration determined by gas liquid chromatography and radioreceptor assay in patients with liver disease with and without overt hepatic encephalopathy. Symbols: ●—no encephalopathy; ▲—clinical encephalopathy; - —acute/subacute hepatic failure. Reproduced with permission from Clinical Science (61).

CONCLUDING PERSPECTIVES

The patterns of VERs in two animal models are consistent with HE due to FHF being associated with increased GABA-ergic tone. Furthermore, the results of pharmacologically antagonizing the GABA/benzodiazepine receptor complex in three animal models suggest that in HE due to FHF, not only is there increased GABA-ergic tone, but (a) an amelioration of encephalopathy can be induced by blockading GABA or benzodiazepine receptors; (b) benzodiazepine receptor antagonists, such as Ro 15-1788, may be of therapeutic value in the management of HE in man; and (c) an endogenous substance with benzodiazepine agonist-like properties may be present. Such a ligand could contribute to the encephalopathy by potentiating the action of GABA.

The observations that the VER pattern in HE is consistent with increased GABA-ergic tone and Ro 15-1788 can induce ameliorations of HE are neither model- nor species-specific. The possible existence of an endogenous benzodiazepine agonist ligand in HE due to FHF is supported by finding benzodiazepine binding activity in CSF and benzodiazepine receptor-antagonist-induced excitation of neurons from rabbits with GalN-induced FHF. Furthermore, the increased sensitivity of neurons from the same model to depression by agonists of the GABA/benzodiazepine receptor complex provides additional evidence for an involvement of this complex and of increased GABA-ergic tone in HE due to FHF.

Whether these findings in models of FHF also apply to satisfactory models of PSE or HE due to chronic liver disease is currently unknown. However, it does appear that two of these findings can tentatively be extrapolated to man. In particular, benzodiazepine binding activity has been detected in the CSF of humans with HE and ameliorations of encephalopathy induced by the benzodiazepine receptor antagonist, Ro 15-1788, have been reported in patients with HE due to FHF, HE associated with cirrhosis and chronic intractable PSE. The reports of Ro 15-1788-induced ameliorations of HE in man are potentially of great interest and significance, but so far they are preliminary and uncontrolled.

The extent to which increased GABA-ergic tone and neural mechanisms postulated in other hypotheses relating to the pathogenesis of HE contribute to the global manifestations of this syndrome are unknown. If increased GABA-ergic tone does play a role in the mediation of the encephalopathy that complicates acute or chronic liver disease, this phenomenon would not be incompatible with substances implicated in other hypotheses such as ammonia, mercaptans, short-chain fatty acids, phenols, dopamine, octopamine, phenylethanolamine and serotonin, also playing roles in the pathogenesis of HE by mechanisms specified in the relevant hypotheses. However, it seems unlikely that any of the substances in this list would directly activate the GABA/benzodiazepine receptor complex. For example, unlike GABA which promotes Cl^- conductance across neuronal membranes from the exterior to the cytoplasm, ammonia has been shown to disinhibit neurons by inhibiting Cl^- extrusion. This effect and the ability of high concentrations of ammonia to increase excitatory neuronal potentials are considered to be the neurophysiologic basis of ammonia-induced seizures (66-70). Furthermore, ammonia has been reported to mediate similar effects to a GABA antagonist on the visual cortex (71). However, recent evidence suggests that ammonia can also induce neural inhibition in some regions of the brain, and that this phenomenon may be related to a decrease in glutamate-mediated excitatory neurotransmission (72-74). Thus, it is possible that ammonia may contribute to HE by decreasing neural excitation. Furthermore, ammonia and other substances such as mercaptans, short-chain fatty acids and phenols could well modulate blood-brain barrier permeability, the composition of neural membranes, the functional status of receptors for neurotransmitters and the neuronal release of neurotransmitters in ways that augment neural inhibition and consequently contribute to the pathogenesis of HE.

If increased GABA-ergic tone occurs in HE, the only candidate substance for inducing this phenomenon at time of writing, other than GABA itself, is a putative endogenous benzodiazepine receptor agonist. The nature and source of such a substance in HE are currently unknown.

REFERENCES

1. Schafer DF, Jones EA. Hepatic encephalopathy and the gamma-aminobutyric acid neurotransmitter system. Lancet 1982; 1:18-20.

2. Jones EA, Schafer DF. Hepatic encephalopathy: A neurochemical disorder. In: Popper H and Schaffner F, eds. Progress in Liver Diseases, Vol VIII. New York: Grune and Stratton, 1986: 525-540.

3. Bassett ML, Mullen KD, Skolnick P, et al. Amelioration of hepatic encephalopathy by pharmacologic antagonism of the $GABA_A$-benzodiazepine receptor complex in a rabbit model of fulminant hepatic failure. Gastroenterology 1987; 93:1069-1077.

4. Jones EA, Mullen KD, Gammal SH. Hepatic encephalopathy. In: Arias IM, Frenkel M, Wilson JHP, eds. Liver Annual/6. Amsterdam: Elsevier Science Publishers, 1987: 396-422.

5. Jones EA, Gammal SH. Hepatic encephalopathy. In: Arias IM, Jakoby WB, Popper H, Schachter D, Shafritz DA, eds. The Liver: Biology and Pathobiology, ed. 2. New York: Raven Press, 1988 (in press).

6. Study RE, Barker JL. Diazepam and (-)—pentobarbital: Fluctuation analysis reveals different mechanisms for potentiation of gamma-aminobutyric acid responses in cultured neurons. Proc Natl Acad Sci USA 1981; 78:7180-7184.

7. Schafer DF, Fowler JM, Munson PJ., et al. Gamma-aminobutyric acid and benzodiazepine receptors in an animal model of fulminant hepatic failure. J Lab

Clin Med 1983; 102:870-880.

8. Jones EA, Schafer DF, Ferenci P, et al. The neurobiology of hepatic encephalopathy. Hepatology 1984; 4:1235-1242.

9. Schafer DF. Hepatic coma: studies on the target organ. Gastroenterology 1987; 93:1132-1134.

10. Schafer DF, Pappas SC, Brody LE, et al. Visual evoked potentials in a rabbit model of hepatic encephalopathy. I. Sequential changes and comparisons with drug-induced comas. Gastroenterology 1984; 86:540-545.

11. Jones DB, Mullen KD, Roessle M, et al. Hepatic encephalopathy: Application of visual evoked responses to test hypotheses of its pathogenesis in rats. J Hepatol 1987; 4:118-126.

12. Baraldi M, Zeneroli ML, Ventura E, et al. Supersensitivity of benzodiazepine receptors in hepatic encephalopathy due to fulminant hepatic failure in the rat: reversal by a benzodiazepine antagonist. Clin Sci 1985; 67:167-175.

13. Gammal SH, Geller D, Skolnick P, et al. Unequivocal amelioration of hepatic encephalopathy (HE) by benzodiazepine receptor antagonists (BZA) in a rat model of fulminant hepatic failure (FHF). Gastroenterology 1987; 92:1734.

14. Scollo-Lavizzari G, Steinmann E. Reversal of hepatic coma by benzodiazepine antagonist (Ro 15-1788). Lancet 1985; 1:1324.

15. Grimm G, Lenz K, Kleinberger G, et al. Ro 15-1788 improves coma in 4 out of 5 patients with fulminant hepatic failure; verification by long latency auditory and somatosensory evoked potentials. J Hepatol 1987; 4 (suppl. 1):S21.

16. Bansky G, Meier PJ, Ziefler WH, et al. Reversal of hepatic coma by benzodiazepine antagonist (Ro 15-1788). Lancet 1985; 1:1324-1325.

17. Bansky G, Meier PJ, Riederer E, et al. Effect of benzodiazepine antagonist in hepatic encephalopathy in man. Hepatology 1987; 7:1103.

18. Ferenci P, Grimm G, Gangl A. Successful longtime treatment of chronic hepatic encephalopathy (HE) with a benzodiazepine antagonist. Hepatology 1987; 7:1064.

19. Mullen KD, Martin JV, Bassett ML, et al. Hepatic encephalopathy: a syndrome modulated by an endogenous benzodiazepine receptor ligand? Hepatology 1986; 6:1221.

20. Mullen KD, Szanter KM, Galloway PG, et al. CSF of patients with hepatic encephalopathy (HE) contains significant benzodiazepine (BZ) binding activity. Correlation with post mortem cortical BZ binding studies. Hepatology 1987; 7:1103.

21. Gammal SH, Basile AS, Mullen KD, et al. Hepatic encephalopathy: Enhanced sensitivity of isolated CNS neurons to a benzodiazepine. Hepatology 1987; 7:1032.

22. Basile AS, Gammal SH, Mullen KD, et al. Hepatic encephalopathy: evidence for the involvement of an endogenous benzodiazepine receptor ligand. Hepatology 1987; 7:1103.

23. MacGillivray BB. The EEG in liver disease. In: Glaser GH, ed. Handbook

of Electroencephalography and Clinical Neurophysiology, Vol 15, part 3. Amsterdam: Elsevier, 1975: 5, 26.

24. Schafer DF, Brody LE, Jones EA. Visual evoked potentials: An objective measurement of hepatic encephalopathy in the rabbit (Abstract). Gastroenterology 1979; 77:A38.

25. Purpura DP. Intracellular studies of synaptic organizations in the mammalian brain. In: Pappas GD, Purpura DP, eds. Structure and Function of Synapses. New York: Raven Press, 1972: 257-302.

26. Bigler ED. Neurophysiology, neuropharmacology and behavioral relationships of visual system evoked after discharges: a review. Biobehav Rev 1977; 1:95-112.

27. Nakayama K. The relationship of visual evoked potentials to cortical physiology. Ann NY Acad Sci 1982; 388:21-36.

28. Schafer DF, Fowler JM, Brody LE, et al. Hepatic coma and inhibitory neurotransmission: the enteric bacterial flora as a source of gamma-aminobutyric acid. Gastroenterology 1980; 79:1052.

29. Skolnick P, Moncada V, Barker JL, et al. Phenobarbital: dual actions to increase brain benzodiazepine receptor affinity. Science 1981; 211:1448-1450.

30. Olsen RW. Drug interactions at the GABA receptor-ionophore complex. Annu Rev Pharmacol Toxicol 1982; 22:245-277.

31. Costa E, Di Chiara G, Gessa GL, eds. GABA and benzodiazepine receptors. Advances in Biochemical Psychopharmacology, Vol 26. New York: Raven Press, 1981.

32. Tallman JF, Paul SM, Skolnick P, et al. Receptors for the age of anxiety: pharmacology of the benzodiazepines. Science 1980; 207:274-281.

33. Paul SM, Marangos PJ, Skolnick P. The benzodiazepine-GABA-chloride ionophore receptor complex: common site of minor tranquilizer action. Biol Psychiatry 1981; 16:213-229.

34. Tallman JF, Gallager DW. The GABAergic system: a locus of benzodiazepine action. Annu Rev Neurosci 1985; 8:21-44.

35. Smialowsky A. The effect of intra-hippocampal administration of gamma-aminobutyric acid (GABA). In: Fonnum F, ed. Amino Acids as Chemical Transmitters. New York: Plenum Press, 1978: 1977-1980.

36. Zeneroli ML, Penne A., Parrinello G, et al. Comparative evaluation of visual evoked potentials in experimental hepatic encephalopathy and in pharmacologically induced coma-like states in rat. Life Sci 1981; 28:1507-1515.

37. Zeneroli ML, Ventura E, Baraldi M, et al. Visual evoked potentials in encephalopathy induced by galactosamine, ammonia, dimethyldisulphide and octanoic acid. Hepatology 1982; 2:532-538.

38. Pappas SC, Ferenci P, Schafer DF, et al. Visual evoked potentials in a rabbit model of hepatic encephalopathy: II. Comparison of hyperammonemic encephalopathy, post-ictal coma and coma induced by synergistic neurotoxins. Gastroenterology 1984; 86:546-551.

39. Zemon V, Kaplan E, Ratliff F. Bicuculline enhances a negative component and diminishes a positive component of the visual evoked cortical potential in the cat. Proc Natl Acad Sci USA 1980; 77:7476-7478.

40. Olsen RW, Snowman AM. [^{3}H]-Bicuculline methochloride binding to low affinity GABA receptor sites. J Neurochem 1983; 41:1653-1663.

41. Squires RF. Benzodiazepine receptors. In: Lajtha A, ed. Handbook of Neurochemistry, 2nd ed., Vol 6. New York: Plenum Press, 1984: 261-306.

42. Squires RF, Casida J, Richardson M, et al. [^{35}S]t-Butylbicyclophorothionate binds with high affinity to brain specific sites coupled with $GABA_A$ and ion recognition sites. Mol Pharmacol 1983; 23:326-336.

43. Akaike N, Hattori K, Domina Y, et al. Bicuculline and picrotoxin block gamma-aminobutyric acid Cl^- conductance by different mechanisms. Experientia 1985; 41:70-71.

44. Havoundjian H, Paul SM, Skolnick P. The permeability of gamma-aminobutyric acid-gated chloride channels is described by the binding of a "cage" convulsant [^{35}S]t-butylbicyclophorothionate. Proc Natl Acad Sci USA 1986; 83:9241-9244.

45. Zaks A, Jones T, Fink M, et al. Treatment of opiate dependence with high dose oral naloxone. JAMA 1971; 215:2108-2110.

46. Blitzer BL, Waggoner JG, Jones EA, et al. A model of fulminant hepatic failure in the rabbit. Gastroenterology 1978; 74:664-671.

47. Jung MJ, Lippert B, Metcalf BW. Gamma-vinyl GABA (4-amino-hex-5-enoic acid), a new selective irreversible inhibitor of GABA-T: effects on brain GABA metabolism in mice. J Neurochem 1977; 29:797-802.

48. Hammond EJ, Wilder BJ. Gamma-vinyl GABA: a new antiepileptic drug. Clin Neuropharmacol 1985; 8:1-12.

49. Lavie P, Peled R, Wollman M, et al. Agonist-like effects of the benzodiazepine receptor antagonist Ro 15-1788. Neuropsychobiology 1987; 17:72-76.

50. Basile AS, Jones EA. Hepatic encephalopathy and the GABA/benzodiazepine receptor/chloride ionophore complex: an update. J Gastroenterol Hepatol 1988 (in press).

51. Conn HO, Lieberthal MM. The Hepatic Coma Syndromes and Lactulose. Baltimore: Williams and Wilkins, 1978.

52. Sherlock S. Diseases of the Liver and Biliary System, ed.7. London: Blackwell Scientific Publications, 1985: 91-116.

53. Zieve L. Hepatic encephalopathy. In: Schiff L, Schiff ER, eds. Diseases of the Liver. Philadelphia: JB Lippincott Company, 1982: 433-459.

54. Duffy TE, Plum F. Hepatic encephalopathy. In: Arias IM, Popper H, Schachter D, Shafritz DA, eds. The Liver: Biology and Pathobiology. New York: Raven Press, 1982: 693-715.

55. Schafer DF, Fowler JM, Jones EA. Colonic bacteria: a source of gamma-aminobutyric acid in blood. Proc Soc Exp Biol Med 1981; 167:301-303.

56. Van Berlo CLH, de Jonge HR, van den Bogaard AEJM, et al. gamma-ami-

nobutyric acid production in small and large intestine of normal and germ-free Wistar rats. Influence of food intake and intestinal flora. Gastroenterology 1987; 93:472-479.

57. Minuk GY, Vergalla J, Ferenci P, et al. Identification of an acceptor system for gamma-aminobutyric acid on isolated rat hepatocytes. Hepatology 1984; 4:180-185.

58. Ferenci P, Schafer DF, Shrager R, et al. Metabolism of the inhibitory neurotransmitter gamma-aminobutyric acid in a rabbit model of acute hepatic failure. Hepatology 1981; 1:509.

59. Ferenci P, Covell D, Schafer DF, et al. Metabolism of the inhibitory neurotransmitter gamma-aminobutyric acid in a rabbit model of fulminant hepatic failure. Hepatology 1983; 3:507-512.

60. Minuk GY, Winder A, Burgess ED, et al. Serum gamma-aminobutyric acid (GABA) levels in patients with hepatic encephalopathy. Hepatogastroenterology 1985; 32:171-174.

61. Levy LJ, Leek J, Losowsky MS. Evidence for gamma-aminobutyric acid as the inhibitor of gamma-aminobutyric acid binding in the plasma of humans with liver disease and hepatic encephalopathy. Clin Sci 1987; 73:531-534.

62. Horowitz ME, Schafer DF, Molnar P, et al. Increased blood-brain transfer in a rabbit model of acute liver failure. Gastroenterology 1983; 84:1003-1011.

63. Bassett ML, Mullen KD, Scholz B, et al. Increased brain GABA uptake in precoma encephalopathy in a rabbit model of fulminant hepatic failure. Hepatology 1985; 5:1032.

64. Martin DL. Carrier-mediated transport and removal of GABA from synaptic regions. In: Roberts E, Chase TM, Tower DB, eds. GABA in Nervous System Function. New York: Raven Press, 1976: 347-387.

65. De Blas AL, Park D, Friedrich P. Endogenous benzodiazepine-like molecules in the human rat and bovine brains with a monoclonal antibody to benzodiazepines. Brain Res 1987; 413:275-284.

66. Lux HD, Loracher C, Neher E. The action of ammonium on postsynaptic inhibition of cat spinal motorneurons. Exp Brain Res 1970; 11:431-447.

67. Iles JF, Jack JJ. Ammonia mediated block of chloride pumping in cat motorneurone. J Physiol (Lond) 1978; 208:20P.

68. Iles JF, Jack JJ. Ammonia: assessment of its action on postsynaptic inhibition as a cause of convulsions. Brain 1980; 103:555-578.

69. Raabe WA. Ammonia and disinhibition in cat motor cortex by ammonium acetate, monofluoroacetate and insulin-induced hypoglycemia. Brain Res 1981; 210:311-322.

70. Raabe W, Lin S. Ammonia. Postsynaptic inhibition and CNS-energy state. Brain Res 1984; 303:67-76.

71. Duffy FH, Burchfiel JL, Snoddgrass SR. The pharmacology of amblyopia. Ophthalmology 1978; 85:489-495.

72. Theoret Y, Davies MF, Esplin B, et al. Effects of ammonium chloride on

synaptic transmission in the rat hippocampal slice. Neuroscience 1985; 14:798-806.

73. Theoret Y, Bossu JL. Effects of ammonium salts on synaptic transmission to hippocampal CA1 and CA3 pyramidal cells in vivo. Neuroscience 1985; 14:807-821.

74. Raabe W. The H-reflex in the encephalopathy due to ammonia intoxication. Exp Neurol 1987; 96:601-611.

ITS THERAPY

7

THE THEORETIC THERAPY OF HEPATIC ENCEPHALOPATHY

HAROLD O. CONN, M.D.

In earlier chapters, many etiologies and several pathogeneses for hepatic encephalopathy have been presented. Using a theoretical approach one can devise a simple model which serves as a rational, generic format for therapy. The weight of evidence indicates that portal-systemic encephalopathy (PSE), the prototype of HE, is caused by the accumulation of potentially toxic substance(s). Such toxins or toxinogens either enter the body via the gastrointestinal tract or are converted by the enteric flora to a toxic substance. These substances escape removal or detoxification by circumhepatic shunting or by impaired metabolism by the damaged liver. The exact nature of the substance is not critical for such a theoretic approach.

One can then postulate a pathogenesis in the form of a biochemical reaction. Equation 1:

$$\text{Substrate} \xrightarrow{\text{Enzyme}} \text{Product}$$

Treatment can then be rationally approached in terms of the components of a biochemical reaction.

First, one can eliminate the substrate (S). Second, one can suppress the enzyme (E) by inhibiting its activity or by destroying the bacteria that produce it. Third, therapy can be designed to remove or to detoxify the toxic product (P). Finally, one can use combinations of all three types of treatment or all three.

For simplicity, let us assume that the potentially toxic substrate is urea. The reaction is shown in Equation 2:

$$\begin{matrix} {}^{\diagup}NH_2 \\ C{=}O \\ {}_{\diagdown}NH_2 \end{matrix} + H_2 02 \xrightarrow{\text{Urease}} NH_3 + CO_2$$

Therapy may be directed at any or all of the components of the reaction.

Let's look at some practical examples. Consider *substrate removal* first. If the precipitant is GI bleeding, stopping the hemorrhage will reduce the substrate. Indeed, it is the most logical approach, since if the bleeding isn't controlled, the patient will be lost anyhow from bleeding, encephalopathy or both.

Indeed, using HE induced by active GI bleeding is an extremely complex model for studying the efficacy of the therapy of HE. In several randomized investigations it is not clear whether the efficacy or failure of anticoma therapy is related to the investigators' management of the bleeding or to the effectiveness or ineffectiveness of the treatment.

Some aspects of GI bleeding deserve clarification. The comagenicity of blood results from its degradation in the intestinal tract. Many potential comagenic substances such as protein and urea are contained in blood, and many others such as ammonia, methanethiol, short-chain fatty acids, phenol and GABA may be derived from its degradation. The amount of such toxic substances produced are not necessarily proportional to the amount of bleeding. If all the blood is vomited or removed from the stomach by gastric aspiration, none can be converted to toxic substances. Similarly, the rate of transit through the alimentary tract may influence the development of encephalopathy. If the transit time is short as a result of the cathartic action of blood in the GI tract or therapeutic attempts to induce catharsis, only small amounts of the toxic substances will be produced and absorbed.

The amount of blood lost can influence the BUN concentration. In a normal person the removal of 500 ml of blood does not noticeably affect the BUN levels, although larger venesections may do so. Similarly, the oral ingestion of 500 ml blood by a normal subject will not alter the BUN level. However, the removal of 500 ml of blood from an individual who then ingests it usually causes an increment in BUN levels. Thus, both the volume of bleeding and the amount of blood retained can both influence the development of HE. Such effects are aggravated in cirrhotic patients.

Dietary protein can contribute to the toxic load in a similar manner and a reduction of protein intake is part of any reduction of substrate as is the generous administration of carbohydrate to minimize protein breakdown.

A similar approach can be made to azotemia, which is a common precipitant of PSE. Treatment of azotemia will depend on the cause of the azotemia. If it is dehydration, the administration of water and electrolytes can correct it. Conceivably, peritoneal dialysis or hemodialysis may be indicated to treat more intractable azotemia.

The *suppression of enzyme activity* is standard therapy of PSE. The most direct approach is antibiotic therapy to kill the bacterial source of the enzymes. This can be accomplished with neomycin or other nonabsorbable aminoglycoside antibiotics, but it can also be accomplished by ampicillin, cephalosporins or other antibiotics that can be administered orally or systemically and that are excreted into the biliary tract.

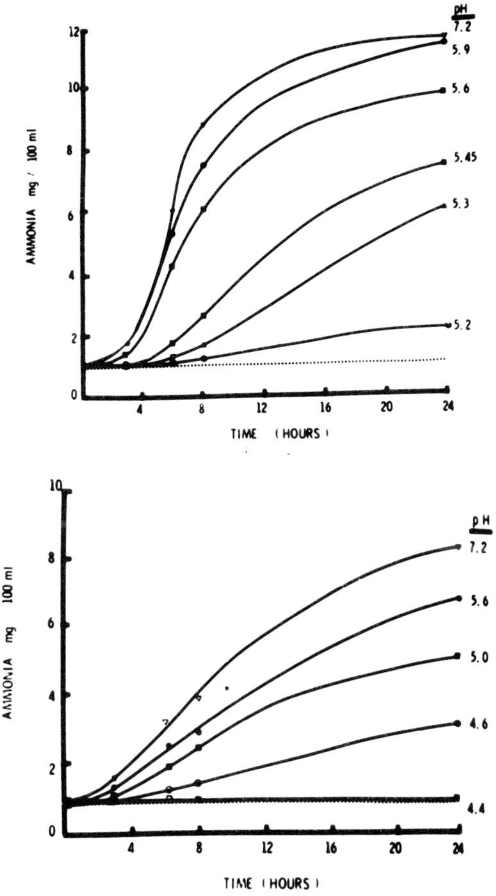

FIGURE 1. Ammonia production from urea by enteric bacteria. Ammonia production by *Proteus mirabilis* (top) and *Escherichia coli* (bottom) from urea at different pHs in static culture. There is little ammonia production below pH 5.3 by *P. mirabilis* and below pH 5.0 by *E. coli*. The ammonia content of the culture medium alone is indicated by the broken line. (Reproduced by permission of authors and publisher (4).

Lactulose, lactitol or other nonabsorbed carbohydrates may make the conditions of the reaction less than optimal. The reduction in intestinal pH below the pH optimum for the hydrolysis of urea decreases the liberation of ammonia from urea (Figure 1) or from protein (1).

One can also use competitive inhibitors of urease such as *nicotinohydroxamate*, which has been shown in a randomized clinical trial to be as effective as neomycin therapy (2) (Figure 2). Would both together be even better?

Third, one can attempt to *eliminate the product.* This can be done mechanically by enemas. It can also be done by acidifying the lumen and trapping ammonia in the gut (Figure 3). Actually, lactulose has several beneficial actions. It can produce an enteric acidosis, which in effect creates an internal pH gradient-dependent dialysis system for the removal of ammonia. Furthermore, lactulose, by reducing pH, stimulates catharsis (3). In addition, lactulose may also induce the incorporation of ammonia into bacterial protein which is then excreted (4). Clearly, lactulose and its therapeutic relatives work on many levels.

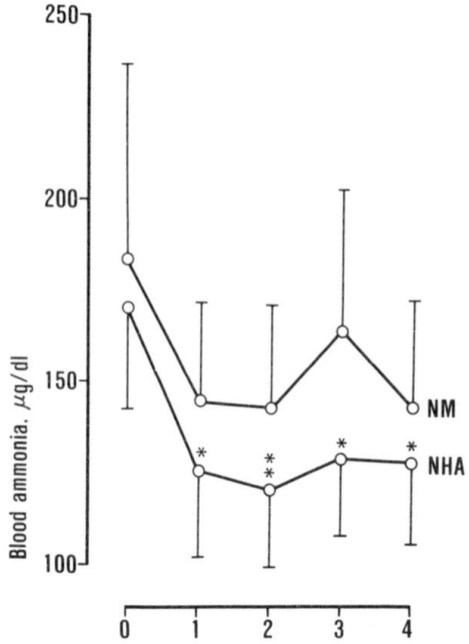

FIGURE 2. Mean venous ammonia levels before and at weekly intervals after neomycin (NM) and nicotinohydroxamic acid (NHA). * = $p<0.05$; ** = $p<0.01$. (Reproduced by permission of the authors and publishers (2).

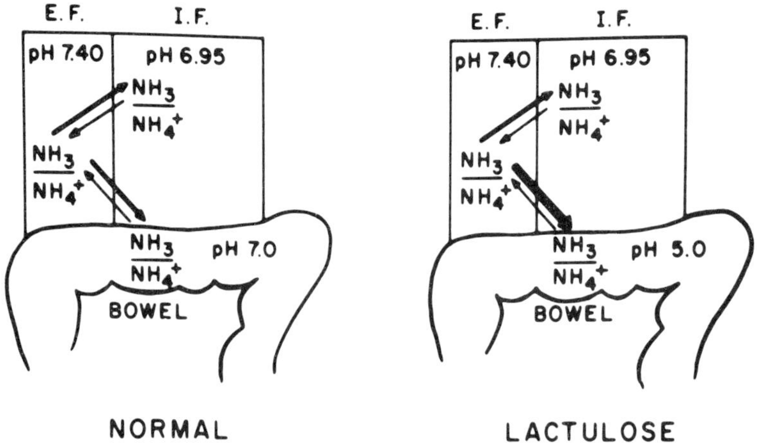

FIGURE 3. Effect of lactulose on nonionic diffusion of ammonia into the intestinal lumen. Normally (shown on the left) the pH of extracellular fluid (EF) is slightly more alkaline than the pH of the intracellular fluid (IF) and than the pH of the lumen of the bowel. The equilibrium favors the diffusion of ammonia from the blood (EF) to the IF and to the bowel (intermediate arrows). In subjects receiving lactulose (shown on the right) the pH of the colonic contents is greatly reduced, the equilibrium is shifted far to the right, and ammonia diffuses into the lumen (heavy arrow). (Reproduced with permission of the authors and the publisher [Conn HO and Lieberthal MM, The Hepatic Coma Syndromes and Lactulose, Baltimore, Williams & Wilkins, 1979].)

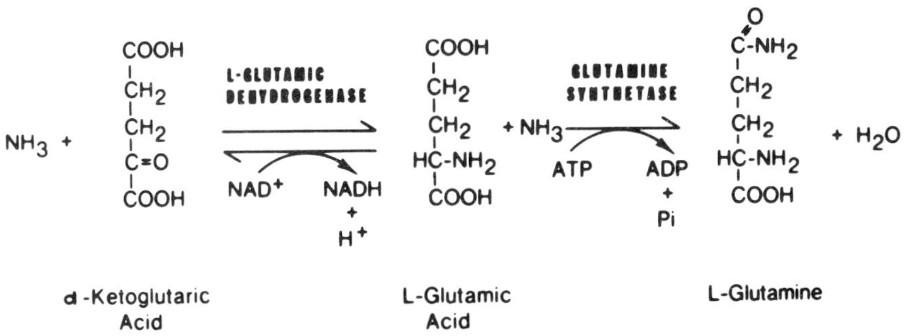

FIGURE 4. Alpha-ketoglutarate-glutamate-glutamine pathway. L-glutamic dehydrogenase catalyzes the amination of alpha-ketoglutaric acid to form L-glutamic acid. This reversible reaction favors glutamic acid synthesis. The reaction is reversible. Glutamine synthetase catalyzes the amidation of L-glutamic acid to form L-glutamine. This reaction is virtually irreversible. (Reproduced with permission of the authors and the publisher [Conn HO and Lieberthal MM, The Hepatic Coma Syndromes and Lactulose, Baltimore, Williams & Wilkins, 1979].)

A series of simple biochemical reactions have been shown to be of value in removing ammonia from the body or incorporating it into less toxic or nontoxic substances.

Sodium *glutamate* (Figure 4), which was in use 30 years ago, may be of value even in these days of other effective therapies (5). *Arginine* can stimulate the synthesis of urea via the urea cycle and is effective in the treatment of PSE provided that the azotemia is not the cause of the PSE (6). *Sodium benzoate* is another such ancillary agent as is *phenylacetylglutamine* (7). Finally, a surprising non-aesthetic approach – the intravenous infusion of *formaldehyde* – may be useful (8). Each molecule of formaldehyde incorporates four molecules of ammonia to form methenamine, which is excreted in the urine (Figure 5). Methenamine is an antibiotic substance, and if a urinary tract infection caused by a sensitive organism is simultaneously present, this may be a fortuitous form of double therapy.

If the substrate were methionine or phenol or GABA instead of urea, the specific therapy administered would differ, but the principles would be the same.

Sometimes conceptual classification of treatment according to the substrate-enzyme-product concept is much less obvious. The amino acid imbalance hypothesis, which is based on the fact that cirrhotic patients have decreased plasma branched-chain amino acid (BCAA) levels and increased aromatic amino acid (AAA) levels in cirrhosis, suggests that increased blood ammonia levels result in increased central nervous system (CNS) glutamine levels (9). The reduction of these increased CNS glutamine levels takes place in part by the exchange with plasma BCAAs and AAAs which share the same carrier system (10). Since plasma BCAA levels are decreased and AAA levels increased in cirrhotic patients with

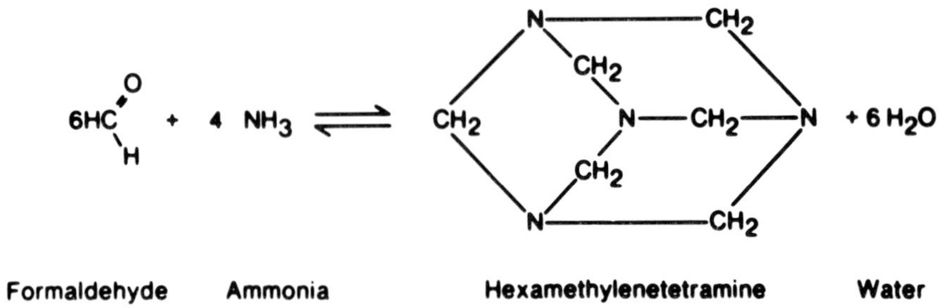

FIGURE 5. The formation of hexamethylenetetramine (methenamine) from formaldehyde and ammonia. Six moles of formaldehyde combine with 4 moles of ammonia. Hexamethylenetetramine is stable in alkaline solution, but at pH less than 6 it releases formaldehyde and ammonia. Formaldehyde intravenously protects against ammonia intoxication induced by ammonium slats and by glycine infusions in experimental animals. (Reproduced with permission of the authors and the publisher [Conn HO and Lieberthal MM, The Hepatic Coma Syndromes and Lactulose, Baltimore, Williams & Wilkins, 1979].)

portal hypertension (11), the exchange favors the accumulation of toxic AAA in the brain (Figure 6). The administration of BCAA is given to correct the imbalance in plasma and ultimately, to reduce the AAA concentration in the CNS (12). Unfortunately, critical analysis of the randomized clinical trials of BCAA therapy in HE do not indicate that it is especially efficacious (13).

Other forms of therapy may be applied to this scheme.

In terms of the substrate-enzyme-product concept, beneficial alterations in diet, such as the administration of vegetable protein (14) or BCAA-enriched supplements of amino acids (15), can be considered to represent reductions in substrate. The explanation for the lesser toxicity of vegetable than of meat protein is not known, but the lower content of ammonia, methionine and AAA in vegetable proteins has been postulated (16). Furthermore, vegetables have a high fiber content and contain indigestible, nonabsorbable oligosaccharides, both of which are carbohydrates that may be metabolized by intestinal bacteria. Such substances, like lactulose, can induce a reduction in intestinal pH, albeit to a lesser degree, that may cause similar but less intense effects than lactulose.

Among the benefits of administering lactulose is the reduction in urea synthesis and pool size (17), which reduces substrate. Its acidifying action a) triggers cathartic activity which reduces substrate and product, b) creates an internal dialysis system which removes ammonia (product) from blood and c) reduces intestinal pH to suboptimal levels for the degradation of urea and protein, thereby suppressing enzyme activity. Thus, lactulose is a true triple-threat therapeutic agent. Lactose administration in patients with lactase deficiency has similar effects as lactulose mediated in the same manner (18).

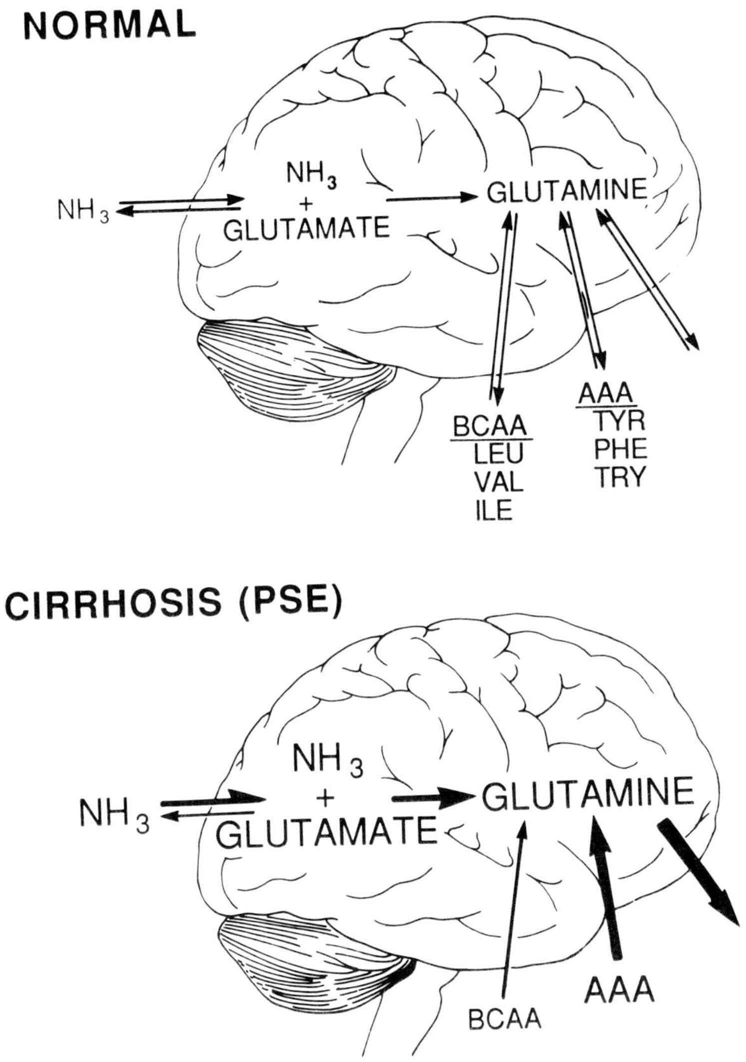

FIGURE 6. Oversimplified diagram of BCAA-Hepatic Encephalopathy Hypothesis. Normal (above). Ammonia that enters the brain is converted to glutamine which exchanges with BCAA and AAA in the plasma which share the same carrier system. In PSE (below) increased blood ammonia levels result in increased glutamine levels in the brain (indicated by larger lettering). The higher concentrations of AAA in the blood than BCAA (indicated by size of the lettering) favors the influx of AAA over BCAA in the exchange for glutamine.

Potassium depletion gives rise to metabolic alkalosis (19) which may be associated with an increased extracellular-intracellular pH gradient that favors the intracellular transport of ammonia (20) and the induction of PSE (Figure 7). Potassium supplementation therapy, which permits potassium ions to replace sodium ions in the intracellular fluid, alters the pH gradient toward normal and, in effect, dialyzes ammonia from the brain. Thus, potassium repletion can be considered to reduce product.

Bromocriptine, a dopamine receptor agonist, is administered in order to restore deficient intracellular amino acids (21, 22). Since the abnormality is the consequence of increased central nervous system glutamine concentrations that are the result of increased ammonia levels, one may consider the exchange of L-dopa for glutamine to represent ultimately a reduction in product.

Sometimes chronic PSE of specific types can be corrected by surgical procedures and their efficacy classified according to the substrate-enzyme-product concept. One such example is the intractable PSE that sometimes follows portal-systemic shunts. It can be reversed by taking down the anastomosis (23) or, presumably, by making the shunt smaller (24). Such a procedure does not decrease substrate or suppress enzyme activity; by decreasing portal-systemic shunting it forces more portal blood to flow through the liver, increasing the clearance of ammonia by the liver and, in effect, decreases product.

Occasionally, patients with intractable PSE are successfully treated with total or hemicolectomy (25) or colon-bypassing procedures (26). Such procedures reduce enzyme activity by decreasing the available space and time for the enzymatic reactions to be carried out.

Peritoneovenous shunts for the treatment of patients with intractable ascites and the hepatorenal syndrome may restore BUN levels to normal and thus ameliorate PSE (27). Such procedures, by increasing the renal excretion of urea, actually reduce substrate.

Patients with ureterosigmoid anastomoses and cirrhosis may develop PSE. Bacteria in the colon hydrolyze the urea to ammonia, which precipitates PSE (28). Externalizing the anastomosis reduces substrate and can prevent further episodes.

Other treatments of PSE can be classified using similar logic (Table 1).

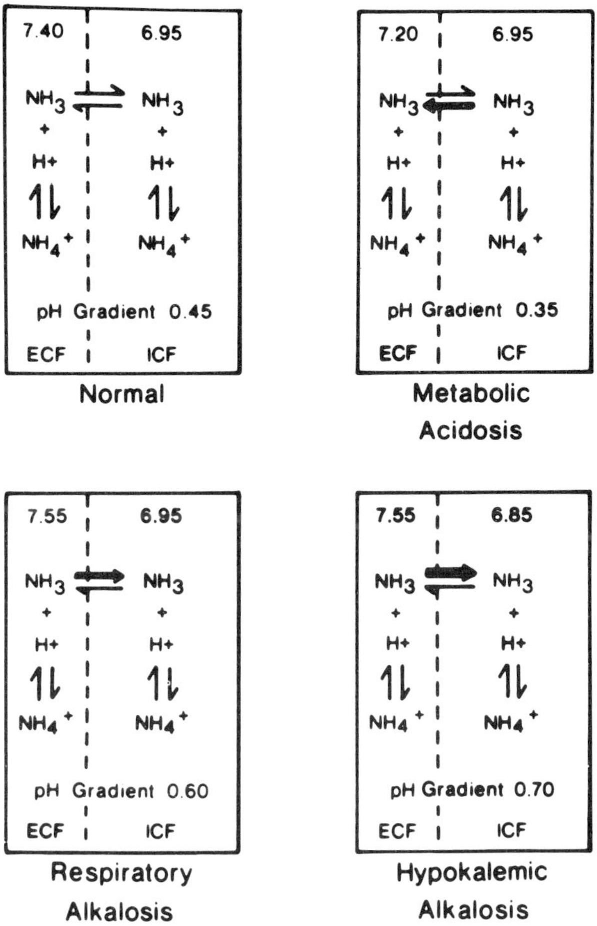

FIGURE 7. Effect of pH gradient on the diffusion of ammonia. The extracellular fluid (ECF) compartment is separated from the intracellular fluid (ICF) compartment by a semipermeable membrane (dotted line). The normal state is depicted in the upper left diagram. Equilibrium exists between NH_3 and NH_4^+ in each compartment and between the NH_3 across the cellular membrane. Metabolic acidosis (upper right) reduces the pH and the pNH_3 of the ECF and the equilibrium is shifted moderately to the left. Respiratory alkalosis (lower left) increases the pH and pNH_3 of the ECF and the equilibrium is shifted moderately to the right. In hypokalemic alkalosis (lower right) there is an increase in the pH and pNH_3 of the ECF and a decrease in the pH and pNH_3 of the ICF, thus greatly increasing the pH gradient and causing a major shift in the equilibrium that favors the diffusion of ammonia from the ECF to the ICF. (Reproduced with permission of the authors and the publisher [Conn HO and Lieberthal MM, The Hepatic Coma Syndromes and Lactulose, Baltimore, Williams & Wilkins, 1979].)

TABLE 1. Theoretic Therapy of Hepatic Encephalopathy

	Examples of specific therapy
1. Substrate (urea) reduction	
1. Hydration	Parenteral fluid
2. Decrease of protein intake	Dietary management
	Vegetable protein diet
3. Control of GI hemorrhage	Management of acute bleeding
4. Correction of renal malperfusion	Blood pressure maintenance
5. Maintenance of blood volume	Transfusion
6. Removal of urea	Dialysis
	Peritoneovenous shunt
	Side-to-side portacaval shunt
7. Suppression of catabolic activity	Carbohydrate-calorie supplementation
8. Suppression of urea synthesis	Lactulose, lactitol, lactose
	High fiber diet.
II. Enzyme inhibition	
1. Suppress bacteria with antibiotics	Oral neomycin
2. Alter conditions of enzymatic reaction	Lactulose, lactitol, lactose
	Acidic enemas
3. Competitive inhibition	Nicotinohydroxamate
4. Surgical alterations	Colectomy or colon bypass
	Take down portacaval shunt
	Externalize ureterosigmoid anastomosis
III. Product removal or utilization	
1. Removal of ammonia	Catharsis
	Lactulose, lactitol, lactose
2. Acidification	Lactulose, lactitol, lactose
	Acid enemas
3. Utilization of product	Arginine
	Glutamate
	Benzoate
	Formaldehyde
	Lactulose, lactitol, lactose
	Branched-chain keto acids
4. Efflux of intracellular ammonia	Branched-chain amino acids
	Bromocriptine
IV. Other mechanisms	
Restore normal plasma amino acid levels	Oral supplementation with BCAA
	Intravenous BCAA

REFERENCES

1. Vince A, Dawson AM, Park N, et al. Ammonia production by intestinal bacteria. Gut 1973; 14:171-177.

2. Hirayama C, Ichida F, Takahashi Y, et al. A controlled clinical trial of nicotinohydroxamic acid and neomycin in advanced chronic liver disease. Digestion 1982; 25:115-123.

3. Bennett A, Eley KG. Intestinal pH and propulsion: an explanation of diarrhoea in lactase deficiency and laxation by lactulose. J Pharm Pharmacol 1976; 28:192-195.

4. Vince A, Killingley M, Wrong OM. Effect of lactulose on ammonia production in a fecal incubation system. Gastroenterology 1978; 74:544-549.

5. Webster LT, Davidson CS. The effect of sodium glutamate on hepatic coma. J Clin Invest 1956; 35:191-199.

6. Reynolds TB, Redeker AG, Davis P. A controlled study of the effects of L-arginine on hepatic encephalopathy. Am J Med 1958; 25:359-367.

7. Batshaw ML, Brusilow S, Waber L, et al. Treatment of inborn errors of urea synthesis. Activation of alternative pathways of waste nitrogen synthesis and excretion. N Engl J Med 1982; 306:1377-1392.

8. Orloff MJ, Peskin GW. The effect of formaldehyde on experimental ammonia intoxication. Surg Forum 1960; 10:295-300.

9. Hourani BT, Hamlin EM, Reynolds TB. Cerebrospinal fluid glutamine as a measure of hepatic encephalopathy. Arch Intern Med 1971; 127:1033-1036.

10. Oldendorf WH, Szabo J. Amino acid assignment to one of three blood-brain barrier amino acid carriers. Am J Physiol 1976; 230:94-98.

11. Morgan MY, Milsom JP, Sherlock S. Plasma ratio of valine, leucine, and isoleucine to phenylalanine and tyrosine in liver disease. Gut 1978; 19:1068-1073.

12. Cerra FB, Cheuhg NK, Fischer JE, et al. Disease-specific amino acid infusion (FO80) in hepatic encephalopathy: a prospective, randomized, double-blind controlled trial. JPEN 1985; 9:288-295.

13. Eriksson LS, Conn HO. Branched chain amino acids in the management of hepatic encephalopathy: an analysis of variants. Hepatology (in press).

14. Uribe M, Marquez MA, Garcia Ramos G, et al. Treatment of chronic portal systemic encephalopathy with vegetable and animal protein diets. A controlled crossover study. Dig Dis Sci 1982; 27:119-126.

15. Horst D, Grace ND, Conn HO, et al. Comparison of dietary protein with an oral branched chain-enriched amino acid supplement with chronic portal-systemic encephalopathy: a double-blind controlled trial. Hepatology 1984; 4:279-287.

16. Uribe M. Dietary management of portal-systemic encephalopathy. In: Conn HO, Bircher J, eds. Hepatic Encephalopathy: Management with Lactulose and Related Carbohydrates. East Lansing, Michigan: Medi-Ed Press, 1988 (in

press).

17. Weber FL Jr, Fresard KM, Lally BR. Effects of lactulose and neomycin on urea metabolism in cirrhotic subjects. Gastroenterology 1982; 82:213-217.

18. Uribe M, Marquez MA, Garcia Ramos G, et al. Treatment of chronic portal-systemic encephalopathy with lactose in lactase-deficient patients. Dig Dis Sci 1980 25:924-929.

19. James IM, Nashat D, Sampson D, et al. Effect of induced metabolic alkalosis in hepatic encephalopathy. Lancet 1969; 2:1106-1108.

20. Stabenau JR, et al. The role of pH gradient in the distribution of ammonia between blood and cerebrospinal fluid, brain and muscle. J Clin Invest 1959; 38:373-378.

21. Uribe M, Farca A, Marquez MA, et al. Treatment of chronic portal-systemic encephalopathy with bromocriptine. A double-blind controlled trial. Gastroenterology 1979; 76:1347-1351.

22. Morgan MY, Jakobovits AW, James IM, et al. Successful use of bromocriptine in the treatment of chronic hepatic encephalopathy. Gastroenterology 1980; 78:663-670.

23. Chandler JG, Fechner RE. Hepatopedal flow restoration in patients intolerant of total portal diversion. Ann Surg 1983; 197:574-583.

24. Sarfeh JL, Rypins EB, Fardi M, et al. Clinical implications of portal hemodynamics after small-diameter portacaval H graft. Surgery 1984; 96:223-229.

25. Piccone SB Jr, Donovan AJ, Yellin AE. Abdominal colectomy for chronic encephalopathy due to portal-systemic shunt. Arch Surg 1983; 118:33-37.

26. Walker JG, Emlyn-Williams A, Craigie A, et al. Treatment of chronic portal-systemic encephalopathy by surgical exclusion of the colon. Lancet 1965; 2:861-866.

27. Wapnick S, et al. Randomized prospective matched pair study comparing peritoneovenous shunt and conventional therapy in massive ascites. Br J Surg 1979; 66:667.

28. Egense J, Schwartz M. Recurrent hepatic coma following uretero-sigmoidostomy. Scand J Gastroenterol 1970; 5:149-152.

8

DIETARY MANAGEMENT OF PORTAL-SYSTEMIC ENCEPHALOPATHY

MISAEL URIBE, M.D.

In patients with advanced liver disease, dietary management is in many cases the key factor in avoiding the precipitation of portal-systemic encephalopathy (PSE). Acute failure of the liver leads to a complete or nearly total metabolic disaster. The liver plays a central role in the transformation, utilization and storage of most nutrients. The liver is, in fact, the central organ in any metabolic scheme. When hepatic failure occurs, myriad enzymes and metabolic processes are deranged and the impact on the body's energy economy may be total. Such great metabolic changes are expressed in the clinical, biochemical and neuropsychiatric abnormalities that characterize fulminant hepatic failure (1). PSE, which is the consequence of portal-systemic shunting rather than hepatocellular failure *per se*, is characterized by many of the metabolic abnormalities of hepatic failure.

In chronic liver disease, adequate nutritional support is an important part of the efforts to sustain hepatic function and to promote hepatic regeneration. Paradoxically, in patients with advanced liver disease and PSE, there is a sharply limited ability to tolerate most nutrients. Glucose and fat tolerance are reduced due to the many hormonal derangements that take place in liver failure (2-6). Most important, however, is the intolerance to dietary protein, which frequently precipitates or uncovers PSE. This is particularly troubling because protein plays the leading role in hepatic regeneration.

RESPONSE TO DIET IN PSE

The overall response to diet in patients with PSE depends on many factors. Studies on diet in PSE are restricted to particular groups of nutrients such as amino acids, which do not reproduce the physiological responses of a specific diet. Interpretation of and extrapolation from these studies are also limited because the *in vivo* response is a complex, multifactorial phenomenon. Such studies are further complicated by our inability to follow the different metabolic pathways of the hundreds of different nutrients ingested.

The responses to diet obey a number of rules that are related to the diet itself and to patients' conditions. Some such factors are shown graphically in Figure 1.

RESPONSE RELATED TO DIET ITSELF

The amount, type and composition of the foods ingested are obviously important factors. Striking variations in the patterns of adherence to a prescribed diet occur, and both intra- and inter-individual variations are common. Nausea, vomiting and anorexia, which are common symptoms of cirrhosis (7), also affect patients' compliance. The fact that in advanced liver disease restriction of protein and sodium is often required may worsen the malnutrition and may further reduce compliance.

The intrinsic content of specific toxins such as ammonia in different foods has been stressed by Rudman (8), although it is not clear whether diet or the intestinal generation of ammonia is more important. The content of fiber and dairy products in a given menu may improve the tolerance to proteins. Both fiber and disaccharides are substrates for colonic bacterial fermentation, the production of fatty acids and acidification. In 1908 Metchnikoff proposed the ingestion of

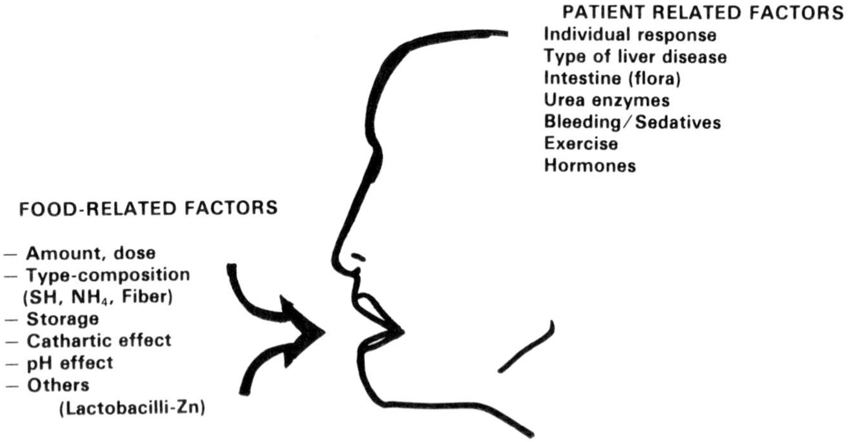

FIGURE 1. Factors effecting response to diet in patients with cirrhosis and portal-systemic encephalopathy

yoghurt to improve human health by means of colonic acidification (9). More recently Macbeth et al. (10) proposed the administration of *Lactobacillus acidophilus* in patients with PSE to modify the colonic ecosystem, to enhance colonic fermentation and acidification.

On the other hand, in lactase deficiency, which affects over two-thirds of the world's population, the administration of lactose (milk sugar) is able to acidify the stools and exert a beneficial effect on PSE (11, 12). This approach to therapy is discussed in Chapter 20.

Finally, other substances in food such as minerals or food preservatives may exert beneficial effects on PSE, e. g., zinc (13) or sodium benzoate (14).

FACTORS RELATED TO PATIENTS

Each patient has a unique response to diet. First, the degree of hepatic decompensation, of portal-systemic shunting and the nutritional status are important. There are a number of other factors that modify the tolerance to diet to variable degrees. Among these are: gastrointestinal motility, the enzymatic and physical integrity of the intestine, the intestinal flora, presence of gastrointestinal bleeding, pancreatic function, the hormonal responses to diet, and even the physical activity of the patient. It has been shown that exercise stimulates ammonia production (15). The variety, complexity and multiplicity of these factors explains the difficulties in understanding and studying the many metabolic changes that are present in PSE.

DIETARY COMPLIANCE

Finally, even though the correct diet is prescribed, great variations in individual compliance are common. Some of the many factors that may alter dietary compliance are shown in Table 1.

TABLE 1. Some Factors Related with Food Compliance

Related to food	Related to patients	Related to environment
Appearance of meals	Sense of taste	Cost
Restrictions (salt, protein, etc.)	Sense of smell	Availability
Side effects (distension, bloating, etc.)	Anorexia	Cooking difficulties
	Nausea	Interactions with drugs
	Vomiting	Cultural
	Ascites	
	Alcoholism	

DIETARY INDICATIONS IN ADVANCED LIVER DISEASE

Vitamins. Malnourished cirrhotic patients have a high incidence of deficiencies of B-complex vitamins. These abnormalities are more frequently seen in alcoholic cirrhosis. Specifically, low blood levels of Vitamin B_{12}, folates, pyridoxine and thiamine are commonly found in cirrhotic patients (16, 17).

Decreased intake of food containing B-complex vitamins in alcoholic patients is common, but chronic alcohol intake also exerts specific detrimental effects on vitamins. Alcohol impairs intestinal absorption of folates and thiamine, interferes with the enterohepatic circulation in the case of folates, promotes the release of vitamins from the liver (B_6 and thiamine), accelerates degradation and systemic clearance of B_6 and increases urinary elimination of B_6. The hepatic storage of vitamins may be reduced in the presence of alcoholic liver disease (18).

Circulating blood levels of water soluble vitamins are below normal in up to half of all patients with cirrhosis. These deficiencies have a wide clinical spectrum, which ranges from asymptomatic cases to pellagra and severe polyneuritis. Although no connection with PSE has yet been established, it seems reasonable to assume that patients with these deficiencies need supplemental B-complex vitamins.

Deficiencies of fat-soluble vitamins, i.e., A, D, E and K, are less frequently found in liver disease. However, in patients with chronic cholestasis, the levels of these vitamins may be reduced. The reason for this abnormality is that the absorption of fat-soluble vitamins is impaired in the absence of bile in the intestine. The main problems of fat-soluble vitamin deficiencies are hemorrhagic disease and bone disease due to decreased Vitamin K and Vitamin D levels, respectively. Specific recommendations for fat-soluble vitamin supplementation are shown in Table 2.

TABLE 2. Fat-soluble Vitamin Deficiencies and Dietary Supplementation in Chronic Cholestasis

Vitamin deficiency	
	Vitamin A - Xerophthalmia (interacts with zinc deficiency)
	Vitamin D - Metabolic bone disease
	Vitamin E - Neuromuscular degeneration
	Vitamin K - Coagulopathy
Supplementation	
	Vitamin A - 10,000-25,000 IU per day water soluble Vitamin A.
	Vitamin D - 5,000-8,000 IU per day of D_2 or 3-5 mg of 25-OH-Vitamin D
	Vitamin E - 50-400 IU per day of oral alpha-tocopherol
	Vitamin K - 2.5-5.0 mg per day of water-soluble derivative of menadione.

TABLE 3. Effect of Zinc Administration on PSE (after Reding et al. [13])

	Zinc (n=8)		Placebo group (n=12)	
	Before	After	Before	After
NCT (in seconds)	55±18	42±16*	56±25	56±25
Blood zinc (mg per dl)	64±21	109±21**	60±18	59±19

* p<0.05, ** p<0.01

Minerals. *Zinc.* Although it has been known for many years that some patients with advanced liver disease have low blood levels of zinc, and that the sense of taste may be impaired as a consequence of this abnormality, only recently has an association between zinc and PSE been proposed. In a very exciting preliminary clinical trial, Reding and coworkers (13) showed that the supplementation of diet with zinc may improve some of the features of PSE. Their proposal was based on the results of a trial performed in 20 patients with mild, chronic PSE. Eight patients received 600 mg qid of zinc acetate for one week and 12 patients received a placebo. The zinc-treated group improved significantly in the time required to perform a trailmaking test (Number Connection Test, NCT) as their blood zinc levels increased (Table 3). Unfortunately, no improvements in other objective parameters of PSE were observed.

There are many reasons, some proven and some only postulated, that suggest that zinc may play a role in PSE. These are summarized in Table 4. However, until more studies are performed to confirm these findings, the use of zinc to treat chronic PSE remains speculative.

Protein. Of the three nutrients, protein, fat and carbohydrate, which provide energy and calories, protein is the most important. It is unfortunate that patients with PSE have limited tolerance to protein, especially to meat. Patients with PSE and protein-calorie malnutrition are in negative nitrogen balance. Deprivation of protein leads to further depletion of liver protein stores, breakdown of cellular

TABLE 4. Effect of Zinc in PSE

- Two of the enzymes are zinc-dependent in the urea cycle.
- In PSE urea cycle enzymes are depressed.
- Impaired absorption and low zinc levels are common in chronic alcoholism.
- Protein restriction inadvertently restricts zinc.
- Vegetable diet may impair zinc absorption.
- Disaccharides (lactose) enhance zinc absorption (the lactose-zinc connection).
- Preliminary trials suggest that zinc may be beneficial for the control of PSE.

(muscle) protein and RNA, and conversion of polysomes to free ribosomes. These events occur mainly in the rough endoplasmic reticulum where albumin is synthesized (17). Up to two-thirds of patients with cirrhosis have protein-calorie malnutrition (19). There are no data on the prevalence of protein-calorie malnutrition in patients with PSE. At our institution, a recent survey (20) demonstrated that 50% of patients with PSE had protein-calorie malnutrition.

By definition cirrhosis is a catabolic disease. Its clinical features include muscle wasting and several biochemical abnormalities such as hypoproteinemia and an abnormal plasma amino acid pattern (21). Several studies have demonstrated that positive nitrogen balance can be achieved in cirrhotic patients at dietary protein intakes of 0.8-1.0 g per kg per day. However, patients with PSE and protein-calorie malnutrition are faced with a nutritional dilemma (Figure 2): they need dietary protein to achieve a positive nitrogen balance, but protein intake often precipitates or accentuates PSE.

The connection between protein intake and the precipitation of PSE was first recognized in dogs in 1893. After constructing an Eck's fistula, Hahn administered a meat load and observed that the animals presented incoordination and changes in behavior. Since then the syndrome has been called "meat intoxication" (22). Discontinuation of meat was followed by the recovery of normal behavior (23). These observations have recently been confirmed (24). The neurologic syndrome associated with gastrointestinal bleeding, described by Gaustad (25) and by Gabuzda et al. (26), was the same syndrome seen in PSE precipitated by the administration of ammonia-containing cation exchange resins. With the advent of

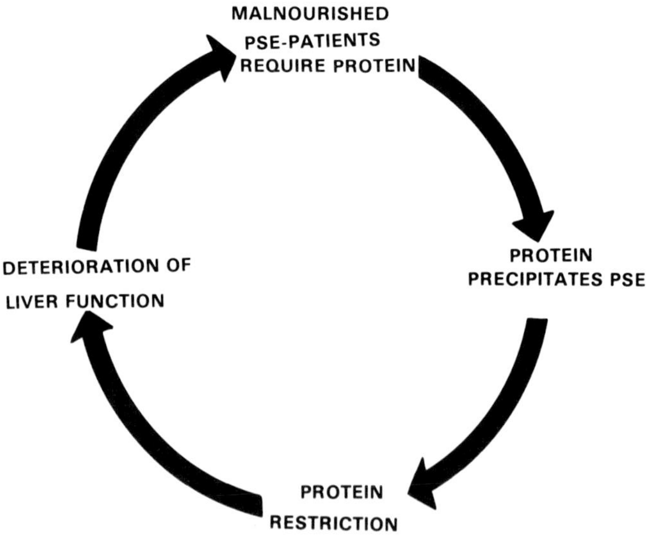

FIGURE 2. The circle of protein restriction leads to progressive deterioration in liver function.

surgical portacaval shunts, the meat intoxication syndrome was observed by McDermott and Adams (27) and Havens and Child (28) in cirrhotic patients who underwent this procedure.

In accord with the previous experiments, recommendations were made to restrict meat intake and to cleanse the intestine to prevent PSE. To date, little change in this basic approach has been made. Ways to improve protein tolerance have only recently been explored either by the oral or intravenous administration of branched-chain amino acids or by supplementation with dietary fiber.

TOLERANCE TO DIFFERENT KINDS OF PROTEIN IN ADVANCED LIVER DISEASE

Blood. Almost 30 years ago, Bessman and Mirick (29) demonstrated that after equivalent doses (74 g) of blood or dairy protein, blood ammonia levels were twice as high after administration of blood. Although no controlled trials were performed, and it is very unlikely that none will ever be performed, most investigators agree that blood protein, gram for gram, is more toxic than meat protein. Based on this belief, gut cleansing is practiced in the presence of gastrointestinal bleeding. This procedure is thought to reduce the generation and absorption of ammonia and other toxins. Most investigators also agree that in case of gastrointestinal bleeding oral diet should be suspended until the bleeding is controlled.

Eggs and Milk. Fenton et al. (30) investigated the effect of 80 g of different proteins in three cirrhotic patients. In this uncontrolled trial, the authors concluded that meat and eggs elevated blood ammonia levels similarly, while milk and cheese-derived proteins increase blood ammonia levels by one-third less than meat or eggs and improve mental state in patients with PSE. Although experience with eggs and milk and cheese protein is limited, most clinicians agree that dairy protein is better tolerated than meat protein by patients with PSE. Dairy proteins stimulate the growth of lactobacilli in the bowel and may influence colonic pH. The beneficial effect of dairy products in PSE is probably more important in patients with PSE and lactase deficiency. (See Chapter 20, "Management of Portal-systemic Encephalopathy with Lactose.")

Meat. Although the role of meat protein in precipitating PSE is undoubted, and restriction of dietary protein reduces the source of nitrogenous toxins, the efficacy of reducing protein intake has never been subjected to a controlled trial. Furthermore, tolerance to meat varies widely between individuals.

Several factors have been implicated with the encephalopathogenicity of meat. Among these are a high content of ammonia and a high capacity of the colonic flora to generate ammonia from meat protein, a high content of aromatic amino acids and sulphur-containing amino acids, a low content of branched-chain amino acids, and a low content of fiber (31).

The mental state of cirrhotic patients can often be titrated by the amount of meat administered. It is important to stress the fact that even when protein intake is restricted to zero, some protein degradation persists. Therefore, as soon as a comatose patient improves, some protein should be administered. A trial with 20 to 30 g of protein per day is advisable in a patient recovering from an acute episode of PSE (32). Continuous carbohydrate administration during protein restriction will minimize endogenous protein breakdown.

Vegetable protein. In addition to the quantity of protein, the nature of the protein seems to be important. In patients with PSE, vegetable protein seems to be better tolerated than meat protein. The beneficial effect of vegetable protein over animal protein in the management of chronic PSE was first suggested by Greenberger et al. (33). They noted that vegetable protein diets resulted in overall clinical improvement, decreased hepatic encephalopathy, decreased arterial ammonia levels, improved intellectual performance and, in one case, markedly improved protein tolerance.

These findings prompted us to compare the effects of two vegetable protein diets containing 40 and 80 g of vegetable protein with a 40 g meat protein diet in patients with chronic PSE (34). Both vegetable protein diets were equal or more effective than the meat protein diet in controlling PSE. Furthermore, vegetable protein diets improved the Number Connection Test times and the electroencephalograms (34) (Figures 3, 4).

During the ingestion of the 80 g vegetable protein diet, the frequency of bowel movements significantly increased from 1.8±1.0 to 3.5±0.5 ($p<0.05$). Of

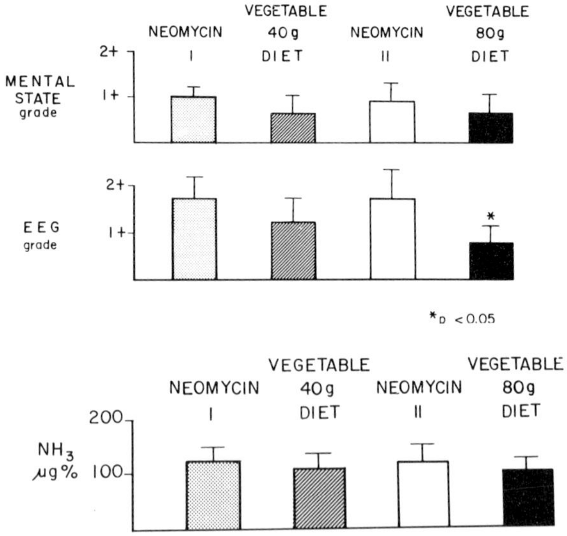

FIGURE 3. Mental state, EEGs and blood ammonia levels after vegetable and meat protein diets in 10 patients with chronic PSE (reproduced with permission, from Reference 34).

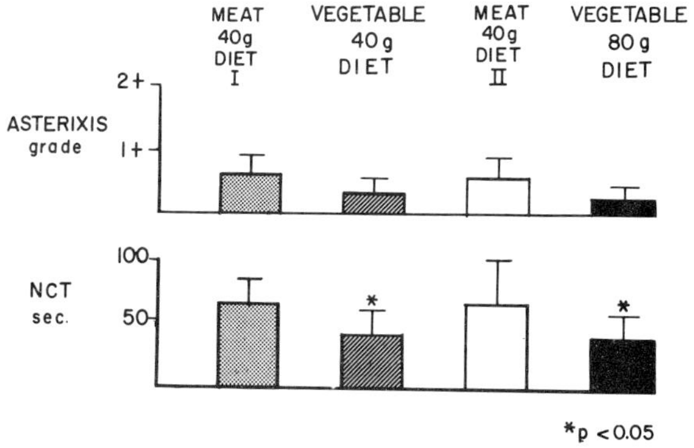

FIGURE 4. Asterixis and Number Connection Tests (NCTs) after vegetable and meat protein diets in ten patients with chronic PSE. Both vegetable protein diets significantly improved the psychometric tests ($P<0.05$).

great interest was the finding of hypoglycemia in two cirrhotic, diabetic patients during treatment with the vegetable protein diets. In these cases, the diet had to be suspended despite improvement in the PSE. This apparent side effect of vegetable protein is related to its content of dietary fiber. Many studies suggest that fiber plays a beneficial role in several metabolic diseases including diabetes mellitus (35, 36). There are also some theoretical reasons why supplementation of diet with fiber may be of benefit in PSE. Some of these are depicted in Figure 5. A summary of recent trials with vegetable protein is shown in Table 5 (37-40).

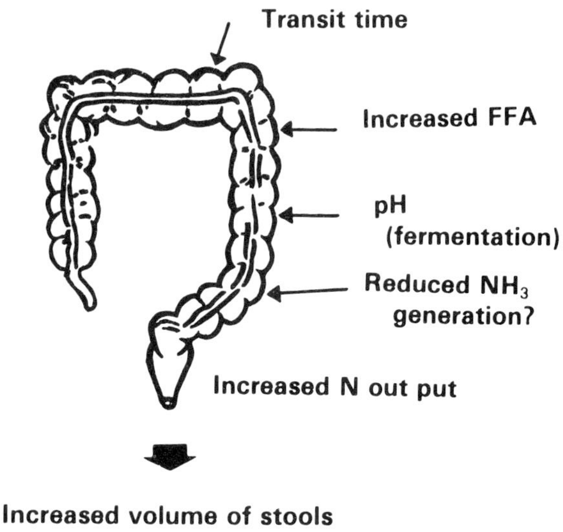

FIGURE 5. Effect of fiber supplementation on colonic function. Fiber induces effects which resemble those obtained with nonabsorbable disaccharides, i.e., it decreases transit time, pH and ammonia generation and it increases free fatty acids (FFA) and ammonia output in the stools.

TABLE 5. Controlled Trials with Vegetable Protein (VP) Diet in Patients with Chronic PSE

Authors	No. of patients	Nature of protein	Dosage of protein (g per day)	PSE parameters improved by VP	Protein tolerance	Plasma amino acid pattern	Overall results
Greenberger et al., 1977 (33)	3	VP vs animal	24-90	NCT, NH_3, PSE Index	Improved	-----	VP beneficial
Uribe et al., 1980 (34)	10	VP vs animal	40-80	Both diets equivalent	Improved	-----	VP beneficial
Bruijn et al., 1981 (37)	8	VP vs animal	40-100	EEG	Improved	unchanged	VP beneficial
Kershavarzian et al., 1984 (38)	6	VP vs animal	——	EEG, mental state	Improved	unchanged	VP better tolerated
Jeppson et al., 1984 (39)	8	VP vs animal	58	Psychometric tests	Improved	unchanged	VP potentially beneficial
Uribe et al., 1985 (41)	8	VP vs animal	0.8 g per kg	No patient deteriorated	Improved	------	VP-beneficial for PSE and diabetes
García-Compean et al., 1987 (42)	20	VP vs animal	0.8 g per kg	NCT, NH_3, PSE Index, N_2 balance	Improved	unchanged	VP-fiber beneficial
Hermann et al., 1987 (40)	6	VP (pectin) vs animal	30	NCT, NH_3 increase fecal N_2	Improved	-----	Dietary fiber (pectin) beneficial

NCT = Number Connection Test

DIETARY FIBER, PSE AND DIABETES

At our institution, which acts as a national referral center for metabolic and nutritional diseases, the association of diabetes and cirrhosis is very high, up to 18%. The frequent concurrence of PSE and diabetes prompted us to evaluate in a controlled trial the effect of vegetable protein diets, which are rich in fiber, in a group of patients with both diseases (41). The study was conducted in a controlled, crossover fashion in eight cirrhotic-diabetic patients with chronic PSE and uncontrolled diabetes. After a basal period of stabilization, the patients received either meat protein (0.8 g per kg per day) plus neomycin and milk of magnesia or the same amount of vegetable protein supplemented with psyllium fiber to reach a daily intake of 35 g fiber per day. The characteristics of both diets are shown in Table 6.

The results of the study demonstrated that both diets were equally effective in controlling PSE (Table 7). No patient deteriorated during the vegetable protein diet, even though neomycin and cathartics were discontinued. The beneficial effect of fiber supplementation in PSE is apparent.

As regards metabolic control of diabetes, fasting glucose levels were 204 ±86 mg per dl after the meat protein diet and 127±8 mg per dl after the vegetable protein diet ($p<0.02$), even though patients received similar amounts of hypoglycemic agents. The individual results are shown graphically in Figure 6.

TABLE 6. Daily Amino Acid Content of Diets Administered (Uribe et al. [41])

	Meat protein diet	Vegetable protein diet
Calories	1600	1558
Protein ((g per day)	43	45
Carbohydrate (g per day)	230	235
Fat (g per day)	56	49
Methionine (g per day)	0.95	0.52
Tryptophan (g per day)	0.51	0.33
Phenylalanine (g per day)	2.0	2.0
Tyrosine (g per day)	1.6	1.1
Valine (g per day)	2.5	2.3
Leucine (g per day)	3.4	3.8
Isoleucine (g per day)	2.2	2.2
BCAA/AAA molar ratio	3.60	3.60
Fiber (g per day)	8.32	15.7
Hemicellulose (Metamucil®) (g per day)	0.0	20.0
Total fiber per day (g)	8.32	35.7

TABLE 7. Effect of Meat Protein and Vegetable Protein+Psyllium Diet in a Group of Cirrhotic-Diabetic Patients (after Uribe [41])

	Basal	MPST*	VPDF**
Mental state (grade)	0.2±0.4	0.2±0.4	0.2±0.4
Asterixis (grade)	0.12±0.5	0.2±0.2	0.0
EEGs (grade)	0.25±0.2	0.4±0.4	0.4±0.4
NH_3 (µg per dl)	151±12	129±35	151±33
NCT (seconds)	67±7	56±15	66±23

* MPST = meat protein + standard therapy (neomycin);
** VPDF = vegetable protein + dietary fiber (psyllium);
NCT = Number Connection Test times.
Note: Results are mean±SD in eight patients.

DOES FIBER DETERMINE TOLERANCE TO NITROGEN IN PSE?

The assumption that fiber may exert a beneficial effect in the treatment of PSE has recently been tested (42). The study was performed in 20 patients with cirrhosis and chronic PSE. After a stabilization period of one week, the two isocaloric (35 kcal per kg per day), isonitrogenous (0.8 g per kg per day) diets were

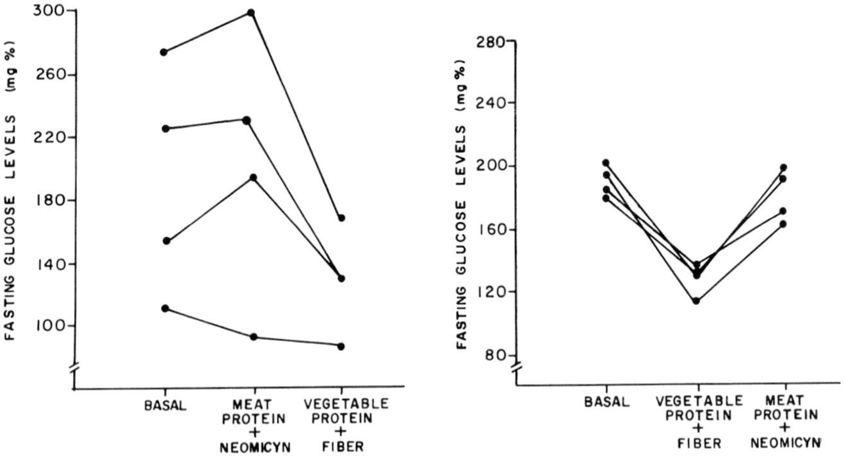

FIGURE 6. Fasting glucose levels in a group of cirrhotic, diabetic patients with PSE who were receiving meat or vegetable protein diets. Fasting glucose levels always decreased after the vegetable-fiber diet (reproduced with permission from Reference 41).

administered for two weeks. The diets were similar in amino acid composition, but were different in fiber content. Ten patients were randomized to receive meat and vegetable protein containing a mean of 28 g of fiber per day. Ten other patients received a similar diet that contained only 12 g of fiber per day. The results (Table 8) demonstrated that fiber was associated with better protein tolerance. In our study, nitrogen balance was similar although fecal elimination of nitrogen was significantly increased by the vegetable protein diet. Both the number and weight of the stools increased with the administration of vegetable protein enriched with fiber. Although in both groups the BCAA/AAA molar ratio was found to be low, improvement in mental state and PSE after fiber supplementation was not associated with changes in the plasma amino acid pattern.

FIBER AND NITROGEN METABOLISM

In a well-designed trial, Weber et al. (43) compared the effects of a vegetable protein diet with a meat protein diet. They studied nitrogen metabolism in a group of six nonencephalopathic cirrhotic patients. The vegetable protein diet contained 4.5 times more fiber than the meat protein diet. The vegetable protein diets produced a fall in urea production rates associated with a fall in the urinary urea output. They also produced an increase in fecal nitrogen output. These investigators confirmed the findings that these changes were not associated with any significant modification in the plasma amino acid pattern. Weber et al. concluded that the effect of vegetable protein diets on nitrogen metabolism can be attributed to the increase in dietary fiber intake.

TABLE 8. Components of PSE after Two Isocaloric, Isonitrogenous Diets, with High and Low Fiber Content (after García-Compean et al. [42])

	High fiber diet n=10	Low fiber diet n=10	p value
EEG improved or unchanged	90%	40%	<0.05
Change in NCT (seconds)	-13±16	2±2.2	<0.05
Change in NH_3 (μg per dl)	-31±8	7±5	<0.05
Change in PSE Index	-8.5±7.8	4.2±1.7	<0.05
Stool weight (g per day)	210±25	149±42	<0.05
Stool N_2 (mg per kg per day)	27±3	5±9	<0.05
Developed acute PSE	0%	20%	NS*

* NS = not significant statistically.

EFFECT OF FIBER IN THE COLON: FERMENTATION AND ACIDIFICATION

It has recently been suggested that fiber administration, like disaccharides, is able to provide substrate for colonic fermentation and that breath hydrogen expiration and plasma acetate levels are equally elevated in volunteers after both lactulose and pectin administration (44). However, the peak time of both hydrogen expiration and plasma acetate levels occurred during the first three hours with disaccharides and after 8 to 10 hours with pectin. Significant increments in hydrogen and acetate levels lasted 6 and 24 hours after the disaccharide and the fiber, respectively. Finally, Jacobs and coworkers in a preliminary study demonstrated that colonic fermentation and colonic acidification occurred after the administration of psyllium fiber (45).

WORLDWIDE TREND TO REDUCE FIBER INTAKE

From the philosophical point of view, it seems unfortunate that over the last two centuries humans have radically changed their alimentary habits and diets (Figure 7). There are few doubts that inhabitants of many "developed" countries in which dietary fiber intake is very low, due in part to modern food processing, suffer

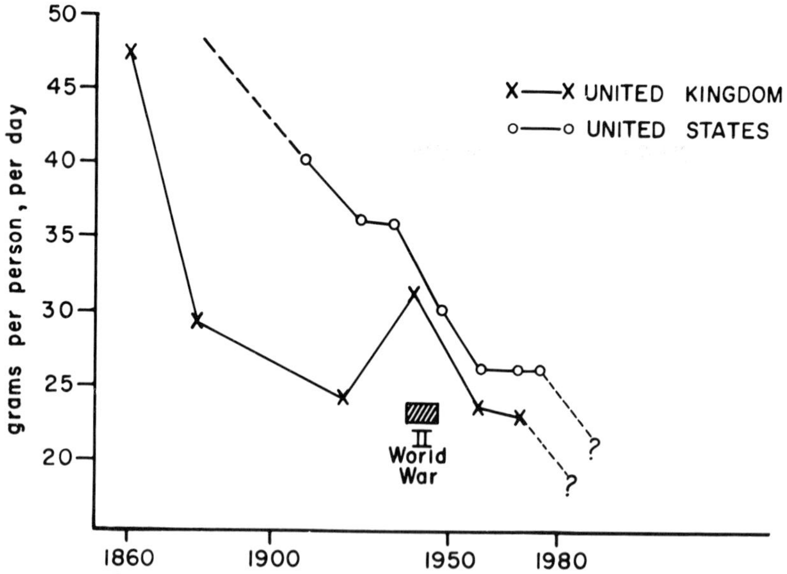

FIGURE 7. Long-term trends in dietary fiber in two developed countries. Current fiber consumed per capita is below 50% of that registered a century ago (47).

TABLE 9. Dietary Fiber Available for Consumption per Capita (1972-1974)

Country	g per day
Mexico	94
Romania	88
Portugal	71
Bulgaria	68
Greece	62
Chile	56
Israel	52
Spain	51
Italy	36
Germany	28
United States	27
France	25
United Kingdom	23
Switzerland	23
Holland	22

Modified from (48).

from a variety of disorders, including obesity, hyperlipidemia, hypertension, diverticular disease, cardiac disease, constipation, and perhaps, even neoplastic diseases like colonic cancer (46,47). Paradoxically, in poor, undeveloped countries in which high fiber diets are consumed, these diseases are less common. Table 9 depicts the amount of fiber available in the menus of developed and undeveloped countries (48).

CONCLUSION

More research must be done with fiber diets to improve the protein tolerance and nutrition in patients with advanced liver disease.

REFERENCES

1. Phillips GB Jr, Gabuzda GJ, Davidson CS. The syndrome of impending hepatic coma in patients with cirrhosis of the liver given certain nitrogenous substances. N Engl J Med 1952; 247:239-246.

2. Soeters P, Fischer JE. Insulin, glucagon, amino acid imbalance, and hepatic encephalopathy. Lancet 1976; 2:880-882.

3. Marchesini G, Bianchi G, Zoli M, et al. Plasma amino acid response to protein ingestion in patients with liver cirrhosis. Gastroenterology 1983; 85:283-290.

4. Marchesini G, Zoli M, Dondi C, et al. Ammonia-induced changes in pancreatic hormones and plasma amino acids in patients with liver disease. Dig Dis Sci 1982; 27:406-412.

5. Marchesini G, Forlani G, Zoli M, et al. Insulin and glucagon levels in liver cirrhosis. Relationship with plasma amino acid imbalance of chronic hepatic encephalopathy. Dig Dis Sci 1979; 24:594-601.

6. Collins JR, Crafford OB. Glucose intolerance and insulin resistance in patients with liver disease. Arch Intern Med 1969; 124:142-148.

7. Galambos JT. The cirrhosis. In: Bockus HL, ed. Gastroenterology, 3rd edition, Vol III. Philadelphia: WHB Saunders, 1976.

8. Rudman D, Smith III RB, Salam AA, et al. Ammonia content of food. Am J Clin Nutr 1973; 26:487-490.

9. Metchnikoff E, Prolongation of life (Essay). New York 1908.

10. Macbeth WAAG, Kass E, MacDermott WV. Treatment of hepatic encephalopathy by alteration of intestinal flora with *Lactobacillus acidophilus*. Lancet 1965; 1:399-402.

11. Uribe M, Marquez MA, Garcia Ramos G, et al. Treatment of chronic portal systemic encephalopathy with lactose in lactase-deficient patients. Dig Dis Sci 1980; 25:924-929.

12. Uribe M. Tratamiento de la encefalopatia hepatica con lactosa. In: Uribe M, Guevara L, eds. Encefalopatia y Coma Hepatico. Mexico: Salvat Ed. 1982.

13. Reding P, Duchateu J, Bataille C. Oral zinc supplementation improves hepatic encephalopathy. Results of a randomized controlled trial. Lancet 1984; 2:493-495.

14. Mendenhall CL, Rouster S, Marshall L, et al. A new therapy for portal systemic encephalopathy. Am J Gastroenterol 1986; 81:540-543.

15. Allen SI, Conn HO: Observations on the effect of exercise on blood ammonia concentration in man. Yale J Biol Med 1960; 33:133-144.

16. Leevy CM, Baker H. Vitamins and alcoholism. Am J Clin Nutr 1968; 21:1328-1368.

17. Achord JL. Malnutrition and the role of nutritional support in alcoholic

liver disease. Am J Gastroenterol 1987; 82:1-7.

18. Hoyumpa A. Alcohol and vitamin metabolism. Syllabus of the postgraduate course "Alcoholism and alcohol induced liver disease": AASLD Chicago. Nov. 5-6, 1981.

19. Merli M, Riggio O, Ipichino S, et al. Amino acid imbalance and malnutrition in liver cirrhosis. Hum Nutr Clin Nutr 1985; 4:249-253.

20. Yanez MA, Palacios N, Uribe M, et al. Estado nutricional de la muestra de poblacion de pacientes con cirrosis hepatica de la Clinica de Higado del instituto nacional de la nutricion (Abstract). Rev Gastroenterol Mex 1986; 51:307.

21. Okuno M, Nagayama M, Takai T, et al. Postoperative total parenteral nutrition in patients with liver disorders. J Surg Res 1985; 39:93-102.

22. Hahn M, Massen O, Nencki M, et al. Die Eck'sche fistelzwischen der unteren hohlvene und der pfortader und ihre foigen fur den organismus. Arch Exper Pathol Pharmackol 1893; 32:161-210.

23. Balo J. Korpassy B. The encephalitis of dogs with Eck fistula fed on meat. Arch Pathol 1932; 13:80-87.

24. Thompson JS, Schafer DF, Haun J, et al. Adequate diet prevents hepatic coma in dogs with Eck's fistula. Surg Gynecol Obstet 1986; 162:126-130.

25. Gaustad V. Transient hepatargy. Acta Med Scand 1949; 135:161-165.

26. Gabuzda GJ, Phillips GB, Davidson CS. Reversible toxic manifestations in patients with cirrhosis of the liver given cation exchange resins. N Engl J Med 1952; 246:124-130.

27. McDermott WV, Adams RD. Episodic stupor associated with the Eck fistula in the human with particular reference to the metabolism of ammonia. J Clin Invest 1954; 33:1-9.

28. Havens LL, Child III CG. Recurrent psychosis associated with liver disease and elevated blood ammonia. N Engl J Med 1955; 252:756-759.

29. Bessman AN, Mirick GS. Blood ammonia levels following the ingestion of casein and whole blood. J Clin Invest 1958; 37:990-999.

30. Fenton JCB, Knight EJ, Humpherson PL. Milk and cheese diet in portal systemic encephalopathy. Lancet 1966; 1:164-166.

31. Uribe M, Guevara L. Encefalopatia hepatica. In: Berenguer, J, ed. Gastroenterologia y Hepatologia, Chapter 51. Barcelona, Espana: Ediciones Doyma, 1986: 715-723.

32. Summerskill WHJ, Wolfe SJ, Davidson CS. The management of hepatic coma in relation to protein withdrawal and certain specific measures. Am J Med 1957; 23:59-76.

33. Greenberger NJ, Carley J, Schenker S, et al. Effect of vegetable and animal protein diets in chronic hepatic encephalopathy. Am J Dig Dis 1977; 22:845-855.

34. Uribe M, Marquez MA, Garcia Ramos G, et al. Treatment of chronic portal systemic encephalopathy with vegetable and animal protein diets. A controlled crossover study. Dig Dis Sci 1982; 27:119-126.

35. Miranda P, Horwitz DL. High fiber diets in the treatment of diabetes

mellitus. Ann Intern Med 1978; 88:482-486.

36. Simpson HCR, Simpson RW, Lousley J, et al. A high carbohydrate, high fiber diet improved all aspects of diabetes control. Lancet 1981; 1:1-5.

37. Bruijn KM, Blendis LM, Zilm DH, et al. Effect of dietary protein manipulations in subclinical portal systemic encephalopathy. Gut 1983; 24:53-60.

38. Keshavarzian A, Meek J, Sutton VM, et al. Dietary supplementation from vegetable sources in the management of chronic portal systemic encephalopathy. Am J Gastroenterol 1984; 79:945-949.

39. Jeppsson B, Kjallman A, Aslund U, et al. Effect of vegan and meat protein diets in mild chronic portal systemic encephalopathy. In: Capocaccia L, Fischer JE, and Rossi-Fanelli F, eds. Hepatic Encephalopathy in Chronic Liver Failure. New York: Plenum Press, 1984: 359-368.

40. Herrman R, Shakoor T, Weber FL. Beneficial effect of pectin in chronic hepatic encephalopathy (Abstract). Gastroenterology 1987; 92:1795.

41. Uribe M, Dibildox M, Malpica S, et al. Beneficial effect of vegetable protein diet supplemented with psyllium plantago in patients with hepatic encephalopathy and diabetes mellitus. Gastroenterology 1985; 88:901-907.

42. Garcia-Compean D, Uribe M. Fiber rather than protein determines tolerance to nitrogen load in chronic portal systemic encephalopathy: a randomized trial (Abstract). Hepatology 1987; 7:1034.

43. Weber FL, Minco D, Fresard K, et al. Effects of vegetable diets on nitrogen metabolism in cirrhotic subjects. Gastroenterology 1985; 89:538-544.

44. Pomare EW, Branch WJ, Cummings JH. Carbohydrate fermentation in the human colon and its relation to acetate concentrations in venous blood. J Clin Invest 1985; 75:1448-1454.

45. Jacobs LR, Domek M, Lonnerdal B, et al. Influence of psyllium fiber supplements on rat colonic mucosal cytokinetics and mineral metabolism (Abstract). Gastroenterology 1987; 92:1450.

46. Roth HP, Meltman MA, eds. Symposium on role of dietary fiber in health (Abstract). Am J Clin Nutr 1978; 31.

47. Bonfield CT. Socioeconomic aspects of a fiber deficient public diet. In: Vahouney GV, Kritchevsky D, eds. Dietary Fiber. Basic and Clinical Aspects. New York: Plenum Press, 1986: 55-68.

48. Brigth See E, McKeown GE. Estimation of per capita crude and dietary fiber supply in 38 countries. Am J Clin Nutr 1984; 39:821-829.

49. Bursey RG. Diet modification and the development of new food products. Ann Intern Med 1983; 98:872-874.

9

COLONIC METABOLISM OF LACTULOSE IN MAN

CH. FLORENT, M.D.

The synthesis of lactulose (ß-1-4 galactosido-fructose) was first reported in 1929. The drug, however, was not used in clinical practice until 1950, when it was given to promote the growth of *Lactobacillus bifidus*. In 1964, Ingelfinger (1) for the first time suggested that lactulose might be beneficial for patients with portal-systemic encephalopathy (PSE). He suggested that lactulose promotes the growth of Lactobacillus species (which contain little urease activity) and decreases the number of putrefactive bacteria.

Bircher et al. in 1966 (2) confirmed that lactulose was actually an effective therapeutic agent in patients with PSE. This was reconfirmed by many other studies. However, the mechanism of action of lactulose remained unclear (3). Different authors have entitled this discrepancy succinctly:

a) Lactulose works, but why? (4);
b) Lactulose: a drug in search of a modus operandi (5);
c) Wrong idea, good results (the lactulose story) (6).

It was suggested that lactulose may induce qualitative and/or quantitative alterations in fecal bacterial flora, that it may have a nonspecific cathartic action, or that it may act by trapping ammonia in the colon in acidified colonic contents. So many studies, so many conflicting results! To understand the mechanism by which lactulose benefits patients with PSE, it is important first to know the fate of this sugar in the human gastrointestinal tract.

Lactulose is a semisynthetic disaccharide (ß-1-4 galacto-fructose). Prior to the intestinal absorption of disaccharides such as lactose (ß-1-4 galacto-glucose), a disaccharidase splits the compound into its two constituent hexoses, which are then absorbed. However, lactulase is lacking in man. This explains the very limited absorption rate of orally administered lactulose in man, which may occur by passive diffusion. After an oral load of lactulose, only 1% appears in the urine of normal subjects. The rate of lactulose absorption is increased in patients with mucosal lesions. Lactulose urinary excretion after lactulose ingestion has been used as an intestinal permeability test.

After an oral load, unabsorbed lactulose exerts osmotic effects in the small bowel and, thereby, induces ileal flow rates that may exceed the critical values above which the right colon is compelled to propel its contents onward. Moreover, the colonic bacterial metabolism of lactulose increases the osmotic load. Each molecule of lactulose releases two hexoses, and each hexose gives rise to two volatile fatty acids. However, the colon absorbs large amounts of volatile fatty acids which stimulate water absorption (7).

Colonic metabolism of carbohydrates in man is quite a complex process. More than 1,000 different bacterial species are involved, and the total bacterial count ranges from 10^{11} to 10^{14} microbes per gram of colonic contents.

Complete knowledge of fecal flora is impossible to obtain at present. Moreover, chronic ingestion of unabsorbable carbohydrates may modify the floral composition and/or its metabolism. As early as 1957, it was suggested that lactulose induced fecal overgrowth of lactobacillus in infants. More extensive studies, however, have failed to find consistent qualitative or quantitative changes in the fecal bacterial flora of subjects treated with lactulose. Finally, it has been noted that the bacterial flora of the right and left sides of the colon are very different, and that fecal flora is probably different from both. *In vitro* and *in vivo* studies confirmed that methane was produced only in the left colon, an area where transit time is very slow. To understand the modification of the colonic flora induced by chronic ingestion of unabsorbable carbohydrates we must think in terms of metabolic activity rather than in terms of bacterial counts.

RATIONALE

Chronic ingestion of lactulose induces a decrease in breath hydrogen (H_2) excretion and marked acidification of the colonic contents. *In vitro* acidification of stools using HCl induces a drop in H_2 production and inhibition of carbohydrate catabolism. From these results, it was concluded that the fall of H_2 production was due to the inhibition of carbohydrate bacterial metabolism by the low colonic pH (8). If this conclusion is true, this situation would lead to an increasing excretion of carbohydrate in the feces and a progressive decrease in the efficiency of lactulose. Likewise, this conclusion is not in agreement with clinical experience in lactase-deficient, preterminal infants given a lactose-containing diet. In such infants H_2 breath excretion does not decrease with time, and even the amounts of malabsorbed lactose calculated from the H_2 production correlate well with lactose intake (9).

These discrepancies incited us to reinvestigate the effects of repeated loads of lactulose on intracolonic metabolism by direct measurement of this sugar and its metabolites in the ileal and cecal fluids and in stools of healthy volunteers (10).

We have studied eight healthy human volunteers, two women and six men, aged 23 to 46 years. All of them were non-methane-producing subjects who had previously undergone a lactose H_2 breath test that was consistent with normal lactose absorption.

All subjects remained on their accustomed diet and received an oral load of 20 g of lactulose twice daily for eight days. This interval will be referred to as the lactulose maintenance period.

a) In four subjects (group A) 24-hour stools were collected on days 1 and 2 (first period) and on days 7 and 8 (second period). Stools were immediately frozen at -20°C for further analysis. Stool weight, pH, carbohydrate (lactulose, galactose, fructose and glucose), ß-galactosidase activity, lactic and volatile fatty acids were measured in total homogenized stools.

b) The four other subjects (group B) were intubated the day before the lactulose maintenance period began (day 0) and on day 7 with a triple-lumen tube weighted by a mercury bag which could be inflated with air through lumen #1 to accelerate progression of the tube in the small intestine. When the mercury bag had reached the cecum, as shown fluoroscopically, the tube progression was stopped by deflating the bag; the subject remained in a semirecumbent position. Lumen #2, the end of which was near the bag, allowed sampling of cecal contents. Lumen #3, which ended 15 cm above lumen #2, was used to collect fluid samples from the distal ileum. On days 1 and 8, subjects ingested 20 g lactulose at 9 a.m. after an overnight fast. Samples of ileal and cecal content were obtained every 30 minutes during the first 4 hours after lactulose ingestion and every hour during the last 4 hours.

Breath hydrogen concentrations were determined in the eight subjects on days 1 and 8, before and at 30-minute intervals for 8 hours after the morning load of lactulose.

Moreover, in subjects of group B, a $^{14}CO_2$ breath test was performed for 4 hours at the same time as a hydrogen breath test by adding 2.5 C_i of 1-^{14}C lactulose.

RESULTS

Basal breath H_2 concentration was low (9.1±2.1 parts per million) (ppm) and did not change after maintenance (9.6±5.4 ppm). Excess breath H_2 declined significantly from 15.2±3 ml per eight hours on day 1 to 8.6±2.3 ml per eight hours on day 8 (60 minutes after the lactulose) ($p<0.05$) (Figure 1). The pulmonary excretion of $^{14}CO_2$ significantly increased from day 1 to day 8, 4 hours after lactulose ($p<0.01$) (Figure 2).

The 24-hour fecal weight, fecal water and carbohydrate (lactulose, galactose, fructose and glucose) outputs tended to decrease between the first and second periods (Table 1). None of the differences is statistically significant, however. Fecal water was constant between the first and second periods at pH 6. The volatile fatty acid concentrations in fecal water and the daily fecal volatile fatty acid outputs were decreased between the two collections, but the differences are not statistically significant (Table 2).

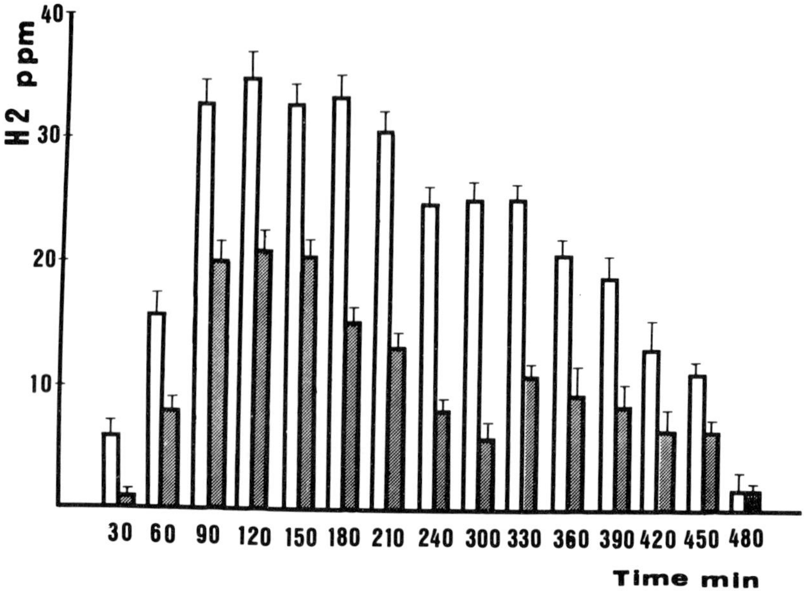

FIGURE 1. Breath H_2 responses to lactulose test doses on day 1 (white columns) and day 8 (hatched columns, after the lactulose maintenance period. n=8 (mean±SEM).

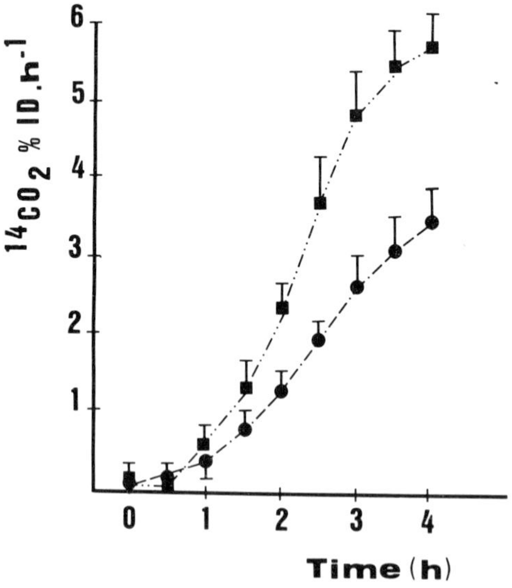

FIGURE 2. Breath $^{14}CO_2$ output after ingestion of 2.5 C_i of ^{14}C-labeled lactulose and 20 g cold lactulose on day 1 (circles) and on day 8 (squares). Bars represent the SEM (ID = ingested dose of ^{14}C-lactulose).

TABLE 1. The 24-hour Stool Weight, Fecal pH and Output of Water and Carbohydrate at the Beginning and at the End of the Lactulose Maintenance Period

	Day 1-2		Day 7-8	
	mean*	range	mean*	range
Stool weight (g per day)	251	48-414	159	89-210
Fecal water (ml per day)	217	34-373	131	74-159
Carbohydrates (mmol per day)	7.3	0.9-16.7	3.0	0.9-4.7
Stool pH	6.3	5.6-7.3	6.1	5.6-7.3

None of the variations between days 1-2 and days 7-8 is statistically significant. * n=4.

TABLE 2. Fecal Concentrations and 24-hour Outputs of Volatile Fatty Acids at the Beginning (Days 1-2) and at the End (Days 7-8) of the Lactulose Maintenance Period. None of the differences is statistically significant.

	Concentration	
	Day 1-2 μmol per gram	Day 7-8 μmol per gram
Total VFA	97.0±17.0	85.2±5.0
Acetic acid	57.0±14.0	53.5±5.5
Propionic acid	12.0±1.5	10.6±1.5
Butyric acid + isobutyric acid	14.8±4.6	13.3±1.8
Isovaleric acid	5.2±0.8	2.8±0.9
Valeric acid	8.0±1.9	5.0±1.9
	24-hour outputs	
	mmol/day	mmol/day
Total VFA	22.8±7.5	11.2±2.0
Acetic acid	14.6±5.2	7.0±1.4
Propionic acid	2.5±0.7	1.4±0.3
Butyric acid + isobutyric acid	3.2±1.3	1.8±0.4
Isovaleric acid	3.0±2.0	0.4±0.1
Valeric acid	1.5±0.6	0.6±0.2

Fecal output of ß-galactosidase increased significantly ($p<0.001$) from 169,000±33,400 to 953,000±366,000 IU per day between the first and the second periods.

Ileal content. The time of lactulose appearance at the ileal sampling site, the peak concentration and the total duration of lactulose recovery were similar on days 1 and 8 (Figure 3). The pH of ileal fluid was always greater than 7.2. Concentrations of galactose and fructose on both days were constantly less than 11 millimoles (mmol), the mean concentration of glucose less than 6 mmol. Similarly, volatile fatty acids and lactic acid concentrations were always less than 11 mmol. This confirmed the absence of ileo-colonic reflux and ileal bacterial overgrowth. The mean osmolalities were 310 and 296 milliosmoles per liter.

Cecal content. In both sampling periods lactulose was recovered from the cecal fluid 30 to 60 minutes after its ingestion. The maximal concentration and the total recovery time decreased significantly ($p<0.02$) between day 1 and day 8. The time courses of lactulose concentration in cecal fluid are shown in Figure 4. The area below the concentration curve has obviously decreased from day 1 to day 8.

Volatile fatty acids. Before lactulose ingestion, neither the total volatile fatty acids nor the distribution of individual fatty acids were different on days 1 and 8 (Table 3) (Figure 5). After lactulose ingestion the total volatile fatty acid and the concentration of acetic acid increased significantly from day 1 to day 8, whereas propionic, butyric, isobutyric, valeric and isovaleric acid concentrations tended to decrease, but the means did not change significantly.

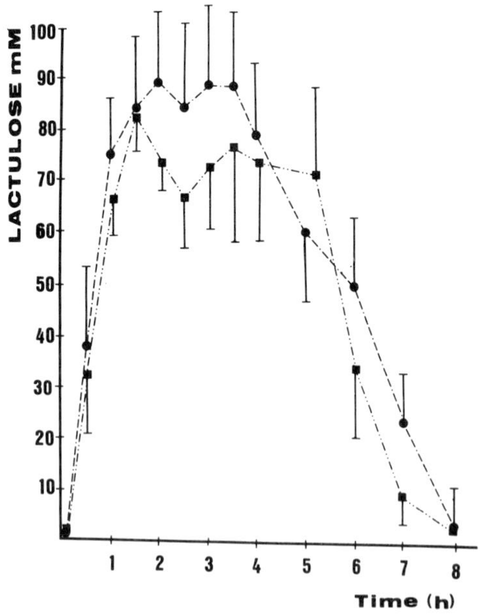

FIGURE 3. Lactulose concentration in ileal fluid after 20 g lactulose ingestion on day 1 (circles) and on day 8 (squares) (mean±SEM).

FIGURE 4. Lactulose concentration in cecal fluid after 20 g lactulose ingestion on day 1 (circles) and on day 8 (squares) after the lactulose maintenance period. n=4 (mean± SEM)

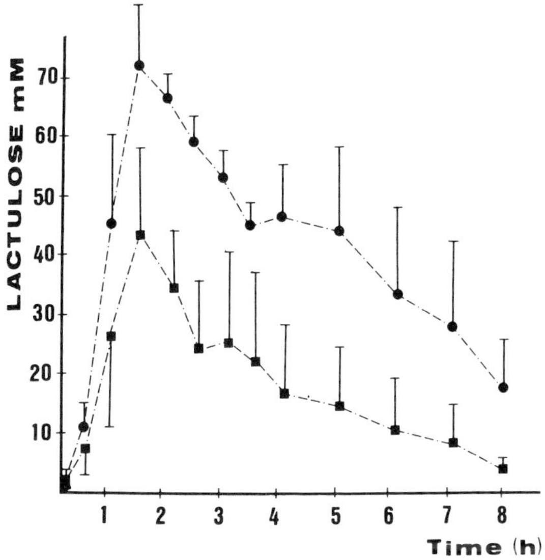

TABLE 3. Total Concentration and Relative Distribution of VFA in Cecal Fluid on Day 1 and Day 8 after the Lactulose Maintenance Period

	Before lactulose ingestion (fasting)				
	Day 1		Day 8		
	mean	range	mean	range	p
VFA mean concentration (mmol)	89.9	39-124	52.8	20-80	NS
Acetic acid (%)	56	39-66	64.1	55-80	NS
Propionic acid (%)	25.5	21-30	22.8	9-30	NS
Butyric and isobutyric acid (%)	10.6	6-15	8.9	6-11	NS
Valeric and isovaleric acid (%)	0.7	0-3	3.9	0-8	NS
	After lactulose ingestion				
VFA mean concentration (mmol)	66.5	49-92	107.8	86-123	0.001
Acetic acid (%)	59.2	53-73	73	63-87	0.001
Propionic acid (%)	26.4	20-32	16.8	9-23	NS
Butyric and isobutyric acid (%)	11.9	7-16	7.8	3-11	NS
Valeric and isovaleric acid (%)	2.5	0-8	2.4	0-4	NS

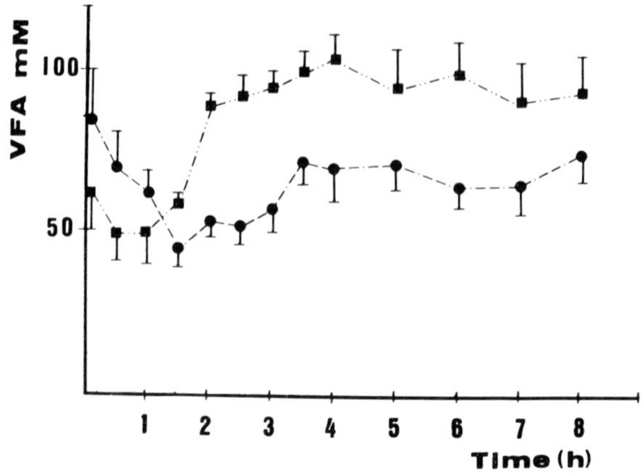

FIGURE 5. Total VFA concentrations in cecal fluid, day 1 (circles), day 8 (squares) (mean±SEM).

pH measurements. Cecal pH before lactulose ingestion was not significantly modified by the lactulose maintenance period. Nadir pH values were lower ($p<0.05$) and occurred earlier ($p<0.05$) on day 8 than on day 1.

The duration of the decrease in pH was shorter on day 8 ($p<0.05$); the pH returned to basal values in all subjects on day 8, but only two of them on day 1 (Figure 6).

Lactic acid. Lactic acid (isomers D and L) concentration curves were very different on days 1 and 8. On day 1, the lactic acid concentration was still increasing at the end of the sampling period, whereas on day 8 the peak concentration occurred at 3 to 4 hours, then decreased (Figure 7). The highest mean concentrations were 27.6 and 49.1 mmol on days 1 and 8, respectively. The area under the curve significantly increased from day 1 to day 8 ($p<0.001$). The ratio between L- and D-lactic acid did not change significantly (1.55±0.11 vs 1.84±0.17).

DISCUSSION

The intracolonic bacterial metabolism of nonabsorbed carbohydrates such as lactulose is a matter of increasing interest. Such metabolism may be a means of caloric salvage and also of adverse effects such as the induction of excess gas production or diarrhea. Relevant to these points, the consequences of a prolonged oral load of nonabsorbable carbohydrates are debated. However, our data clearly

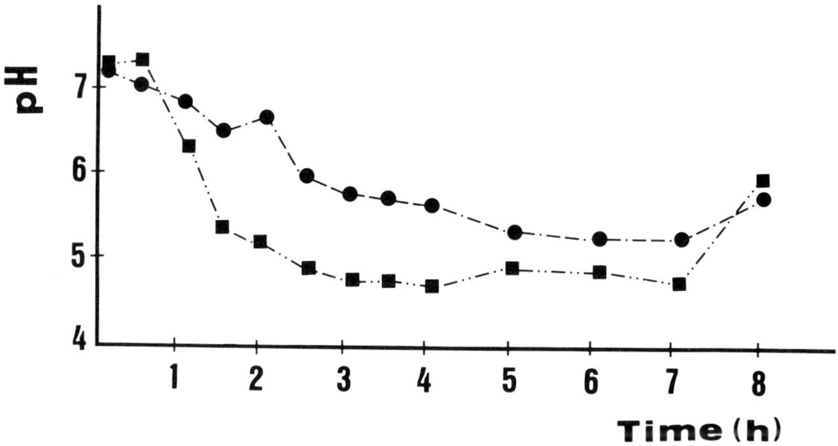

FIGURE 6. Mean cecal pH after 20 g lactulose ingestion on day 1 (circles) and day 8 (squares). n=4.

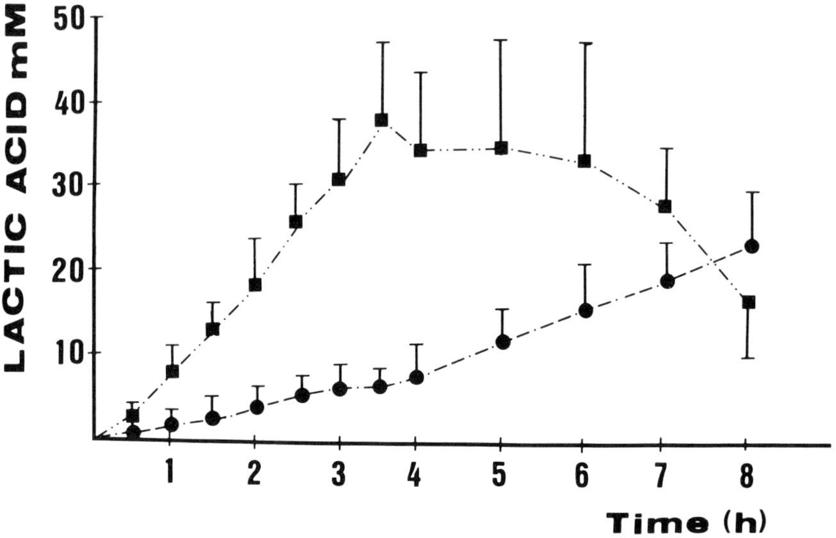

FIGURE 7. Lactic acid (D + L) concentrations in cecal fluid after 20 g lactulose ingestion on day 1 (circles) and day 8 (squares). n=4 (mean±SEM).

show that a chronic load of lactulose induces changes in colonic bacterial metabolic pathways that result in greater efficiency of the bacterial digestion of the carbohydrate. The modifications of volatile fatty acids and the faster and greater drop of cecal pH favor the growth of lactic acid-producing bacteria such as Lactobacillus, Bifidobacterium and Eubacterium species. These microorganisms are able to maintain an intracellular pH of 6.5 even in the presence of an extracellular pH of 3.5 or less. At such an acidic pH they remain good producers of ß-galactosidase. The catabolism of carbohydrates by these bacteria increases acetic and lactic acid production, which is responsible for a marked decrease in H_2 production.

To determine whether or not this adaptation inhibits lactulose-induced diarrhea, we performed a second study.

METHODS

Studies were performed in 12 healthy volunteer subjects (five women and seven men, aged 23 to 27 years). Six of them were methane-producing subjects. All had previously had a lactose breath test that was consistent with normal lactose absorption. The subjects remained on their accustomed diets and were studied during two test periods, separated by eight days, during which 20 g lactulose was taken twice daily (lactulose maintenance period). At both test periods, the subjects ingested 60 g lactulose and 10 g polyethylene glycol 4,000 (PEG) diluted in 350 ml water. H_2 breath excretion was measured for 12 hours following the lactulose ingestion.

a) In eight subjects (group A), 24-hour stools were collected on dry ice for 12 hours following the 60 g lactulose oral load, and thereafter for three days. Stools were frozen and stored until analysis. Stool weight, dry matter, pH, carbohydrate and PEG outputs were measured on total homogenized stools.

b) The four other subjects (group B) were intubated on the day before the ingestion of the 60 g lactulose load with a triple lumen tube weighted by a mercury bag which could be inflated with air (lumen 1). The bag was placed in the cecum under fluoroscopy. The second tube, which ended 10 cm above the bag, was used to collect ileal fluid (0.5 ml per minute), and the third tube, which ended 15 cm above tube 2 was used to infuse ^{14}C PEG as a dilution marker at a rate of 0.25 ml per minute. Ileal sampling was performed at 30-minute intervals. Colonic transit times were assessed after the bolus injection of 2.5 microcuries of ^{57}Co-cobalamin into the cecum along with breath H_2 concentrations.

RESULTS

In the subjects of group A, breath H_2 excretion before adaptation (73.0±10 ml per 12 hours) was significantly higher than that after adaptation (42.7±12.0 ml per 12 hours) ($p<0.05$). In the six methane-producing subjects, methane pulmonary

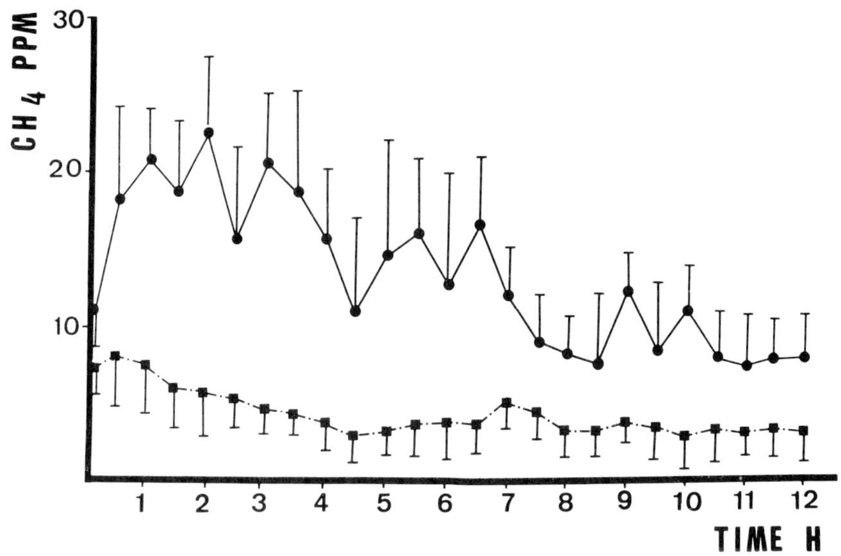

FIGURE 8. Breath CH_4 pulmonary excretion in 6 methane-producing subjects after lactulose 60 g oral load; before (circles) and after (squares) lactulose maintenance. PPM = parts per million.

excretion decreased from day 1 to day 8 ($p<0.05$) (Figure 8).

Ileal content and colonic transit time. Water flow rates before adaptation (2146±188 ml per 12 hours) were not significantly different from those after adaptation (2101±257 ml per 12 hours) (Figure 9). Mean maximal ileal outputs reached 12.4±2 and 12.6±1.9 ml per minute, (range 9.2-18.3 ml per minute). Lactulose ileal concentrations and ileal flow rates were similar in the two periods (53±3 vs 53±2 g per 12 hours) (Figure 10). Ileal flow rates of water were linearly related to those of lactulose ($p<0.05$). In the four intubated subjects, the colonic transit time of ^{57}Co-cobalamin increased significantly after the lactulose maintenance period (85±26 vs 315±47 per minute [$p<0.05$]), whereas the recovered percentage of ^{57}Co-cobalamin in stools decreased significantly (65±12 vs 9±6% per 12 hours) ($p<0.01$) (Figure 11).

Feces. After the lactulose maintenance period, the number of stools and the fecal weight decreased significantly ($p<0.01$) (Figure 12); (stool frequency: 5.9±1.2 vs 2.1±0.4 stools per 12 hours; stool weight: 614±116 vs 298±90 g per 12 hours). The recovered percentage of ingested PEG (Figure 13) and the fecal lactulose output decreased significantly ($p<0.02$) after the lactulose maintenance period (recovered PEG: 31±9 vs 14±5.6% per 12 hours; lactulose output 12.9±4.4 vs 4.3±1.5 g per 12 hours. Stool weight correlated with fecal lactulose output ($r=0.96$, $p<0.001$).

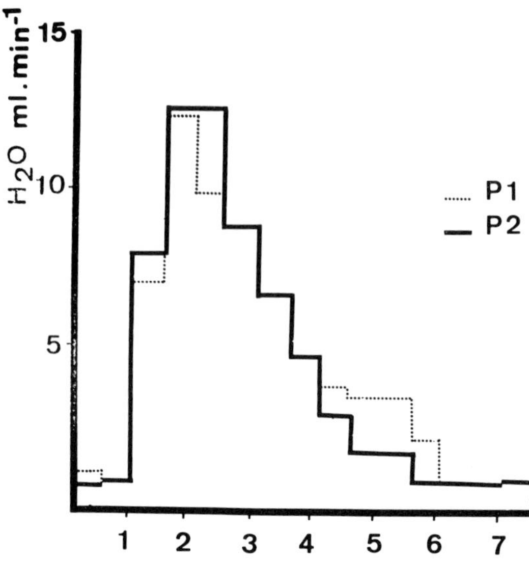

FIGURE 9. Water ileal flow rates after lactulose 60 g oral load: before (dotted line) and after (continuous line) maintenance period. n=4.

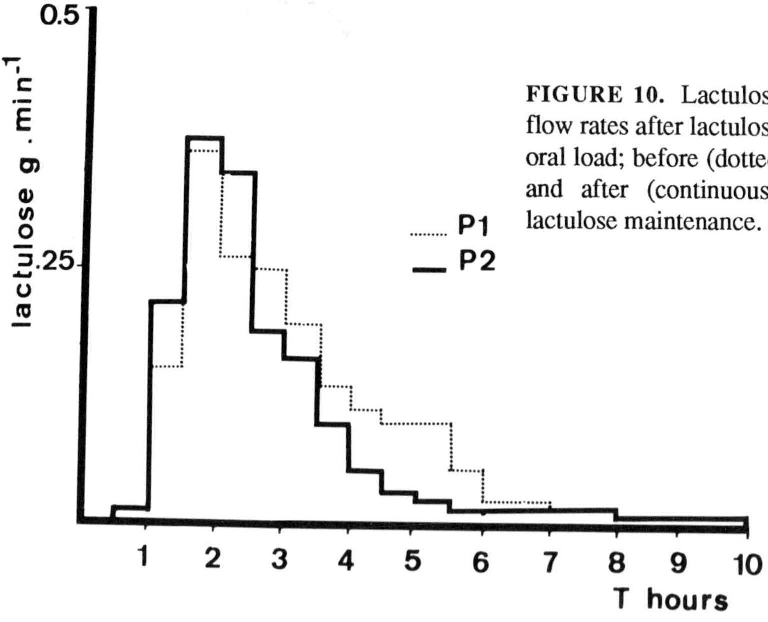

FIGURE 10. Lactulose ileal flow rates after lactulose 60 g oral load; before (dotted line) and after (continuous line) lactulose maintenance. n=4.

FIGURE 11. [57]Co fecal outputs before (open columns) and after (hatched columns) lactulose maintenance. P = 12 hours after 60 g lactulose oral load (test period). n=4. Group B.

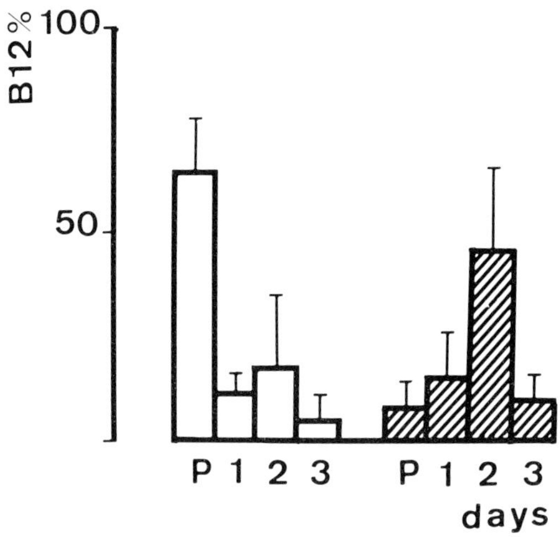

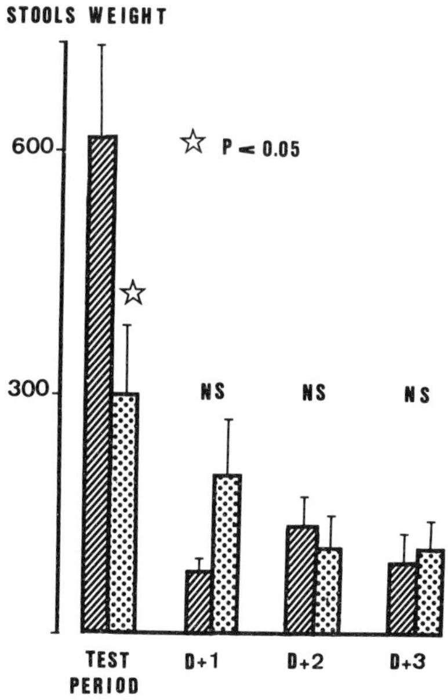

FIGURE 12. Stool weight during the test period and the three following days, before (hatched columns) and after (black spotted columns) lactulose maintenance. n=8. Group A.

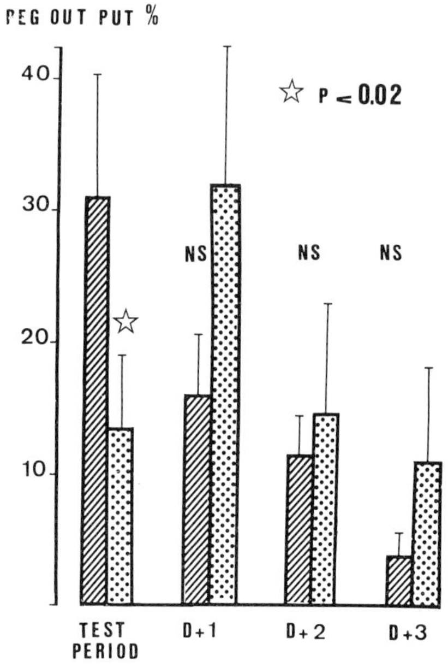

FIGURE 13. Fecal PEG output after 60 g lactulose oral load; before (hatched columns) and after (dotted columns) lactulose maintenance. n=8. Group A.

Clinical symptoms. During the two periods all subjects complained of excessive flatus. Bloating and abdominal girth increased significantly ($p<0.05$) after the lactulose maintenance period, whereas cramping decreased.

DISCUSSION

Chronic lactulose ingestion in nondiarrhea-producing amounts (20 g bid) results in a progressive decrease of diarrhea and abdominal pain. A larger dose of lactulose, however, still causes the symptoms. This improvement is not associated with changes in the small intestinal transit time or the delivery rate into the cecum. Changes in breath H_2 and decreases in lactulose fecal excretion suggest that colonic adaptation may involve different pathways of bacterial metabolism of lactulose. In the first test period, the fecal excretion of lactulose varied from one subject to another (0.3 to 27.6 g per 12 hours). Since the osmolality of excreted carbohydrates is low, our preliminary results could not explain the increase of stool weight. In animals, the acidification of the cecal fluid induces colonic cell injury, which suggests that the bacterial adaptation observed may be deleterious.

CONCLUSION

These investigations clearly show that chronic lactulose administration changes not only the colonic environment, but also the metabolic pathways and/or the population levels of the colonic flora. Beneficial effects of lactulose in the treatment of portal-systemic encephalopathy may be related to the production in excess of some bacterial metabolites and/or to the reduction of some deleterious metabolites.

REFERENCES

1. Ingelfinger F. Editorial comments. In: Beeson PB, ed. Year Book of Medicine. Chicago: Year Book Medical Publishers, 1964-1965: 591-592.

2. Bircher J, Muller J, Guggenheim P, et al. Treatment of chronic portal-systemic encephalopathy with lactulose. Lancet 1966; 1:890-893.

3. Weber FL. The use of lactulose in the treatment of portal-systemic encephalopathy. In: Spiller AG, ed. Nutritional Pharmacology. New York: 1981: 217-253.

4. Hubel KA. Lactulose works, but why? Gastroenterology 1973; 65:349-351.

5. Conn HO. Lactulose: a drug in search of a modus operandi. Gastroenterology 1978; 74:624-626.

6. Haemmerli UP, Bircher J. Wrong idea, good results (the lactulose story). N Engl J Med 1969; 281:441-442.

7. Ruppin H, Bar Meir S, Soergel K, et al. Absorption of short chain fatty acids by the colon. Gastroenterology 1980; 78:1500-1507.

8. MacLean WC, Fink BB. Lactose malabsorption by premature infants: magnitude and clinical significance. J Pediatr 1980; 97:383-388.

9. Perman JA, Molders S, Olson AC. Role of pH in production of hydrogen from carbohydrates by colonic bacterial flora: studies in vivo and in vitro. J Clin Invest 1981; 67:643-650.

10. Florent Ch, Flourie B, Leblond A, et al. Influence of chronic lactulose ingestion on the colonic metabolism of lactulose in man. J Clin Invest 1985; 75:608-613.

10

BRANCHED-CHAIN AMINO ACIDS IN THE TREATMENT OF HEPATIC ENCEPHALOPATHY

L. SIW ERIKSSON, M.D.

The enigma of hepatic encephalopathy has frustrated hepatologists all over the world for decades. A number of substances, found in increased concentrations in cirrhotic patients, have been named as hypothetical etiological agents. These include ammonia, mercaptans, short-chain fatty acids, false neurotransmitters and, quite recently, GABA (1). However, none of these has been proven to be the sole villain in hepatic encephalopathy.

The "false neurotransmitter theory" was formulated in 1971 by Fischer and Baldessarini (2). Based on neuromuscular symptoms in patients with hepatic coma (increased muscle tone, brisk tendon reflexes and tremors) which resemble those observed in patients with Parkinson's disease, a dysfunction of dopaminergic central neurons, possibly involving replacement of less active or "false" neurotransmitters was suggested (3). This theory later involved the deranged amino acid pattern in patients with chronic liver disease, and therapeutic trials to normalize the plasma amino acids were performed. In the late 1970s and early 1980s, a number of enthusiastic but uncontrolled case reports stated the efficacy of branched-chain amino acid treatment (5-9). Unfortunately, the controlled clinical studies published so far do not support this view.

BACKGROUND

Patients with chronic liver disease show a typical amino acid pattern in plasma as well as in whole blood. The concentrations of the three branched-chain amino acids (BCAA), valine, leucine and isoleucine are decreased, while the levels of the aromatic amino acids (AAA), tyrosine, phenylalanine and tryptophan, are increased (10, 11). In the brain, tyrosine and phenylalanine are converted to the neurotransmitters dopamine and norepinephrine; tryptophan is the precursor of serotonin. It has been suggested that an excessive uptake of these amino acids would block the enzyme, tyrosine hydroxylase, used for converting tyrosine to dopa (12). The production of norepinephrine and dopamine could then theoretically be reduced and, instead, tyrosine and phenylalanine would be metabolized to tyramine, octopamine and phenylethanolamine (4). Structurally similar to dopamine and norepinephrine, these substances could, therefore, act as "weak" or "false" neurotransmitters. In fact, Fischer and Baldessarini found increased amounts of octopamine and phenylalanine in the brain and heart of rats with acute hepatic coma and elevated urinary excretion of octopamine in cirrhotic patients with hepatic encephalopathy (2).

The aromatic and the branched-chain amino acids are taken up by the brain across the blood-brain barrier via the same transport carrier system (13). Therefore, they could compete with each other across the blood-brain barrier. If this were true, an increase in the circulating levels of the branched-chain amino acids might restore a normal or more normal ratio of BCAA to AAA and decrease the brain uptake of aromatic amino acids.

Administration of BCAA has been found to decrease the blood levels of several amino acids, above all, the aromatic amino acids and methionine, in both healthy subjects and patients with cirrhosis (11). The brain uptake of amino acids has also been studied in a group of cirrhotic patients in the basal state after an overnight fast and during intravenous infusion of a pure branched-chain amino acid solution (11). This was shown by measuring the arterial-jugular venous concentration differences. In the basal state, the patients demonstrated a significantly increased uptake of tyrosine while the uptake of the branched-chain amino acids was no different in the patients as compared to a group of healthy controls. During the infusion the uptake of BCAA increased in both patients and controls. This rise was even greater in the patients so that the uptake of leucine was significantly higher in the patients than in the controls. In contrast, the uptake of the aromatic amino acids, in particular that of tyrosine, reverted essentially to zero. This study supported the concept that branched-chain amino acid solutions might be of benefit to the encephalopathic patient.

A vast number of uncontrolled studies have also suggested the efficacy of branched-chain amino acid solutions in patients with acute hepatic coma (5-9). However, in view of the fact that the rate of spontaneous recovery after standard hospital measures may be as high as 70%, it is difficult to prove a positive effect of BCAA without carefully controlled studies. BCAAs have been used in three clinical disorders: acute hepatic coma, chronic encephalopathy and subclinical encephalopathy. Finally, they have been discussed as a means of improving nitrogen balance in patients with or without hepatic encephalopathy. The results of the controlled studies in these different situations will be discussed.

BCAA IN THE TREATMENT OF ACUTE HEPATIC ENCEPHALOPATHY

A number of controlled clinical trials have been reported in abstract form. So far, however, only six randomized, controlled, clinical studies have been published in peer-reviewed journals. Data from these studies, as described in the respective publications, are given in Table 1.

In 1982, Rossi-Fanelli and coworkers (14) published a study in which 34 patients with hepatic coma of grade III to IV were randomized to receive 4-day courses of either a BCAA solution with 20% dextrose (17 patients) or lactulose via a nasogastric tube (17 patients). Twelve patients in the BCAA-treated group and eight in the lactulose group regained consciousness during the study period, a difference which did not achieve statistical significance. Three and four patients, respectively, died from factors unrelated to the treatment regimen (gastrointestinal bleeding, hepatorenal failure and acute liver failure). The main drawback of this study is that it was not blinded, and electroencephalograms and trailmaking tests were performed in only a few patients.

One year later, the first double-blind study, which compared BCAA to glucose, was published by Wahren et al. (15). Altogether 50 patients were studied of which 25 received a BCAA solution (40 g BCAA per day) in 5% glucose and 25 patients received 5% glucose until "wake up" or for a maximum of five days. Both groups received nutritional support by intravenous infusions of carbohydrate and fat in equal caloric proportions. Improvement was seen in 14 and 12 of the patients treated with BCAA and placebo, respectively. In the BCAA group, 10 of the patients died in the course of the study as compared to 5 of 25 in the placebo group. Thus, the infusion of BCAA did not improve cerebral function or decrease mortality despite a decrease in the plasma concentrations of the aromatic amino acids and an increase in the ratio between BCAA and AAA.

In 1985, a similar conclusion was reached by Michel and coworkers (16), who compared the effect of a commercially available conventional amino acid mixture and a modified solution enriched in BCAA. Again, all patients were given calories by a combined infusion of glucose and lipid emulsion. Neither improvement in encephalopathy nor reduction of mortality was seen in the BCAA group, although the ratio of plasma AAA to BCAA was corrected.

A fourth study by Cerra and associates (17) is more complex. In this double-blind trial 75 patients were randomized for treatment either with neomycin or an amino acid solution containing 36% BCAA (FO80 or Hepatamine®). The BCAA group was given placebo tablets and the neomycin group received 25% glucose plus 4 g of neomycin per day. The study continued for 14 days with a 7-day follow-up period. Oral intake of food generally started on days 5 and 6 of the study and increased continuously thereafter. The results during the first four days of the study, when the patients were given only the trial substances and no food, are

TABLE 1. Controlled Clinical Trials with BCAA in Patients with Acute Hepatic

Study	No. of patients	Double-blind	Control substance
Rossi-Fanelli et al., 1982	34	No	Lactulose
Wahren et al., 1983	50	Yes	Glucose
Cerra et al., 1985	59	Yes	Neomycin
Michel et al., 1985	70	No	Amino Acids
Fiaccadori et al., 1985*	48	No	Lactulose
Strauss et al., 1987	29	No	Neomycin

* A third group received both BCAA and lactulose and improved in 100% of cases.

partly excluded from the evaluation of the data. The patients who died during the first four days are regarded as "drop outs" and are not taken into consideration when the conclusions of the study are drawn. Moreover, those patients who did not show any improvement in encephalopathy during the first four days were crossed over from their initial treatment group to the other. The final outcomes, however, were calculated as if these patients had continued to receive the first treatment modality. Another problem with this study is that deaths during the seven days after completion of the study period were regarded as part of the trial. Table 2 shows the mortality data in the two groups for the different time periods. In this table the crossover patients, four in the BCAA group and seven in the neomycin group, are excluded since it is not clear to which group they should belong. However, of the patients crossed over from neomycin to BCAA, four died during BCAA treatment as compared to one of the four patients crossed over from BCAA to neomycin.

From Table 2 it can be seen that the mortality during the actual treatment period is similar in the two groups. Eleven patients in the BCAA and nine in the neomycin group died during treatment. The major difference between the groups as reported by the authors occurs in the week after the study when the patients died from liver failure, sepsis and bleeding. Thus, it is evident that FO80 had no true advantage over neomycin with regard to mortality. Similarly, when looking at the number of patients who improved, disregarding the degree of improvement (which is difficult to discern from the article), 24 of the BCAA-treated patients (67%) as compared to 19 in the neomycin group (68%) improved (treated patients minus crossover and deaths in both groups). These corrected results are not statistically significant.

Coma as Reported by the Authors

Improvement		Mortality	
BCAA %	Control %	BCAA %	Control %
70	47	18	23
56	48	40	20
77	45	17	55
33	34	19	20
94	62	-	-
87	87	14	13

In 1986, two controlled studies were published, neither of which was double-blind. Fiaccadori and coworkers (18) randomized 48 patients to one of three different treatments: 16 received lactulose, 16 were given a BCAA-enriched amino acid solution and 16 patients received lactulose together with the amino acid solution. The treatment continued for seven days. In each group, 10, 15, and 16 patients, respectively, improved with regard to the "clinical assessment." However, no differences were observed between the groups when more objective investigations such as EEG and Number Connection Tests were analyzed. The mortality is not presented by the authors. In Brazil, Strauss et al. (19) treated 32 episodes of grade I to III hepatic encephalopathy in 29 patients. Sixteen episodes were treated with neomycin and as many with FO80. Fourteen episodes in each group improved during treatment and the mortality was similar in the two groups (two and three patients died in these groups, respectively).

TABLE 2. Reappraisal of Mortality Data from Cerra et al., 1985

	Patients included	Excluding crossover	Mortality		
			Day 0-4	Day 5-14	After study
BCAA	40	36	9	2	2
Neomycin	35	28	6	3	9

These six studies differ in regard to the control substances, the therapeutic solutions and also in regard to the etiology and severity of the cirrhosis. It is therefore difficult to make direct comparisons between the studies. However, if, in spite of this, all studies are taken together, the "wake up" rate during BCAA infusions tends to be higher (68±9%) than during control treatment (58±8%). The difference is not significant. The mortality was not influenced by the treatment; 24±5% of the patients died during BCAA administration and 22±3% during control treatment (Figure 1). These figures demonstrate both the inability of BCAA solutions to improve the patients with acute hepatic coma, and the overall inadequacy of standard therapy in such patients.

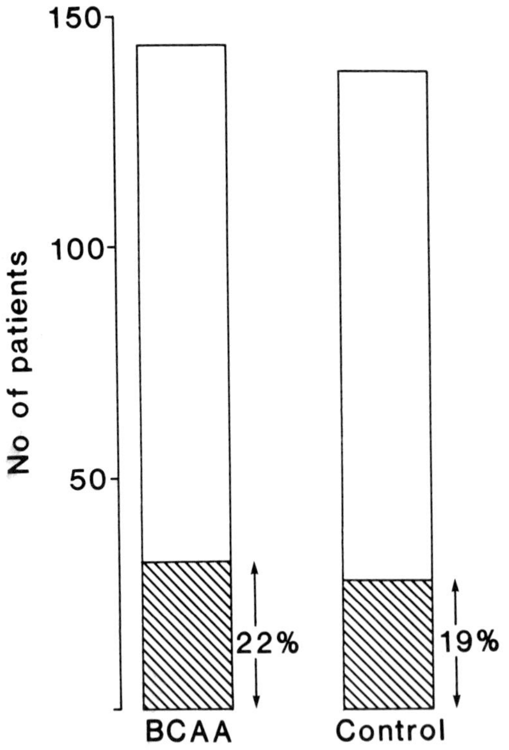

FIGURE 1. Effects of BCAA on mortality in acute hepatic encephalopathy. The height of the bars denote the total number of patients in the six studies while the hatched parts show the number of patients that died during the study periods. (The crossover patients in the study by Cerra et al. (17) are excluded as discussed in the text).

BCAA IN THE TREATMENT OF CHRONIC ENCEPHALOPATHY

So far, four controlled studies involving BCAA administration have been conducted in patients with cirrhosis and chronic hepatic encephalopathy (Table 3). As was the case with the acute encephalopathy, the therapeutic substances differed from pure BCAA to BCAA-enriched protein diets and in the control substances (carbohydrate, protein). The study periods varied in length from one week (with a gradual increase of oral protein intake) to three-month periods.

Three of the studies were performed as crossover studies. In one by Eriksson et al. (20) seven patients ingested 30 g branched-chain amino acids or placebo during two consecutive 14-day periods. Neither clinical observations, psychometric tests nor electroencephalograms showed a significant difference in patients' responses to BCAA as compared to placebo. In another crossover study by Schäfer et al. (21), eight patients with cirrhosis and mild chronic hepatic encephalopathy (grade I or II) received 45 g per day of a protein mixture enriched in BCAA, the same daily amount of milk protein or an isocaloric carbohydrate mixture in three alternate, 3-month periods. The patients were treated as outpatients; intake was controlled by a relative or recorded by the patient. All patients tolerated BCAA-protein well, but during the intake of milk protein (which contained 20 g of lactose), several patients suffered from dyspepsia, bloating and diarrhea. The Number Connection Tests tended to be completed faster during BCAA treatment than during the previous treatment period, but the difference did not reach statistical significance. Electroencephalograms, ammonia concentrations and plasma amino acid levels did not change during BCAA ingestion as compared to the previous test period.

Thus, in neither of these studies did BCAA administration improve the encephalopathy. A drawback in both studies is the lack of comparative protein intake. Eriksson et al. (20) used carbohydrate as control. Schäfer et al. (21), although using protein as one of the control diets, chose a protein that gave side effects so severe that the test period had to be shortened or the amount of protein had to be decreased.

A third carefully conducted study was performed on only four patients (22). The patients were randomly given a casein diet or a casein diet supplemented with BCAA during two 11-day periods in a crossover manner. During the BCAA period the molar ratio between the BCAA (leucine + isoleucine + valine) and the AAA (tyrosine + phenylalanine) increased significantly, but no changes were observed in clinical status, psychometric tests nor EEG between the two study periods. Moreover, the nitrogen balance did not differ between the two treatments.

A fourth randomized, controlled study by Horst et al. compared dietary protein with an oral branched-chain enriched amino acid supplement in two groups of nonencephalopathic or minimally encephalopathic patients (23). All patients received 20 g per day of dietary protein for one week during basal assessment.

TABLE 3. Controlled Clinical Trials with Oral BCAA in Cirrhotic Patients. Effect on Chronic Hepatic Encephalopathy and/or Nitrogen Balance

Study	Type	No. of patients (days)	Study periods (g)	Basal protein (g)	Amount (%) of BCAA	Amount of control substance (g)	BCAA and control encephalopathy (g)	Effects on nitrogen balance
Schäfer (21)	Crossover	8	28-56	40-50	45 (34%)	45 Milk protein	No difference	Not done
Eriksson (20)	Crossover	7	14	40-60	30 (100%)	30 Carbohydrate	No difference	Not done
McGhee (22)	Crossover	4	11	20	30 (28%)	30 Casein	No difference	No difference
Horst (23)	Two groups	26	21	20	20-60 (35%)	20-60 Dietary protein	BCAA tolerated signif. better without PSE	No difference
Christie (29)	Crossover	8	6	40	60 (50%)	60 Casein	PSE-index improved on control substance; no change with BCAA	No difference
Millihan (28)	Crossover	8	6	Not given	0.6g/kg BW (% not given)	0.6 g/kg BW Enteral diet	Not done	No difference

Thereafter, 20 g of dietary protein or of BCAA were added weekly until a total intake of 80 g of protein per day was attained, or until the patients developed grade II encephalopathy. Seven of the 20 patients in the protein group and one of 17 in the BCAA group developed encephalopathy of grade II or greater ($p<0.05$). At the end of the study the mental state, asterixis and portal-systemic encephalopathy index were better in the BCAA-treated patients than in the patients that received dietary protein. Nitrogen balance improved in both groups. The authors concluded that oral BCAA supplements could induce positive nitrogen balance to approximately the same degree as an equivalent amount of dietary protein, but without inducing encephalopathy as frequently.

BCAA IN SUBCLINICAL ENCEPHALOPATHY

With the development of psychometric testing it has been shown repeatedly that a large fraction of cirrhotic patients have some degree of cerebral impairment in the absence of overt encephalopathy (24). Verbal capacity is often preserved and subtle encephalopathy may go undetected. Since this subclinical or latent encephalopathy may be a problem for patients with specific skills, it may be of value to treat such patients. In a carefully conducted, crossover study, 22 patients with cirrhosis and subclinical encephalopathy were studied during one week on a BCAA-supplemented diet, and one week on a diet of casein given in equal amounts (25). Electroencephalograms and a series of 15 psychometric tests were performed before and at the end of the test periods. Significant improvement was demonstrated in some specific tests measuring psychomotor functions, attention and practical intelligence during BCAA treatment. However, the overall mental state, designated as "fitness to drive" was not influenced by the treatment. Similar results were achieved by Sieg and coworkers (26). In a crossover design they studied the effect of BCAA compared to a carbohydrate placebo in 14 patients, only three of whom had encephalopathy (grade I). They found no difference in mental state or in the PSE Index between the test periods, but their psychometric tests were limited to the Number Connection Tests.

In conclusion, the addition of BCAA may be of some value in patients with subclinical encephalopathy. It is difficult to understand why it would improve latent but not overt encephalopathy.

DOES BCAA IMPROVE NITROGEN BALANCE?

From *in vitro* studies it has been suggested that BCAAs, primarily leucine, stimulate protein synthesis and diminish protein catabolism (27). It is therefore plausible that BCAA administration may improve nitrogen balance.

Apart from the two studies mentioned previously (22, 23) on chronic encephalopathic patients in which nitrogen balance was measured, three other controlled studies that compare the effect of BCAA and dietary protein on nitrogen balance have been published (28, 29, 30) (Table 3). In one of these (28), nitrogen fluxes were studied using ^{15}N, ^{13}C-leucine in eight cirrhotic patients and five healthy controls during two 6-day periods on conventional or BCAA-enriched protein diets. The results demonstrated that carbon and nitrogen fluxes, oxidation, synthesis and deamination were higher when the conventional diet was fed than in the fasted patients. The BCAA enrichment further increased fluxes and oxidation but did not stimulate protein synthesis nor decrease protein breakdown. Leucine metabolism was similar in the cirrhotic patients and in the healthy controls, and the authors conclude that "leucine-enriched formulas increase oxidation to CO_2 without improving protein synthesis" (28).

Normal nitrogen balance was measured by Christie et al. (29) in a randomized, double-blind, crossover study in eight malnourished cirrhotic patients. Again, a BCAA-enriched diet was compared to a casein-based diet. Balance data were similar between the two treatment periods and the patients tolerated approximately 75 g daily of either diet. In contrast to the study previously described (23), the neurologic status improved during the casein diet but not during the BCAA-enriched diet.

In 36 compensated cirrhotic patients without clinical signs of encephalopathy, Rocchi et al. (30) compared the nutritional effect of a pure BCAA solution with that of amino acid solutions that contained 35% and 26% BCAA. The patients were divided into four groups: twelve received BCAA, (0.5 g per kg per day); seven received twice the amount (1.0 g per kg per day); seven were given 0.8 g per kg per day of a selective amino acid solution (35% BCAA); and ten patients received 0.5 g per kg of an ordinary amino acid solution (26% BCAA). Carbohydrate and lipids were given orally in isocaloric amounts to all patients during the five days of study. In the basal state, nitrogen balance was negative in all four groups, and this was not altered by a small amount of the pure BCAA (0.5 g per kg). The other three infusions resulted in significantly improved nitrogen balance by the fifth day of the study. Although these increments were most pronounced during the infusion of 1 g BCAA per kg, they did not differ statistically from that of the selective amino acid solution (35% BCAA). Moreover, the latter was similar to the nitrogen balance seen during infusion of the standard solution (26% BCAA). All patients tolerated the solutions well; the authors concluded that the study demonstrated the "good tolerance and protein-sparing effect of low doses of commercially available standard amino acids..."

SUMMARY

The controlled, randomized clinical trials hitherto published do not favor the use of BCAA in patients with cirrhosis and portal-systemic encephalopathy. In acute hepatic coma, amino acid infusions did not restore mental state to normal or reduce mortality. In patients with chronic encephalopathy, three of four studies have demonstrated similar efficacy of BCAA-enriched and control diets on the cerebral dysfunction. Studies of nitrogen balance have failed to show that BCAA has a more positive effect on protein regulation than does ordinary protein. Only in patients with subclinical encephalopathy does BCAA seem to have a positive effect. Whether the latter merely reflects the paucity of investigations so far conducted and the small number of patients studied, or implies that BCAA may be of some value in a carefully selected subgroup of patients with subclinical encephalopathy, is still an unsettled question.

REFERENCES

1. Jones EA, Schafer DF, Ferenci P, et al. The GABA hypothesis of the pathogenesis of hepatic encephalopathy: current status. Yale J Biol Med 1984; 57:301-316.

2. Fischer JE, Baldessarini RJ. False neurotransmitters and hepatic failure. Lancet 1971; 2:75-79.

3. Fischer JE, Horst WD, Kopin IJ. Beta-hydroxylated sympathomimetic amines as false neurotransmitters. Br J Pharmacol 1965; 24:477-484.

4. Fischer JE, Baldessarini RJ. Pathogenesis and therapy of hepatic coma. In: Popper H, Schaffner, F, eds. Progress in Liver Disease, Vol V. New York: Grune and Stratton, 1976: 363-397.

5. Delin A, Hagenfeldt L, Hallberg D, et al. Behanding av leverkoma med balanserad aminosyralösning. Läkartidningen 1978; 75:50-58.

6. Fischer JE, Rosen HM, Ebeid AM, et al. The effect of normalization of plasma amino acids on hepatic encephalopathy in man. Surgery 1976; 80:77-91.

7. Freund H, Dienstag J, Lehrich J, et al. Infusion of branched chain enriched amino acid solution in patients with hepatic encephalopathy. Ann Surg 1982; 196:209-220.

8. Pellegrino F, Zola C, Ginelli F. L'impiego delle soluzioni selettive di aminoacidi nel trattamento pre- e post-operatorio dei cirrotici. Minerva Chir 1980; 35:439-444.

9. Freund H, Yoshimura N, Fischer JE. Chronic hepatic encephalopathy. Long-term therapy with a branched chain amino acid enriched elemental diet. JAMA 1979; 242:347-349.

10. Iber FL, Rosen H, Levenson SM, et al. The plasma amino acids in patients with liver failure. J Lab Clin Med 1957; 50:417-425.

11. Sato Y, Eriksson S, Hagenfeldt L, et al. Influence of branched chain amino acid infusion on arterial concentrations and brain exchange of amino acids in patients with hepatic cirrhosis. Clin Physiol 1981; 1: 151-165.

12. Wurtman RJ, Larin F, Mostafapour S, et al. Brain catechol synthesis:

control by brain tyrosine concentration. Science 1974; 185:183-186.

13. Olendorf WH, Szabo J. Amino acid assignment to one of the three blood-brain barrier amino acid carriers. Am J Physiol 1976; 230:94-98.

14. Rossi-Fanelli F, Riggio O, Cangiano C, et al. Branched chain amino acids vs lactulose in the treatment of hepatic coma. A controlled study. Dig Dis Sci 1982; 27:929-935.

15. Wahren J, Denis J, Desurmont P, et al. Is intravenous administration of branched chain amino acids effective in the treatment of hepatic encephalopathy? A multicenter study. Hepatology 1983; 3:475-480.

16. Michel H, Bories P, Aubin JP, et al. Treatment of acute hepatic encephalopathy in cirrhotics with a branched-chain amino acids enriched versus a conventional amino acids mixture. A controlled study of 70 patients. Liver 1985; 5:282-289.

17. Cerra FB, Cheung NK, Fischer JE, et al. Disease-specific amino acid infusion (FO80) in hepatic encephalopathy: a prospective, randomized, double-blind, controlled trial. JPEN 1985; 9:288-295.

18. Fiaccadori F, Ginelli F, Pedretti G, et al. Branched-chain enriched amino acid solutions in the treatment of hepatic encephalopathy: a controlled trial. Ital J Gastroenterol 1985; 17:5-10.

19. Strauss, E, dos Santos WR, daSilva EC, et al. Treatment of hepatic encephalopathy: a randomized clinical trial comparing a branched chain enriched amino acid solution to oral neomycin. Nutr Supp Svcs 1986; 6:18-21.

20. Eriksson LS, Persson A, Wahren J. Branched chain amino acids in the treatment of chronic hepatic encephalopathy. Gut 1982; 23:801-806.

21. Schäfer K, Winther MB, Ukida M, et al. Influence of an orally administered protein mixture enriched in branched chain amino acids on the chronic hepatic encephalopathy (CHE) of patients with liver cirrhosis. Z Gastroenterol 1981; 19:356-362.

22. McGhee A, Henderson M, Millikan WJ, et al. Comparison of the effects of hepatic aid and a casein modular diet on encephalopathy, plasma amino acids, and nitrogen balance in cirrhotic patients. Ann Surg 1983; 197:288-293.

23. Horst D, Grace ND, Conn HO, et al. Comparison of dietary protein with an oral, branched chain enriched amino acid supplement in chronic portal systemic encephalopathy: a randomized controlled trial. Hepatology 1984; 4:279-287.

24. Rikkers L, Jenko P, Rudman D, et al. Subclinical hepatic encephalopathy: detection, prevalence, and relationship to nitrogen metabolism. Gastroenterology 1978; 75:462-469.

25. Egberts EH, Schomerus H, Hamster W, et al. Branched chain amino acids in the treatment of latent portosystemic encephalopathy. A double-blind placebo-controlled crossover study. Gastroenterology 1985; 88:887-895.

26. Sieg A, Walker S, Czygan P, et al. Branched chain amino acid enriched elemental diet in patients with cirrhosis of the liver. A double blind crossover trial. Z Gastroenterol 1983; 21:644-650.

27. Buse MG, Reid SS. Leucine. A possible regulator of protein turnover in muscle. J Clin Invest 1975; 56:1250-1261.

28. Millikan WJ, Henderson JM, Galloway JR, et al. In vivo measurement of leucine metabolism with stable isotopes in normal subjects and in those with cirrhosis fed conventional and branched chain amino acid enriched diets. Surgery 1985; 98:405-413.

29. Christie ML, Sack DM, Pomposelli J, et al. Enriched branched chain amino acid formula versus a casein based supplement in the treatment of cirrhosis. JPEN 1985; 9:671-678.

30. Rocchi E, Cassanelli M, Gibertini P, et al. Standard or branched-chain amino acid infusions as short-term nutritional support in liver cirrhosis? JPEN 1985; 9:447-451.

LACTULOSE

11

THE PHARMACOLOGY OF LACTULOSE

MILTON M. LIEBERTHAL, M.D.

The key to the success of lactulose as a therapeutic agent lies in certain pharmacologic phenomena: a) that it is a synthetic disaccharide that does not occur naturally; b) that there are no enzymes in humans or animals that are capable of metabolizing it; and c) that it is poorly absorbed from the small intestine. As a result, lactulose flowers in a colonic venue.

LACTULOSE ABSORPTION IN HEALTHY SUBJECTS

The disaccharidases that split naturally-occurring disaccharides into their hexose moieties, which are then absorbed, do not include a *lactulase*. Preparations of small intestine from puppies (1), from human infants (1), and from human adults (2), have shown no detectable lactulase activity. There is, however, a very little absorption of orally administered lactulose; it appears to take place by a passive mechanism. After an oral dose, from 1% to 3% has been found in the urine of infants and adults (3-5).

ABSORPTION IN INFANTS

As measured by the lactose/L-rhamnose urinary excretion ratio during continued infusion of milk containing both sugars, healthy infants of gestational age 31 to 36 weeks proved to have a period of enhanced permeability to lactulose during the first week of life (6). The lactose/L-rhamnose excretion ratio was significantly higher on postnatal day 2 than on days 9 or 16 when a mature pattern of permeability could be seen. Asphyxia of the infant or sepsis blunted this change. Healthy preterm infants of gestational age 26-29 weeks showed a mature pattern of permeability.

Lactulose is present in small amounts in many heat processed milk products (7) (Table 1), where it is formed from lactose. These products appear to contain approximately 100-250 mg of lactulose per 100 ml (Hendrickse RG: personal communication, 1978).

By colorimetric measurement, the amounts of lactulose in 12 lots of evaporated milk averaged 660 mg per 100 ml. A 2:1 ratio between lactose and lactulose has been found in canned milk (11). Lactulose is not found in fresh cow's milk or in the carbohydrate supplements ordinarily added to infant formulas (8). There is no lactulose in breast milk (9).

ABSORPTION IN ADULTS

Studies of six normal adults also showed that lactulose is not metabolized or absorbed in significant amounts in the small intestine, and absorption in the colon of lactulose and its degradation products is negligible (3). Lactulose was detected in the urine 2 hours after the ingested dose. In four subjects, maximum excretion occurred in 4 hours, and in the remaining two between 4 and 8 hours. One other subject took 16 hours to complete lactulose excretion, and no lactulose was detected in the urine of any subject after 24 hours. The total amount of lactulose excreted in

TABLE 1. The Presence of Sugars in Natural and Processed Milks

Milk	Lactose	Lactulose	Glucose	Galactose	Mannose	Maltose	Fructose	Other
Breast milk	+	0	+	+	+	0	+	a,b
Cow's milk	+	0	+	+	+	0	0	c
Enfamil	+	+	N.S.	N.S.	0	N.S.	N.S.	0
Similac	+	+	+	+	+	N.S.	+	b
Lactum	+	+	N.S.	N.S.	N.S.	N.S.	N.S.	0
Evap. milk	+	+	+	+	+	+	+	b

[a] Unidentified aldohexose; [b] arabinose, ribose; [c] sedoheptulose, fucose; N.S., not stated. Based on the findings of Adachi and Patton (7) and Gryboski et al. (8, 9).

This table and other tables in this chapter are reproduced by permission from Conn HO and Lieberthal MM: The Hepatic Coma Syndromes and Lactulose.©1979 The Williams and Wilkins Co., Baltimore (10).

the urine was less than 1% in five subjects, and 2.8% in the sixth.

Similar observations on two healthy men given approximately 20 g of lactulose gave similar results (Table 2). Japanese workers have also confirmed the limited small intestinal absorption of lactulose and its excretion in the urine (12).

In normal adults, intestinal permeability to lactulose in hypertonic solution made by adding various solutes (sucrose, glucose, mannitol, glycerol, urea, or sodium chloride) is also increased as the concentration of the solute is increased (4).

EFFECT ON BLOOD GLUCOSE LEVELS

The effect of lactulose syrup and its constituent carbohydrates on blood glucose levels was determined in four healthy volunteers (13). Within 40 to 60 minutes after ingestion of the lactulose syrup, the blood glucose levels increased an average of 12 mg per 100 ml. Twenty minutes after the ingestion of a fructose-galactose control solution, the blood glucose rose an average of 38 mg per 100 ml, a significant difference.

Another study, this one in five subjects with impaired glucose tolerance, likewise showed no appreciable increase in blood glucose levels after lactulose (14). None of the tested subjects was taking insulin or oral hypoglycemic agents. Blood glucose levels were determined before and at 30, 60, 90, and 150 minutes after doses of pure lactulose, lactulose syrup, galactose, glucose and lactose (Figure 1). The average increment in blood glucose was only 3.6 mg per 100 ml 30 minutes after ingestion of lactulose. All the other sugars produced a sharp rise of at least 42 mg per 100 ml, averaging 64.3 mg per 100 ml, in blood glucose concentration.

It seems quite clear from these observations that lactulose is not absorbed to any significant degree, nor is it metabolized to its constituent monosaccharides in the small intestine, as happens in the colon as the result of bacterial degradation (15). If it had been, blood glucose levels would have sharply increased.

TABLE 2. Excretion of Lactulose in Urine after a 20-g Dose * (10)

Subject	0-4.5 hours (mg)	4.5-24 hours (mg)	Total (mg)	% Dose
1	70	50	120	0.6
2	138	19	157	0.8

*Administered as the syrup, containing 0.67 g per ml

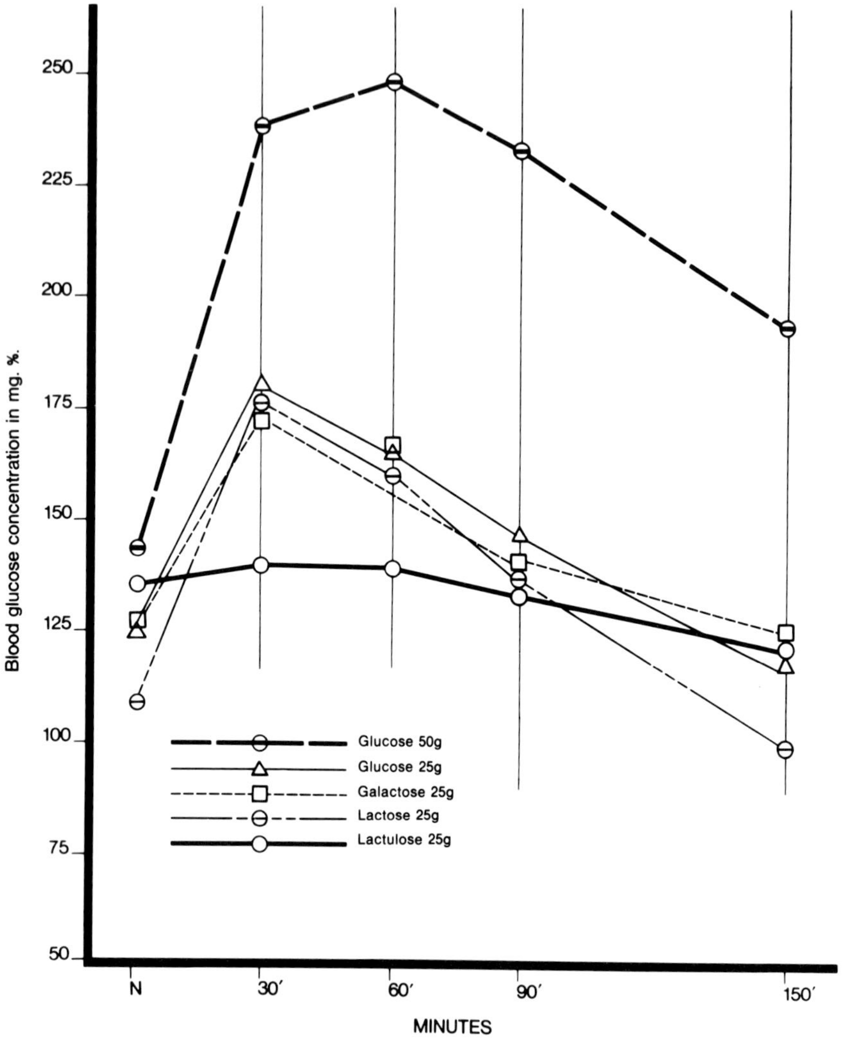

FIGURE 1. Blood glucose curves in five untreated diabetic patients. Test doses of glucose (25 and 50 g), galactose (25 g), lactose (25 g) and lactulose (25 g) were administered. Only the lactulose failed to cause a sharp rise in blood sugar. (Reprinted by permission from Conn HO and Lieberthal MM: The Hepatic Coma Syndromes and Lactulose ©1979 The Williams & Wilkins Co., Baltimore.)

TABLE 3. Urinary Levels of Lactulose in Rats Following Oral Administration (10)

Rat no.	Lactulose syrup (0.67 g per ml)	Lactulose found in urine in mg 0-2	2-4	4-8 (hours)	8-24	Total 24 hr
1	Lactulose 0.33 g	n.d.	0.75	0.75	0.75	2.25
2	Lactulose 0.33 g	n.d.	0.75	0.75	0.75	2.25
3	Lactulose 0.32 g	1.00	1.00	0.75	0.45	3.20
4	Water 0.47 ml	n.d.	n.d.	n.d.		n.d.

n.d. = not detectable

ABSORPTION IN ANIMALS

Female baboons and male and female rats were given various doses of lactulose syrup orally, and serum and urine samples were obtained. Less than 1% of the ingested dose was subsequently detected in the urine of the baboons (14). Lactulose was also tested for by different methods in the urine (Table 3) and in the serum (Table 4) of rats. Less than 1% of the ingested dose appeared in the urine in this species, too. In another experiment on four female rats, ^{14}C-lactulose was administered after cannulation of their bile ducts and ligation of their small intestines proximal to the cecum. Radioactivity in the liver and bile ducts over the 6 hours

TABLE 4. Serum Levels (μg/ml) in Rats Following Oral Administration of Lactulose (10)

Rat No.	Lactulose syrup (0.67 g per ml)	At 1 hour	At 3 hours	At 6 hours	At 24 hours
1	Water 2.87 ml	n.d.	n.d.	n.d.	n.d.
2	Water 2.80 ml	n.d.	n.d.	n.d.	n.d.
3	Lactulose 1.53 g	20	10	50	n.d.
4	Lactulose 1.56 g	30	20	10	n.d.
5	Lactulose 1.86 g	30	10	10	n.d.
6	Lactulose 1.76 g	35	15	15	n.d.

n.d. = not detectable

following the ingested dose was extremely low. Radioactivity in the small intestine, on the other hand, averaged 78.58% of the ingested dose. This suggested that a relatively small amount of lactulose absorption from the intestine had taken place.

There is some evidence to suggest that lactulose may inhibit the absorption of glucose, at least in rats (16). Japanese workers perfused a segment of rat jejunum with equiosmolar lactulose in a glucose-containing solution and found that the absorption of glucose was reduced by 40%.

EXSORPTION

It is interesting to note here, parenthetically, that while intestinal mucosa allows selected intestinal contents to pass through it into the circulation, it also functions as a barrier that prevents the contents of the blood from diffusing into the intestinal lumen. However, in the rabbit, that barrier is only partially effective in preventing lactulose, and certain other substances, from passing out of the plasma into the intestinal lumen by a process called "exsorption" (17). The rate of exsorption from plasma to intestinal lumen for lactulose in rabbits has been found to be directly related to its plasma concentration and molecular weight (18). In the human, the plasma content of lactulose following therapeutic doses is so small that the process of exsorption probably does not take place.

LACTULOSE ABSORPTION IN DISEASED CHILDREN

Several studies have been done to measure the absorption of lactulose in celiac disease. In one such study, 12 normal children, 4 children with active celiac disease and 3 children with celiac disease in remission, were given lactulose syrup (0.67 g lactulose per ml) in doses of 5, 10, or 20 g per square meter of body surface (5) (Table 5). In 6 hours, 0.04% to 2.01% of the lactulose was recovered in the urine of all 19 children, as determined by gas chromatography. The amount recovered was not affected by the presence or absence of celiac disease. From 0.07% to 1.38% of the ingested lactulose had been recovered in 24 hours.

These studies seem to indicate that less than 3% of orally ingested lactulose appears in the urine of normal or celiac children, even when the dose is as large as 20 g per square meter of body surface.

British workers studied intestinal permeability to lactulose in children with atopic eczema and food allergy. In one such study (19), the percentage excretion of the oral dose of L-rhamnose was no different in 20 children with atopic eczema from that in 10 normal and 8 skin disease controls. However, the ratio of percentage excretion of the oral dose of lactulose to percentage excretion of the oral dose of rhamnose was significantly elevated in the children with eczema compared with both control groups. The results implied an increase in macromolecular

TABLE 5. Excretion of Lactulose in the Urine in Controls, in Children with Active Celiac Disease, and in Children with Celiac Disease in Remission (10)

Patients and dosages (per m² of body surface)	Excretion of lactulose in urine (% of dose)					
	6 hours			24 hours		
	No. of subjects	Range	Mean	No. of subjects	Range	Mean
Normals						
5 g	3	0.56-0.88	0.70	3	0.70-1.17	0.91
10 g	6	0.04-0.42	0.22	6	0.07-0.73	0.43
20 g	3	0.08-0.57	0.28			
Active celiac disease (flat mucosa)						
5 g	1		0.98	1		1.06
10 g	1		0.63	1		1.38
20 g	2	0.40-0.52	0.46			
Celiac disease in remission (normal mucosa)						
20 g	3	0.32-2.01	1.29			

Adapted from Muller et al (5).

permeability in atopic eczema. In another study (20), no difference in intestinal permeability to lactulose was found between ten children with active atopic eczema and clinically proven food allergy and ten healthy children controls. When two children from the active atopic eczema group and another eight children, whose eczema was exacerbated by either a tartrazine or milk challenge, were investigated further with a hypertonic load plus an antigen challenge, only two showed an increased permeability to lactulose. Whether an increase in macromolecular permeability explains food allergies and skin responses remains unclear.

Ten cystic fibrosis children were found to have increased intestinal permeability to lactulose and rhamnose (21). The same was true of 48 male subjects with diabetes mellitus (22), suggesting that caution must be used in interpreting the rhamnose-lactulose test of mucosal functions in diabetic patients.

LACTULOSE ABSORPTION IN DISEASED ADULTS

Certain disease states in adults, such as tropical sprue, are associated with increased permeability of the intestine to lactulose. In a study comparing lactulose permeability in five tropical sprue patients with nine patients with tropical diarrhea and no malabsorption and 16 healthy control subjects (23), urinalysis demonstrated that intestinal permeation of lactulose was increased and that of rhamnose decreased in the tropical sprue group compared with the normal controls (Table 6). The difference was enhanced when lactulose was administered as a hyperosmotic solution.

The same findings regarding lactulose absorption in celiac children do not hold for adults with celiac disease. It has been shown that celiac adults excrete almost twice as much lactulose in the urine after a hyperosmolar loading dose as they do after an isosmolar load (24). Untreated celiac adults absorb less mannitol and more lactulose than controls (25). Absorption returned toward normal on

TABLE 6. Absolute Values for 5-hour Urinary Lactulose and Rhamnose Excretion in the Three Groups*

Group	No. of patients	5-hour urinary excretion percentage of dose			
		Lactulose		Rhamnose	
		From iso-osmotic solution	From hyper-osmotic solution	From iso-osmotic solution	From hyper-osmotic solution
Tropical sprue	5	0.52 (0.36-0.92)	1.62 (0.90-3.14)	2.60 (1.0-4.4)	3.46 (1.6-4.5)
Tropical diarrhea	9	0.31 (0.08-0.64)	0.70 (0.20-1.94)	9.09 (4.3-15.8)	9.70 (4.1-18.7)
Control	16	0.30 (0.10-0.50)	0.45 (0.22-0.81)	11.64 (6.5-16.4)	9.44 (4.3-15.8)

* Mean and range are shown for each measurement as percentage of oral dose. Reproduced by permission from Cook GC, Menzies IS: Intestinal absorption and unmediated permeation of sugars in post-infective tropical malabsorption (tropical sprue) ©Digestion (S. Karger AG, Basel) 1986; 33:109-116.

treatment. It was concluded that the mucosa in celiac disease is more "leaky" than normal.

When the intestinal permeability to lactulose was studied in patients with ulcerative colitis, no difference from normal controls was detected (26). Patients with Crohn's disease of the ileum, on the other hand, exhibited increased absorption compared to normal controls. As might be expected, absorption of lactulose in patients with *colonic* Crohn's disease was not significantly higher than in normals.

Cytotoxic chemotherapy virtually doubled the intestinal permeability to lactulose in nine patients with nonintestinal lymphoma (27). The increased permeability rapidly resolved when treatment ceased.

It might be noted here that the significance of increased intestinal permeability in man is really unknown. There is no evidence up to this point that such increase has a role in the etiology of any disease, certain diseases of so-called allergic origin being possible exceptions (28).

The small amount of lactulose absorbed under any of the circumstances described above does not appear to be metabolized within the body. Very close to 100% of intravenously administered lactulose has been recovered in the urine (29). After unconventionally large doses of lactulose, blood concentrations have reached 3 mg per dl, but after the usual therapeutic doses of 10 to 20 g, blood concentrations have been undetectable or in the range of 0.2 mg per dl (3, 4). It is not surprising, therefore, that no systemic effects have been detected as the result of the absorption of such small amounts of lactulose from the intestine.

LACTULOSE DEGRADATION

Contrary to the inadequacies of mammalian species in this regard, bacteria are able to metabolize lactulose. The site of their degrading action has been shown to be in the colon, mostly the right colon. Exceptions to this localization occur when bacterial colonization of the small intestine is encountered, as happens sometimes in cirrhosis and certain other disorders. Otherwise, in the now proven absence of any enzyme capable of metabolizing lactulose in the human small intestine (1, 2, 30), lactulose reaches the colon unchanged. There it is metabolized by intestinal flora into low molecular weight organic acids (13, 15). The principal organisms performing this function are gram-positive cocci and bacilli, especially clostridium, lactobacilli, and streptococci (Table 7). Lactic acid has proven to be the principal metabolite in lactulose metabolism (13).

Observations made with a radiotelemetry device on normal adults taking 40 to 60 ml of lactulose syrup daily showed a sharp drop in pH in the right colon (31). In the ten subjects tested, the median pH changed from 7.0 in the lower small intestine to 4.8 in the right colon ($p<0.002$) (Figure 2). It was presumed that the bacterial fermentation of lactulose took place where the pH drop was greatest. The median pH then rose to 6.7 as the intestinal content reached the left colon. When

TABLE 7. Breakdown of Lactulose by the Most Frequently Occurring Bacteria in the Colon

Organisms utilizing >20% lactulose	Percentage utilization after 48 h cultivation	Gas production (on a scale + to +++)
Bacteroides oralis[a]	21.0	-
Bacteroides vulgatus[a]	21.0	+
Bifidobacterium bifidum	30.5	-
Clostridium perfringens (8)	33.6-43.1	+++
Lactobacillus casei sub. casei	33.5	-
Lactobacillus sp. (4)	21.1-47.3	-
Organisms utilizing 5-20% lactulose		
Bacteroides distasonis[a] (3)	11.5-19.5	-
Bacteroides fragilis (6)	9.0-13.5	+
Bacteroides ovatus (2)	5.0-8.1	+
Bacteroides thetaiotaomicron (3)	5.0-8.0	+
Bacteroides uniformis (3)	9.4-13.5	+
Bacteroides vulgatus[a]	9.8	+
Clostridium butyricum (3)	7.5-19.0	++
Clostridium cadaveris (2)	5.0-17.5	++
Clostridium difficile (2)	5.0-13.8	++
Enterobacter aerogenes	12.0	+
Escherichia coli	5.0	+
Klebsiella aerogenes	9.6	-
Lactobacillus acidophilus (2)	10.0-13.1	-
Peptostreptococcus anaerobius	13.2	-
Proteus mirabilis	10.0	++
Proteus vulgaris	11.6	++
Staphylococcus aureus	16.1	++
Streptococcus faecalis	7.0	-
Streptococcus intermedius	6.0	+
Streptococcus sp.	6.6	+
Streptococcus viridans	8.8	+

* Number of strains shown in parentheses if more than one used.

[a] Galactose and/or fructose found in the culture medium after growth.

Adapted from Sahota, Bramley and Menzies (15).

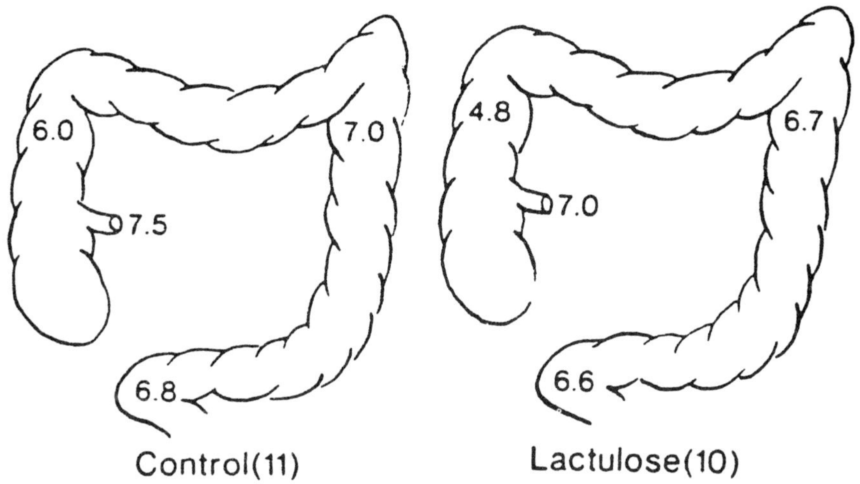

FIGURE 2. Mean values of pH along the intestinal tract in basal state and after lactulose. Lactulose in moderate dosage reduced pH in the cecum, but only slightly elsewhere. pH values are median levels determined by radiotelemetry capsule (after Bown et al. [31]). (Reprinted by permission from Conn HO and Lieberthal MM: The Hepatic Coma Syndromes and Lactulose ©1979 The Williams & Wilkins Co., Baltimore).

larger doses of lactulose are administered, as is the case in the treatment of portal-systemic encephalopathy, the drop in pH is usually maintained throughout the colon and the stool (32-35).

BACTERIAL METABOLISM OF LACTULOSE

The degradation of lactulose to its acid metabolites is considered to be the result of ß-galactosidase action, which is followed by lactic acid fermentation (10) (Figure 3). Mixed acid fermentation, characteristic of most enteric bacteria, then takes place. Most of their substrate goes through a fermentation characterized by the splitting of pyruvate to an acetyl group and formate, the remainder being disposed of through a lactic fermentation (36). Formic acid, acetic acid, and ethanol are formed from pyruvic acid, shown on the metabolic map in Figure 4.

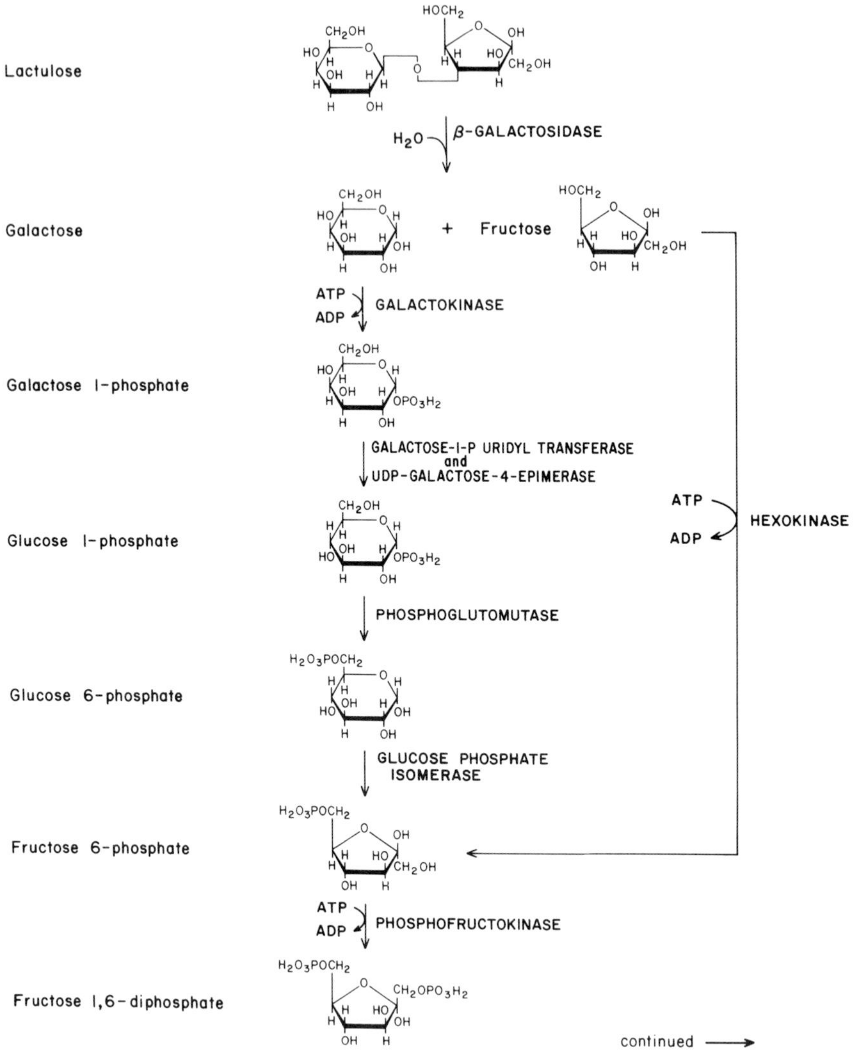

FIGURE 3. The bacterial degradation of lactulose. The metabolism of lactulose involves ß-galactosidase action followed by lactic acid fermentation. The steps in this process were graciously constructed by Robert Hook, Ph. D., of the Drug

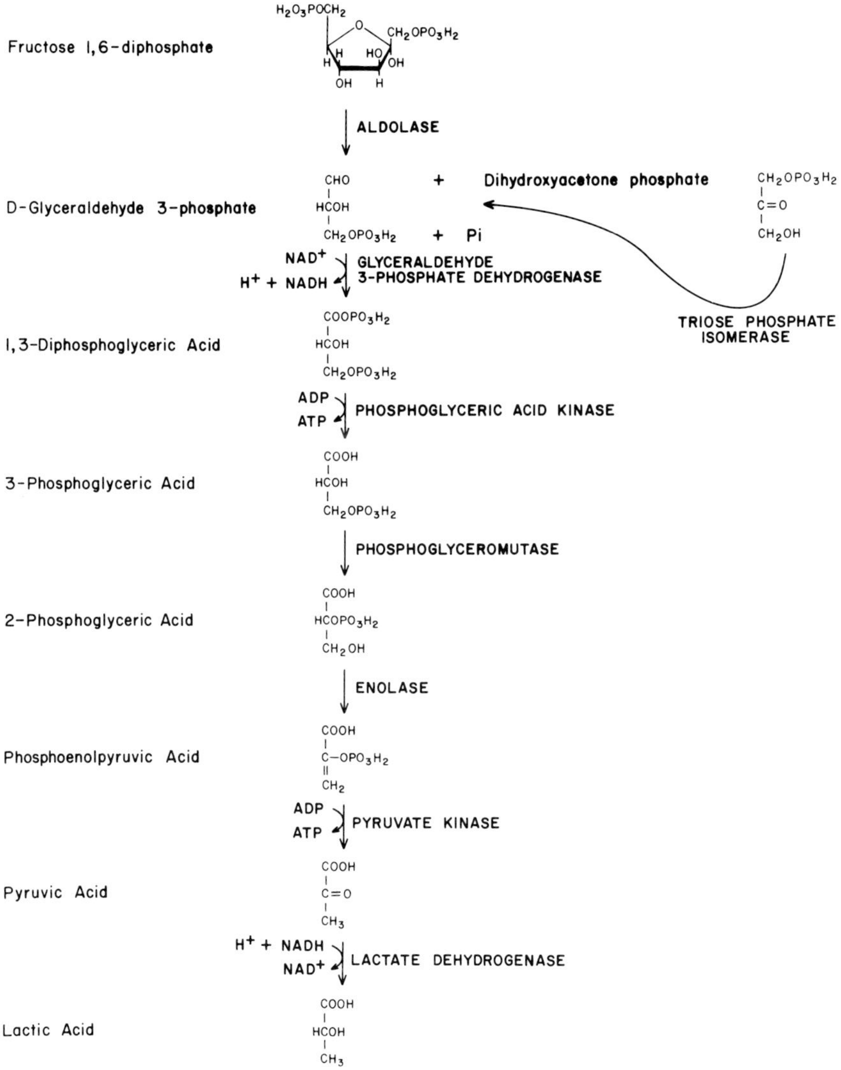

(FIGURE 3, continued) Metabolism Section, Merrell Dow Laboratories. (Reprinted by permission from Conn HO and Lieberthal MM: The Hepatic Coma Syndromes and Lactulose ©1979 The Williams & Wilkins Co., Baltimore).

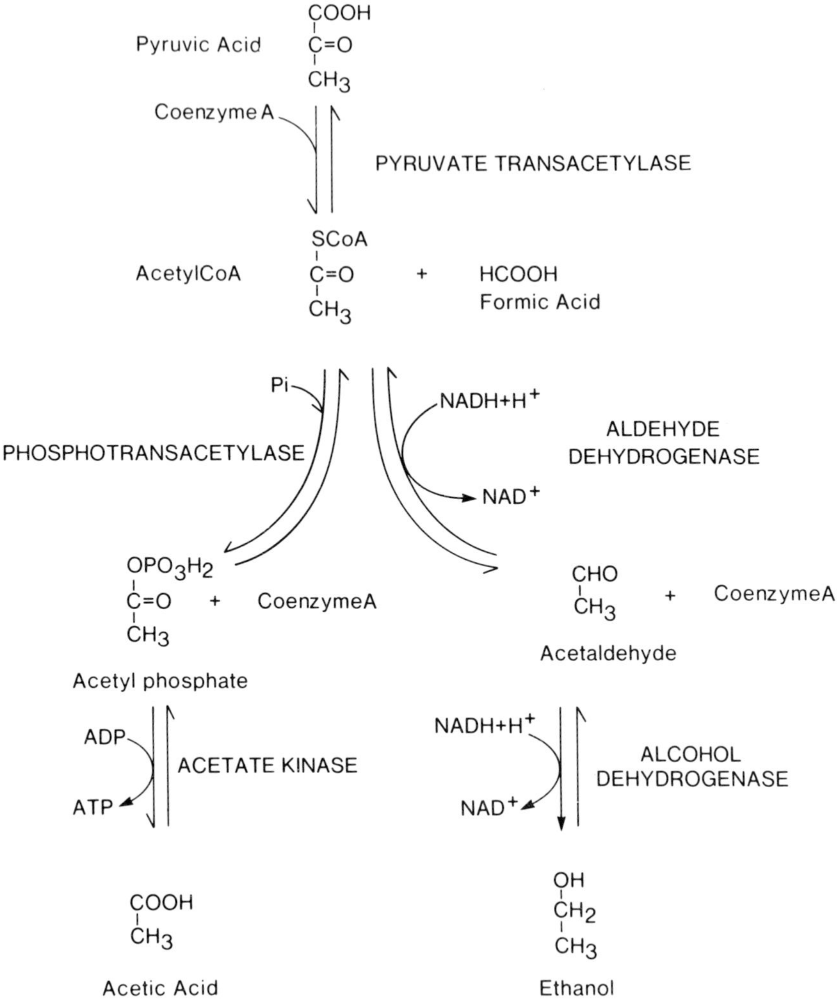

FIGURE 4. The final steps in the bacterial degradation of lactulose. Pyruvic acid is converted to formic and acetic acids. The acids occur in much smaller amounts than the principal metabolite, lactic acid. This schema is based on a bacterial metabolic map devised by Robert Hook, Ph. D. (Reprinted by permission from Conn HO and Lieberthal MM: The Hepatic Coma Syndromes and Lactulose ©1979 The Williams & Wilkins Co., Baltimore).

POTENTIAL OR ESTABLISHED THERAPEUTIC EFFECTS OF LACTULOSE

Effect of Lactulose on Excretion. Since lactulose is not metabolized in the small intestine, it is essentially unabsorbed. As a result, lactulose reaches the colon unchanged, there to be promptly metabolized by various colonic bacteria. It remains only to record what happens as the result of that encounter.

Very early in the studies of lactulose, it was noted that the metabolites of lactulose, lactic and pyruvic acids, have laxative effects (37), consisting of an increase in the frequency of defecation and softening of the stool. No effect on motor function of rabbit intestine or on the intestinal nervous system of cats and dogs could be found to explain these effects. It was also noted that lactulose relieved constipation in a very satisfactory manner without becoming habit-forming.

The part the acidification of colonic contents might be playing in this laxative effect was suggested by studies of the effect of pH on intestinal propulsion in guinea pigs (38) (Table 8). It was noted that a lowered pH increased propulsive waves, independent of the acid used (Figure 5). It has been presumed that the same effect occurs in the human colon. Further, the acid metabolites of lactulose appear to increase osmotic pressure in the colon four-fold (39, 40). The resulting increase in water content increases the bulk of the colonic contents, which, coupled with the smooth-muscle stimulating acidity, is apparently responsible for lactulose-induced laxation.

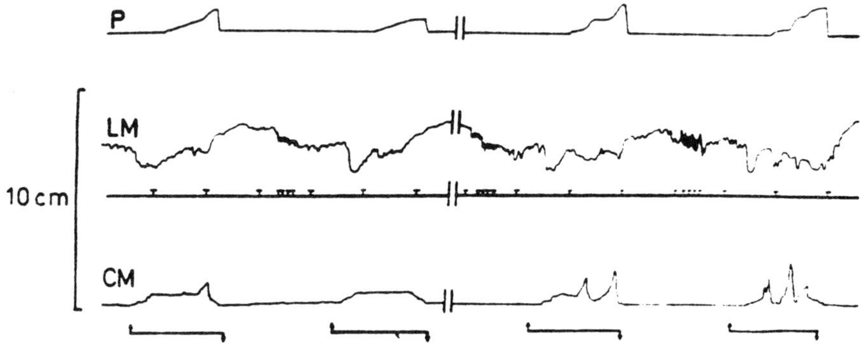

FIGURE 5. The effect of acid on the propulsive waves (P) in guinea pig intestine. When acid solution was infused at the break in the tracing, the area under the propulsive waves representing propulsive activity increased substantially. Longitudinal muscle (LM) and circular muscle (CM) were stimulated to a lesser degree. (Reprinted with permission from Bennett A and Eley KG: Intestinal pH and propulsion: an explanation of diarrhoea in lactase deficiency and laxation by lactulose. J Pharm Pharmacol © 1976; 28:192-195.)

TABLE 8. Effect of pH on Muscle Activity of Guinea Pig Intestine (10)

			Effect in ileum on		
Infused solution*	% concentration	Resulting intraluminal pH (ileum)	Propulsion	Circular muscle activity	Longitudinal muscle activity
Lactic acid	0.05-0.5	3-6	Increased by 21%	Increased	Increased
Sodium lactate		No effect	Reduced by 23%	Decreased	No effect
Lactulose	0.4-4	No effect	Reduced by 14%	Decreased	No effect
HCl	0.012	3-5	Increased by 33%	Increased	Increased
HCl	0.5	4.6	Increased	Increased	Temporary increase
Bicarbonate-free Krebs (control)		No effect or reduced	No effect	No effect	No effect
Bicarbonate-free Krebs, acidified to pH 5					

Based on the data of Bennett and Eley (38).
* Solutions were infused intraluminally in the ileum at the rate of 2.25 to 18 ml per h^1.

Effect on Intestinal Absorption. Lactulose was shown to cause a steatorrhea which proved to be reversible during a 3- to 6-day recovery period (41). Stool fat averaged 26.3 g per day in three cirrhotic patients who received 30-35 ml of lactulose syrup three times daily for ten days. Two obese control subjects averaged 9 g of fecal fat on the same regimen. Stool frequency, fecal sodium excretion, and fecal potassium excretion all rose. Stool pH fell. There were no changes in serum electrolytes or fecal nitrogen excretion. Fecal bile acid excretion rose 93% in the two patients in whom this was measured, and fecal sterols rose 27%.

An increase in bile acid excretion is perceived as a distinct benefit by many clinicians. The quantity of bile acids in the enterohepatic circulation helps control the synthesis of cholesterol by a negative feedback mechanism. The greater the loss of bile acids in the stool, the lower the body stores of cholesterol. When 62 hypercholesterolemic subjects (serum cholesterol >280 mg per 100 ml) were given 30 to 60 ml lactulose for one month, a 20.7% decrease in mean serum cholesterol

	Effect in colon on				
Stimulant effect compared to control	Resulting intraluminal pH (colon)	Propulsion	Circular muscle activity	Longitudinal muscle activity	Stimulant effect compared to control
Significant (2 $p<0.006$) compared to bicarbonate-free Krebs	3.5-5	Increased by 27%	Increased	Little effect	Significant (2 $p=0.004$) compared to sodium lactate
Not significantly different		Inhibited by 29%			
Not significantly different					
Significantly different (2 $p=0.004$)	4.3-4.8	Increased 45-47%	Increased	Little effect	
	5.7	Increased	Increased	No effect	

levels ($p<0.01$) occurred in 51 subjects and a decrease of similar significance was seen in the other 11 subjects after a second month of treatment (42). This cholesterol-lowering effect is not specific for lactulose, however. A hydrophilic colloid has been shown to have the same effect, presumably also by increasing fecal bile acid excretion (43).

Lactulose ingestion may also affect the cholesterol content of bile (44). Ten healthy women took from 39 to 60 g of lactulose daily for six weeks. Bile was collected by duodenal intubation before and immediately after the six weeks. All subjects showed a fall in the percentage of deoxycholic acid (mean 28.4±SEM 3.7 to 15.6±2.4; $p<0.002$) and a rise in the percentage of chenodeoxycholic acid (mean 33.2±3.2 to 42.9±2.9; $p<0.001$). The mean percentage of cholic acid did not change significantly (Figure 6). Bile was initially supersaturated with cholesterol in most subjects and became less saturated with cholesterol in all but one (mean saturation index 1.40±0.11 to 1.19±0.07; $p<0.005$) (Figure 7). These data support the idea that

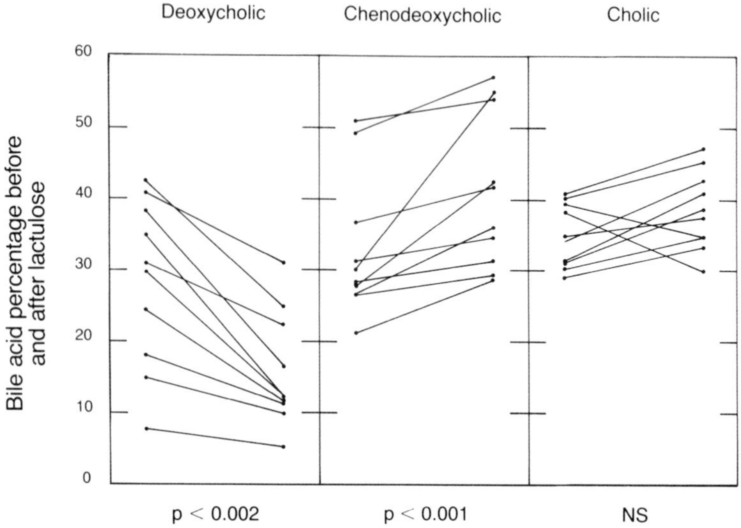

FIGURE 6. Effect of lactulose administration on biliary percentages of deoxycholic acid, chenodeoxycholic acid, and cholic acid. (Reprinted by permission from Thornton JR and Heaton KW. Do colonic bacteria contribute to cholesterol gall-stone formation? Effects of lactulose on bile. © 1981 Br Med J; 282:1018-1019.)

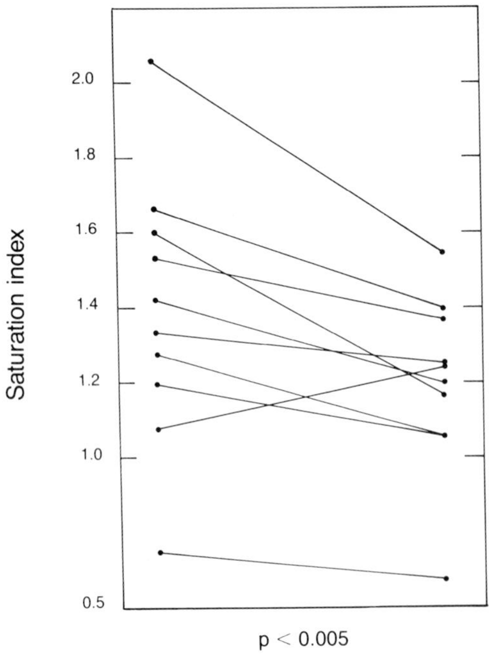

FIGURE 7. Effect of lactulose administration on bile cholesterol saturation index. (Reprinted by permission from Thornton JR and Heaton KW. Do colonic bacteria contribute to cholesterol gall-stone formation? Effects of lactulose on bile. © 1981 Br Med J; 282:1018-1019.)

TABLE 9. Effect of Lactulose on Fecal Bile Acids and Cholesterol Metabolism

	Lactulose (8 pts)		Control (8 pts)	
	Before	After	Before	After
Bowel movements (n./24h)	0.8	1.6	0.7	0.8
Fecal wet weight (g/24h)	128	177	136	141
Fecal pH	6.4	6.0	6.3	6.2
Cholesterol absorption (%)	—	40.2	—	46.6[a]
Fecal bile acids (mg/24h)	358	566[b]	388	365
Fecal neutral sterols (mg/24)	868	917	796	814
% primary fecal bile acids	10.8	18.6	9.2	8.9
Sterol balance (mg/24h)[c]	726	993[b]	694	665

[a] $p<0.02$; [b] $p<0.01$; [c] Sterol balance = (fecal bile acids + fecal neutral sterols) - dietary cholesterol. Adapted from Salvioli and Lugli (45).

the supersaturation of bile with cholesterol due to colonic bacterial activity can be reduced by lactulose administration. Presumably, a decrease in the incidence of cholesterol gallstones would follow.

A more recent study (45) confirmed the increase in fecal bile acid excretion that follows lactulose administration. Sixteen male subjects aged 67 to 75 years, free of metabolic or gastrointestinal disease, were placed on a constant diet containing 500 mg cholesterol for 30 days. On day 15, half of them were given 18 g lactulose in three daily administrations. The other eight acted as controls. Results of the evaluations of fecal bile acid excretion, neutral sterols, sterol balance, and fecal characteristics before and after lactulose are shown in Table 9. Absorption of exogenous cholesterol was evaluated at the end of treatment by the double isotope method. These investigators concluded that lactulose modifies the metabolism of cholesterol and bile acids in the intestine.

Effect on Endotoxin. When lactulose was fed to rats over a period of four to eight days preceding the intravenous administration of 0.5 g per kg of galactosamine, the liver damage that normally follows because of systemic endotoxemia of intestinal origin did not occur (46). This *in vivo* demonstration of the antiendotoxin effect of lactulose suggested its possible usefulness in certain clinical situations, such as some liver diseases, shock states, and gram negative sepsis, in which endotoxemia is of pathogenetic significance. However, the experimental model used in this study has been criticized (47).

In a later study, the incidence of endotoxemia and bacteremia was evaluated in 30 pigs with ischemic hepatic necrosis treated with hemodialysis (48). Twenty pigs pretreated with lactulose and magnesium sulfate for bowel cleansing failed to develop the preterminal endotoxemia experienced by the other ten pigs treated only with oral magnesium sulfate for bowel cleansing. The preterminal endotoxemia and bacteremia did not significantly influence survival. The authors felt that the prevention of endotoxemia was the result of the bowel cleansing effect of the two drugs, resulting in a diminished number of endotoxin-producing intestinal bacteria.

The clinical usefulness of these observations was subsequently underscored by a prospective study of the role of lactulose in preventing endotoxemia in patients with obstructive jaundice (49). Twelve patients with obstructive jaundice (plasma bilirubin level >100 mmol per L) undergoing surgery were given oral lactulose (30 ml every 6 hours as the syrup) for three days preceding operation and 12 patients with obstructive jaundice of similar intensity acted as controls. Blood aspirated from a peripheral vein before and after operation and analyzed for endotoxin levels and portal blood aspirated during operation revealed significantly fewer episodes of endotoxemia (plasma endotoxin level >100 mg per ml) in both operative portal and postoperative systemic blood samples in the lactulose group compared to the control group. Further, the incidence of postoperative acute renal failure, which is considered to be associated with the presence of endotoxins in the systemic circulation, was lower in the lactulose-treated group. In the control group, three patients had preoperative and six patients had postoperative renal impairment as measured by 24-hour creatinine clearance. In the lactulose group, two patients had preoperative and only one patient had postoperative renal impairment. The difference between the two groups was significant. In another part of this same work, this time performed on jaundiced rats receiving both endotoxin and lead acetate, the mortality among those pretreated with lactulose was 25% in contrast to the 83% mortality among rats not pretreated. The difference was significant ($p<0.05$). In an associated *in vitro* experiment, lactulose produced a 400-fold decrease in the measurable level of endotoxin.

Apparently, lactulose has a direct and clinically valuable antiendotoxin effect.

CONCLUSION

It is rare to find a substance whose pharmacology is so intimately relevant to the disease states for which it is most commonly administered, namely chronic constipation and portal-systemic encephalopathy. The absence of small intestinal absorption of lactulose itself, and its minimal effect on small intestinal secretion and absorption of other substances make it an ideal drug for long-term use. The drop in pH and increase in osmotic pressure confined to the colon constitute an exaggeration of the physiologic mechanism for laxation in the normal human as currently perceived. Moreover, the further dose-related increase in colonic acidity adds the key effect that converts the colon from an organ responsible for ammonia generation to an organ into which ammonia is dialyzed, with resulting relief of portal-systemic encephalopathy.

TOXICOLOGY

Every marketable drug worth its salt has a certain benefit-to-risk ratio that expresses whether its efficacy outweighs its complications. The possible spectra obviously cover a wide range. In one direction, there are the categories of little benefit, no complications; moderate benefit with some complications; or great benefit and severe complications. In the other direction, there are the categories of great benefit, minimal complications; moderate benefit, moderate complications; and little benefit, severe complications. The disease for which treatment is being given obviously dictates which benefit-to-risk ratio is acceptable. In the case of lactulose, the great benefit, minimal risk category continues to be appropriate, as many studies in animals and humans indicate.

Animal Studies. *Acute toxicity* (short-term administration) studies to determine the LD_{50} levels of lactulose syrup (administered via stomach tube) for rodents and dogs (50, 51) were carried out on fasting or newborn animals and calculated by the graphical method of Litchfield and Wilcoxin (52). The LD_{50} levels appeared to be similar for the mouse and hamster (Table 10). Emesis was produced in dogs at a dose of 25 ml per kg in 1 to 2 hours post-dosing. There were no clinical signs at the dose of 15 ml per kg.

An attempt to obtain LD_{50} for lactulose syrup in a baboon (51) was unsuccessful, again because the animal couldn't retain the large volume (130 ml

TABLE 10. Determination of LD_{50} of Lactulose (10)

Species	Sex	Wt in g	No. per group	No. of groups	Dose (ml/kg)	LD_{50} (ml/kg)	(95%conf. limits) (ml/kg)
Mice (Swiss)[a]	F	18-24	10	7	10-50	48.8	(47-51)
Rats (Wistar)	F	106-210	10	3	10-30	>30.[b]	
Hamster (Syrian)[c]	M,F	54-80	10	5	10-50	41.3	(35-49)
Dogs (mongrel)	M,F	11-13	2	2	15-25	>25.[d]	
Guinea pigs (albino)	F	500-700	7	1	"massive"[e]	>15	

[a] Decreased activity, ataxia, and tremors. Death in 70 min to 24 hr from respiratory failure.

[b] Statistical LD_{50} values not obtained due to large volumes involved.

[c] Depression, ataxia, prostration and death in from 80 min to several days from respiratory failure.

[d] Emesis occurred in 1-2 hr after 25-ml/kg dose. Statistical LD_{50} values not obtained due to large volumes involved.

[e] Each dose was different, given within a 6-hr period by gavage in sufficient volume to distend the stomach to its maximum.

3 times over a 4-hour period) necessary to complete the calculation. The baboon vomited twice and became comatose for a period, developed diarrhea and mild dehydration, but did recover. It appeared unlikely that the LD_{50} could be determined for this species, and it was assumed to be in excess of 37 ml per kg.

By way of comparison, the usual lactulose dose for the human is 40 to 100 g daily (60-150 ml of the syrup or 0.6-1.5 g per kg of body weight) divided into four doses. In the experimental animals shown in Table 10, the LD_{50} runs from 50 to 150 times greater than the total daily dose, based solely on body weight. Actually, due to the low toxicity of lactulose, the determination of the LD_{50} proved to be impossible in four of the animal species tested, which many clinicians will find very comforting. However, comprehensive LD_{50}s were not done.

Chronic toxicity (long-term administration) studies have also been carried out in rats, dogs, pigs and baboons. The periods of observation ranged from four weeks to two years. One toxicity study of 80 young Sprague-Dawley rats (90-120 g) over a 3-month period failed to find any toxic change due to lactulose treatment of up to 40 ml per kg per day in any of the treated animals (51). Weight, and hematologic and blood chemistry determinations showed no significant differences between the treated animals and controls. All the rats that died during the study (four of the controls and six treated animals) revealed evidence of chronic respiratory infection at autopsy.

Another two-year toxicity study of 25 male and 25 female Sprague-Dawley rats gave similar results (53). No changes were found attributable to lactulose treatment, which was added to the diet at concentrations up to 15%. Weekly examinations of the eyes showed no evidence of adverse effect. No cataracts appeared during the two years of observation. No evidence of carcinogenicity was found.

A two-year study was also carried out involving 20 beagle dogs administered lactulose syrup at a once-a-day daily dose of 4 or 12 ml per kg by intubation (54). The lactulose-treated dogs occasionally vomited and usually had watery or soft stools. The majority of treated dogs exhibited excessive shedding and regrowth of hair at various times during the experiment. The controls did not exhibit this phenomenon, which was attributed to a marginally disturbed nutritional state on the basis of the vomiting and loose stools. Body weights, however, were not affected. All dogs were sacrificed and autopsied at the conclusion of the study. Aside from some misplaced test material in the lungs of six dogs, no differences from controls attributable to lactulose treatment were found.

Twelve 10-day-old piglets were also used for subchronic (5-week) studies of lactulose toxicity (55). In addition to the usual clinical appearance and hematologic findings, a comparison was made between the influence of the addition to the diet of 10% (v/w) of lactulose (as a dry powder) and the addition of 10%(v/w) of lactose. Diarrhea occurred in both groups during the first three weeks of treatment. Food consumption in grams of dry matter and body weight gain were

TABLE 11. Lactulose Influence on Weight, Feed Consumption, and Food Efficiency in Piglets (10)

Experimental period	On lactose			On lactulose		
	Growth (g)	Feed consumed (g)	Food efficiency*	Growth (g)	Feed consumed (g)	Food efficiency*
1st week	382	985	2.58	710	1137	1.60
2nd week	1163	1641	1.41	995	1482	1.49
3rd week	1950	2195	1.13	2285	2170	0.95
4th week	3790	3747	0.99	3747	4050	1.08
5th week	4798	6008	1.25	4500	4811	1.07

* Defined as feed consumption per g of weight increase.

calculated at weekly intervals. "Food efficiency" was then calculated as the grams of feed consumed per gram of weight increase. Over the period of observation, there was slight food efficiency difference in favor of the lactulose-added diet (Table 11). Body weight gain was not affected by either diet, nor were there any gross or microscopic pathologic findings at autopsy in any of the animals.

The final animal species studied for chronic (6 months) lactulose toxicity consisted of 18 young baboons fed lactulose in doses that ranged from 2 to 3 times to 10 to 15 times the average therapeutic dose in man (20-30 g per day) (51). Body weights and general condition were examined weekly. Blood chemistry values were obtained six times during the study. The usual battery of hematologic determinations was obtained, plus bromsulphalein tests. Urines were examined and all animals were autopsied. All animals except one remained healthy. That one was a control animal that died during the first week. Autopsy failed to establish a cause. Hematologic and blood chemistry findings were within normal limits. Six animals given high doses of lactulose syrup had small amounts of sugar in the urine. At the end of the study, only three of them still showed some sugar. There were no findings at autopsy that were related to lactulose treatment.

An 18-month carcinogenicity study in the CD-1 mouse treated with either 3% or 10% (v/w) lactulose syrup was also carried out. No clinical signs related to treatment or evidence of carcinogenicity were shown (56).

Thus, rats, dogs, pigs and baboons tolerated and survived relatively massive doses of lactulose syrup when compared to projected therapeutic doses in the human. It is to be hoped that other species fare as well.

Toxicity of nonanalyzed by-products of lactulose syrup was tested by comparing them with the toxicity of lactulose syrup, pure lactulose and distilled water (57). The nonanalyzed by-products comprise 3.1% of lactulose syrup and were separated from the principal components of the syrup, lactulose, lactose and galactose, by repeated column chromatography. The separated fraction was finally shown to consist of at least five components. Tagatose, a ketohexose isomer of levulose was identified as one component, but the other components remain unidentified sugars. Testing of the by-products was done in female, albino, Swiss mice and no toxic effects were suffered at any dose level.

Teratogenic effects of lactulose administration were tested for in mice (58), rats (59, 60) and rabbits (61), the three most commonly used species for this type of study. Observations were made on the number of fetuses, placement in the uterus, number of stillborn, number of live births, implantation and resorption sites, weight at birth and malformations. Four groups of 20 female mice each received 6 ml lactulose syrup per kg, 12 ml lactulose syrup per kg, 12 ml isosmotic glucose solution per kg, or served as untreated controls. There were no alterations or adverse effects that could be attributed to lactulose administration. Two groups of Sprague-Dawley rats were also studied, using the same criteria for evidence of teratogenic effect. No such effect attributable to lactulose was identified. The same results were obtained in the teratogenicity studies conducted with New Zealand white rabbits. About half the group of 16 rabbits that received 6 ml lactulose syrup per kg developed some diarrhea, and two rabbits died of nondosing causes. There was some inhibition in body weight gain. The doses of lactulose did not appear to be associated with any embryotoxic teratogenic effects.

Actually, the question of teratogenic effect from lactulose syrup is moot as far as its use in the treatment of portal-systemic encephalopathy is concerned. Cirrhosis is characterized by amenorrhea, oligomenorrhea, and nonovulatory cycling in the female (62) and impotence in the male (63). The incidence of pregnancy is understandably very low when such patients are involved. The delivery of viable infants is even lower.

HUMAN STUDIES

Observations on the occurrence of side effects and adverse reactions have been made on both normal humans and patients with portal-systemic encephalopathy complicating cirrhosis of the liver.

One unpublished study involved 75 healthy, male, prisoner volunteers (64). Twenty-nine lactulose-treated and 18 placebo-treated subjects completed the study which lasted three months. Subjects received a daily dose of 30 ml of lactulose syrup (20 g of lactulose) or glucose as a placebo. The most commonly reported side effects were flatulence, complained of by 96% of the placebo group and 98% of the lactulose group, and diarrhea. Flatulence occurred more often in the lactulose group (43 of 83 days) than in the placebo group (28 of 83 days). Diarrhea was also more frequent in the lactulose group than in the placebo group. Other nonspecific gastrointestinal side effects, which included nausea, anorexia, cramping and rectal burning, occurred in 41.7% of the lactulose group and 16% of the placebo group. The difference was significant ($p<0.05$). No abnormal physical findings attributable to lactulose administration were identified. No related eye changes took place. An eosinophilia was found in the tested groups—both treated and controls—but this was found to be endemic in the general prison population and of no special significance in terms of lactulose toxicity. Various other laboratory determinations of hematologic and chemical elements showed no differences between treated and control subjects. Actually, the side effects noted in this prison population were those related to the desired laxative effects of lactulose, and are ordinarily managed by dose reduction.

An unpublished study of intestinal absorption and electrolyte secretion resulting from lactulose administration was carried out in four healthy, obese subjects and five cirrhotic patients (65). In general, values for fecal excretion tended to increase during lactulose administration (Table 12), whereas urine D-xylose and Vitamin B_{12} decreased. The same trends were noted in both the obese and cirrhotic subjects. No adverse effects were noted.

Suspecting that the increased excretion of nitrogen during lactulose treatment might well be beneficial, German and Japanese investigators have administered lactulose syrup to patients with impaired renal function. In one study of eight patients with chronic renal failure (66), lactulose treatment resulted in increased excretion of nitrogen in the stool from 1.3 to 2.34 g per day ($p<0.05$) and

TABLE 12. Effect of Lactulose on Excretion and Absorption (10)

Excretion	Unit of measure	No. of subjects	Average during control period	Average during lactulose period*	% of change
Fecal					
Sodium	mEq/day	8	3.4 (0.8-8.2)	13.0 (3.6-29.7)	282
Potassium	mEq/day	8	13.9 (3.6-32.1)	19.8 (4.2-42.0)	42
Nitrogen	g/day	8	1.9 (0.3-7.0)	3.6 (1.2-13.8)	89
Fat	g/day	9	6.4 (3.7-11.1)	17.6 (10.4-39.0)	175
Neutral sterols	mg/day	8	518.0 (273-980)	876.0 (373-2267)	69
Bile acids	mg/day	8	154.0 (80-248)	257.0 (143-410)	67
Urinary					
D-xylose	g/5 hr	6	7.2 (3.3-8.5)	6.5 (3.9-10.6)	-11
Vitamin B_{12}	%/24 hr	7	16.9 (6.9-24.0)	12.0 (4.8-20.0)	-29

* The highest single reading obtained on lactulose therapy was used in the calculation of averages.

decreased excretion in the urine from 9 to 7.8 g per day. Serum urea fell significantly from 28.3 to 21.2 mmol per L ($p<0.005$). The Japanese study (67) involved 15 patients with chronic renal failure who received an initial dose of 30 ml of lactulose, later raised to 45 ml in four patients and to 60 ml in nine. Most of the patients passed soft stools. The results indicated that lactulose decreased the serum concentration of urea, guanidinosuccinic acid, methylguanidine and phosphate, and suggested that lactulose might be useful for the therapy of chronic renal failure.

The initial case report in 1977 of severe hypernatremia associated with the administration of lactulose in the treatment of a cirrhotic patient with portal-systemic encephalopathy seemed to be more the result of diarrhea for which no dose modification was ordered than of the lactulose *per se* (68). Since that article, additional episodes of hypernatremia have been reported from Japan, the United States and Canada (69-72). In each of the 23 patients, the hypernatremia seemed to be associated with an excess loss of hypotonic fluid in the stools in excess of sodium, resulting in contraction of extracellular fluid volume and hypernatremia. Increased administration of intravenous fluids and discontinuation of lactulose were corrective in most instances. One of the studies (70) showed that the mortality among 20 patients whose sodium level exceeded 145 mEq per L was 41%. The mortality among the 50 who remained eunatremic was 14%. Unfortunately, it is not possible to draw precise conclusions from this series since the patients fell into the broad category of "hepatic failure" when other causes may be responsible for the hypernatremia, such as insufficient antidiuretic hormone (ADH), lack of renal tubular response to ADH, mineralocorticoid effect, or even primary hypernatremia.

Regardless, it seems quite clear that lactulose therapy in cirrhotic patients should be monitored by observations of stool frequency and consistency and serum sodium levels.

Serum D-lactic and L-lactic acid levels were determined after oral lactulose administration in ten patients with histologically proven cirrhosis (73). Oral lactulose, 30 ml three times daily, was given until stool pH was lower than 5.5. No alteration in blood pH occurred. Serum L-lactic acid levels rose slightly. No D-lactic acid was detected in the blood at any time. However, another report (74) called attention to the fact that lactic acid, a breakdown product of lactulose, may be reabsorbed in the colon if the patient is unable to pass any stools, and thus cause lactic acidosis. The patient presented to illustrate this series of events was a 31-year-old man who had adynamic ileus secondary to uremic enteropathy. Inability to empty the bowel is unusual when therapeutic doses of lactulose are administered. It seems unlikely that this scenario could become common or clinically important.

The most commonly reported side effects are gastrointestinal in origin and consist of gaseousness which is usually transient, diarrhea, abdominal pain and vomiting. In one review of 198 patients treated with lactulose (10) reported in the literature from 1968 to 1974 by a variety of investigators, 47 were recorded as having gaseousness, 32 abdominal pain, 27 diarrhea, and 1 vomiting. Subsequent reports have done little to change this general impression.

SUMMARY

All in all, lactulose survives the many diligent searches for untoward effects remarkably well. Those that do occur with any regularity are associated with degradation of carbohydrate in the colon and are dose related, by and large. The diarrhea that may occur is really an overdose response rather than an intrinsic side effect. Diarrhea is not necessary for the success of treatment with lactulose, and the hypernatremia reported in association with lactulose therapy is more likely due to the loss of fecal fluid than to lactulose treatment *per se*. No reports of damage to heart, liver or kidneys, to blood-forming organs, or to hormone relationships have appeared. Side effects that were anticipated years ago to be in the offing (10) when increased usage of lactulose took place have so far failed to materialize.

Valuable contributions to the form and substance of this chapter were cheerfully provided by Michael Palfreyman, PhD, and John Yarrington, DVM, PhD, and are herewith gratefully acknowledged.

REFERENCES

1. Tanaka F. Experimental and clinical studies on digestion, absorption and utilization of lactulose. Bull Kobe Med Coll 1962; 212:328-338.
2. Dahlqvist A, Gryboski JD. Inability of the human small-intestinal lactase to hydrolyze lactulose. Biochim Biophys Acta 1965; 10:635-636.
3. Carulli N, Salvioli GF, Manenti F. Absorption of lactulose in man. Digestion 1972; 6:139-145.
4. Laker MF, Menzies IS. Increase in human intestinal permeability following ingestion of hypertonic solutions. J Physiol 1977; 265:881-894.
5. Muller M, Walker-Smith J, Shmerling DH, et al. Lactulose: a gas-liquid chromatography method of determination and evaluation of its use to assess intestinal mucosal damage. Clin Chim Acta 1969; 24:45-49.
6. Beach RC, Menzies IS, Clayden GS, et al. Gastrointestinal permeability changes in the preterm neonate. Arch Dis Child 1982; 57:141-145.
7. Adachi S, Patton S. Presence and significance of lactulose in milk products: a review. J Dairy Sci 1961; 44:1375-1393.
8. Gryboski JD, Zillis J, Ma OH. A study of fecal sugars by high voltage electrophoresis. Gastroenterology 1964; 47:26-31.
9. Gryboski JD, Boehm JJ. Lactulosuria in the neonate: a preliminary report. Pediatrics 1965; 35:340-341.
10. Conn HO, Lieberthal MM. The Hepatic Coma Syndromes and Lactulose. Baltimore: The Williams and Wilkins Co., ©1979.

11. Gerritsen T, Lemli L, Ptacek LJ, et al. The presence of lactulose in the urine of infants with lactosuria. Pediatrics 1963; 32:1033-1038.

12. Hinohara Y, Zuzuke S. Studies on absorption and excretion of lactulose in man. Oyo Yakuri 1974; 8:417-420.

13. Hoffmann K, Mossel DA, Korus W, et al. Investigations on the mode of action of lactulose (ß-galactosido-fructose) in the human intestine. Klin Wochenschr 1964; 42:126-130.

14. Liem KS. Biochemical report on the absorption of lactulose. N.V. Philips-Duphar, Clinical Research Department, Weesp, Dec. 1966, Report no. 5/56874. Project Report A-71-42, on file, Merrell Dow Pharmaceuticals Inc., Cincinnati, OH 45242-9553.

15. Sahota SS, Bramley PM, Menzies IS. The fermentation of lactulose by colonic bacteria. J Gen Microbiol 1982; 128:319-325.

16. Hosaka H, Tokunaga K, Sakumoto I, et al. The influence of lactulose on intestinal absorption. Gastroenterol Jpn 1972; 7:316-317.

17. Code CF. The semantics of the process of absorption. Perspect Biol Med 1960; 3:561-562.

18. Axon ATR, Creamer B. The exsorption characteristics of various sugars. Gut 1975; 16:99-104.

19. Atherton DJ, Heddle RJ, Boulton P. Intestinal permeability in atopic eczema. Br J Dermatol 1984; 3 (suppl 26):34-35.

20. DuMont GCL, Beach RC, Menzies IS. Gastrointestinal permeability in food-allergic eczematous children. Clin Allergy 1984; 14:55-59.

21. Forget PP, Leclercq J, Van Cutsem JL. Lactulose - rhamnose intestinal permeability in children with cystic fibrosis (Abstract). Dig Dis Sci 1986; 31:293S.

22. Mooradian AD, Morley JE, Levine AS, et al. Abnormal intestinal permeability to sugars in diabetes mellitus. Diabetologia 1986; 29:221-224.

23. Cook GC, Menzies IS. Intestinal absorption and unmediated permeation of sugars in post-infective tropical malabsorption (tropical sprue). Digestion 1986; 33:109-116.

24. Menzies IS. Absorption of intact oligosaccharide in health and disease. Biochem Soc Trans 1974; 2:1042-1047.

25. Ukabam SO, Cooper BT. Small intestinal permeability to mannitol, lactulose, and polyethylene glycol 400 in celiac disease. Dig Dis Sci 1984; 29:809-816.

26. Ukabam SO, Clamp JR, Cooper BT. Abnormal small intestinal permeability to sugars in patients with Crohn's disease of the terminal ileum and colon. Digestion 1983; 27:70-74.

27. Parrilli G, Iaffaioli RV, Capuono G, et al. Changes in intestinal permeability to lactulose induced by cytotoxic therapy. Cancer Treat Rep 1982; 66:1435-1436.

28. Cooper BT. Small intestinal permeability in clinical practice. J Clin Gastroenterol 1984; 6:499-501.

29. Wheeler PG, Menzies IS, Creamer B. Effect of hyperosmolar stimuli and coeliac disease on the permeability of the human gastrointestinal tract. Clin Sci Molec Med 1978; 54:495-501.

30. ten Ham EJ. Biochemical experiments with lactulose. NV. Philips-Duphar Research Laboratories, Report no. 55641/28/1962. Project Report A-71-12, on file Merrell Dow Pharmaceuticals Inc., Cincinnati, OH 45242-9553.

31. Bown RL, Gibson JA, Sladen GE, et al. Effects of lactulose and other laxatives on ileal and colonic pH as measured by a radiotelemetry device. Gut 1974; 15:999-1004.

32. Conn HO, Leevy CM, Vlahcevic ZR, et al. Comparison of lactulose and neomycin in the treatment of chronic portal-systemic encephalopathy: a double-blind controlled trial. Gastroenterology 1977; 72:573-583.

33. Elkington SG, Floch MH, Conn HO. Lactulose in the treatment of chronic portal-systemic encephalopathy. A double-blind clinical trial. N Engl J Med 1969; 281:408-412.

34. Fessel JM, Conn HO. Lactulose in the treatment of acute hepatic encephalopathy. Am J Med Sci 1973; 266:103-110.

35. Atterbury CE, Madrey WC, Conn HO, et al. Neomycin-sorbitol and lactulose in the treatment of acute portal-systemic encephalopathy. A controlled, double-blind clinical trial. Am J Dig Dis 1978; 23:398-406.

36. Davis BD, Dulbecco R, Eisen HN, et al. Microbiology. New York: Harper and Row, 1967: 60-62.

37. Mayerhofer F, Petuely F. Investigations regarding the regulation of the intestinal activity in adults with the aid of lactulose (bifidus factor). Wein Klin Wochenschr 1959; 71:865-869.

38. Bennett A, Eley KG. Intestinal pH and propulsion: an explanation of diarrhoea in lactase deficiency and laxation by lactulose. J Pharm Pharmacol 1976; 28:192-195.

39. Avery GS, Davies EF, Brogden RN: Lactulose: a review of its therapeutic and pharmacological properties with particular reference to ammonia metabolism and its mode of action in portal-systemic encephalopathy. Drugs 1972; 4:7-48.

40. Pertsiounis S, Egger G, Bircher J. Radiological "quantitation" of osmotic effect. From: Symposium on Lactulose, Baden near Vienna, Austria, September 8, 1969.

41. Lim EC, Rubulis A, Faloon WW. Effect of lactulose upon intestinal absorption (Abstract). Gastroenterology 1971; 60:782.

42. Conte D, Bardella MT, Bernardi R, et al. Hypocholesterolemic effect of lactulose in man. Panminerva Med 1977; 19:1-4.

43. Lieberthal MM, Martens RA. Lowered serum cholesterol following the ingestion of a hydrophilic colloid. Am J Dig Dis 1975; 20:469-474.

44. Thornton JR, Heaton KW. Do colonic bacteria contribute to cholesterol gall-stone formation? Effects of lactulose on bile. Brit Med J 1981; 282:1018-1019.

45. Salvioli G, Lugli R. Effects of lactulose on cholesterol and bile acid metabolism. Ital J Gastroenterol 1986; 18:65.

46. Liehr H, Englisch G, Rasenack U. Lactulose - a drug with antiendotoxin effect. Hepatogastroenterology 1980; 27:356-360.

47. van Vugt H, van Gool J, Thomas LLM. Galactosamine hepatitis, endotoxemia, and lactulose. Hepatology 1983; 3:236-240.

48. de Groot GH, Schalm SW, Batavier P, et al. Incidence of endotoxemia in pigs with ischemic hepatic necrosis treated by hemodialysis. Prevention of endotoxemia with lactulose. Hepatogastroenterology 1983; 30:240-242.

49. Pain JA, Bailey ME. Experimental and clinical study of lactulose in obstructive jaundice. Br J Surg 1986; 73:775-778.

50. Jones SM, Chudkowski M. A summary of the acute oral toxicity studies with W5489 (lactulose) in the mouse, rat, hamster and dog. Report number 1943, Warner Lambert Research Institute, 1966. Project Report A-71-52, on file, Merrell Dow Pharmaceuticals Inc., Cincinnati, OH 45242-9553.

51. Toxicological studies on Duphalac Syrup. Report to Crookes Laboratories Ltd., Basingstoke, Hants. Philips Roxane Laboratories Inc. Project Report A-72-57, on file, Merrell Dow Pharmaceuticals Inc., Cincinnati, OH 45242-9553.

52. Litchfield JT Jr, Wilcoxin F. A simplified method of evaluating dose-effect experiments. J Pharmacol Exp Ther 1949; 96:99-113.

53. Two year chronic oral toxicity study of lactulose on rats (1967). International Bio-Research, Inc., St. Louis and Hannover-Andersten, Germany. Project Report A-71-51, on file, Merrell Dow Pharmaceuticals Inc., Cincinnati, OH 45242-9553.

54. Grady KS, Gibson JP, Newberne JW. Report on the chronic (2-year) oral toxicity study with lactulose in dogs. Project Report T-74-40. Unpublished data on file at Merrell Dow Pharmaceuticals Inc., Cincinnati, OH 45242-9553.

55. de Groot AP. Investigation into any harmful effect of lactulose. I. Comparison of lactulose syrup with lactulose in a growth test with baby piglets. Central Institute of Food Research, Utrecht. Report no. R1162, 1960. Project report A-71-43, on file, Merrell Dow Pharmaceuticals Inc., Cincinnati, OH 45242-9553.

56. Carcinogenicity study in the mouse. Project Report T-78-19. Unpublished data on file at Merrell Dow Pharmaceuticals Inc., Cincinnati, OH 45242-9553.

57. Kemp A. Comparative acute oral toxicity of the "non-analyzed byproducts" from the preparation of Duphalac, Commercial Duphalac, pure lactulose, and distilled water, in the female mouse. Report no. 56645/2/69 Philips-Duphar, Weesp. February 1969, Project report A-71-50, on file, Merrell Dow Pharmaceuticals Inc., Cincinnati, OH 45242-9553.

58. Teratological study of lactulose on mice (1967). International Bio-Research, Inc., St. Louis and Hannover-Andersten, Germany. Project Report A-71-49, on file, Merrell Dow Pharmaceuticals Inc., Cincinnati, OH 45242-9553.

59. Teratological study of lactulose on rats (1966). International Bio-Research, Inc. St. Louis and Hannover-Andersten, Germany. Project Report A-71-48, on file,

Merrell Dow Pharmaceuticals Inc., Cincinnati, OH 45242-9553.

60. Effect of lactulose on the reproduction of rats. International Bio-Research Inc., St. Louis and Hannover-Andersten, Germany. Project Report A-71-47, on file, Merrell Dow Pharmaceuticals Inc., Cincinnati, OH 45242-9553.

61. Palmer AK, Fletcher MA. Effect of Duphalac Syrup upon pregnancy of the New Zealand white rabbit (1967). Huntingdon Research Center, Huntingdon, England. Project Report A-71-53, on file, Merrell Dow Pharmaceuticals Inc., Cincinnati, OH 45242-9553.

62. Haemmerli UP. Jaundice during pregnancy. The liver in normal pregnancy. In: Schiff L, ed. Diseases of the Liver, ed. 4. Philadelphia: J.B. Lippincott Company, 1975: 1336-1353.

63. Conn HO. Cirrhosis. In: Schiff L, ed. Diseases of the Liver, ed. 4. Philadelphia: J. B. Lippincott Company, 1975: 867.

64. Bodi T. A safety evaluation of lactulose in normal subjects. Unpublished data on file, Merrell Dow Pharmaceuticals Inc., Cincinnati, OH 45242-9553.

65. Faloon WW. The effect of lactulose upon intestinal absorption and electrolyte excretion. Unpublished data on file, Merrell Dow Pharmaceuticals Inc., Cincinnati, OH 45242-9553.

66. Wizemann V, Spring M, Rink W, et al. Lactulose in chronic renal failure: action on aromatic amines and phosphate (Abstract). Kidney Int 1983; 24 (suppl. 16):S341.

67. Miyazaki M, Aoyagi K, Tojo S. Lactulose therapy for chronic renal failure. Nippon Jinzo Gakkai Shi 1984; 26:1091-1098.

68. Kaupke C, Sprague T, Gitnick GL. Hypernatremia after the administration of lactulose (Correspondence). Ann Intern Med 1977; 86:745.

69. Ito M, Sawa H, Higashiyama S, et al. Hypernatremia during the treatment with lactulose. Mie Med J 1981; 31:321-326.

70. Nelson DC, McGrew WRG, Hoyumpa AM. Hypernatremia and lactulose therapy. JAMA 1983; 249:1295-1298.

71. Nanji AA, Lauener RW. Lactulose-induced hypernatremia. Drug Intell Clin Pharm 1984; 18:70-71.

72. Lusk JA. Hypernatremia due to lactulose. Bull Mason Clin 1986; 40:90.

73. Gitlin N, Popma JJ, Mann LT, et al. Serum D-lactic acid and L-lactic acid levels after oral lactulose administration (Abstract). Clin Res 1983; 31:31A.

74. Mann NS, Russman HB, Mann SK, et al. Lactulose and severe lactic acidosis (Correspondence). Ann Intern Med 1985; 103:637.

12

CLINICAL PHARMACOLOGY OF LACTULOSE

JOHANNES BIRCHER, M.D., AND DIETER ULLRICH, M.D.

The purpose of this review is to focus on some pertinent basic aspects of the clinical pharmacology of lactulose. Attention to this topic is particularly relevant, because in several respects lactulose is an unusual drug. Although its purpose is the treatment of an abnormality of the central nervous system, its main site of action is within the gut. Furthermore, neither the precise pathogenesis of portal-systemic encephalopathy (PSE) nor the exact mode of action of lactulose is really understood. Consequently, the pharmacology of lactulose has not been investigated in the conventional manner. Nevertheless, much experimental and clinical data have been accumulated over the years and they suggest that lactulose is a fascinating hybrid of a nutrient and a drug.

PHARMACOKINETICS OF LACTULOSE

Although there seems to be no enzyme for hydrolysis of lactulose in the human intestinal mucosa (1-3), many bacteria are able to metabolize it (4-7). Since most of these bacteria are located in the colon (8-11), it is generally agreed that lactulose is not hydrolyzed in the small intestine. With a molecular radius of 0.52 nm (12), only minute amounts of lactulose are passively absorbed and almost all of the dose is transported intact to the colon (13-18).

It is reasonable to assume that in humans no enzymes exist that can metabolize the minute amount of lactulose that is absorbed from the intestine, although formal evidence for this assumption is difficult to ascertain (1, 2). Correspondingly, the lactulose that appears in the urine generally is thought to be the amount absorbed. When measured by chromatography, the median recovery in urine was 0.8% of the dose with a range of 0.4% to 2.8% (18). Most of the excreted lactulose appears within eight hours of ingestion; the half-life of urinary elimination ranges between 0.6 and 2.5 hours with a median of 1.5 hours (18). In another study using an enzymatic assay, 0.21±0.06% was recovered in the urine within 6 hours (19). Only in premature infants and in inflammatory bowel disease were larger amounts excreted. Consequently, lactulose may be used as a tool for the investigation of small intestinal permeability (20-30).

Lactulose concentrations in ileal and cecal fluid have been measured by Florent et al. (6) after a 20 g oral dose. For the ileum a mean appearance time of 45 minutes (range 30 - 60 minutes) was estimated. The mean peak concentration of lactulose was 110 mmol (83 - 130) after 170 minutes (60 - 270). Lactulose administration (20 g b.i.d.) for eight days did not appreciably alter these numbers. In the cecum, the mean appearance time was 60 minutes (30 - 90), the mean peak concentration was 88 mmol (73 - 112) and the mean peak time 105 minutes (90 - 135). Interestingly, after eight days on lactulose, the mean peak concentration was reduced to 46 mmol (16 - 91; $p<0.02$), whereas times of appearance and of peak concentration were unchanged.

Small bowel transit time has also been investigated using the hydrogen breath test. Once the sugar has reached the cecum, the mass of bacteria available for hydrolysis and the surface for absorption are enormous. Consequently, it is assumed that the formation of molecular hydrogen and its exhalation in breath are almost immediate (31-35). Even if these assumptions are valid, it must be realized that the method gives an idea about small bowel transit time only for the most rapidly passing fraction of the dose. In normal adult subjects, transit times of 93±6.6 (36), 117±42 (37), 72.6±5 (38), 85±18 (39) and 85±19 minutes (40) have been measured, with a range of 30 to 130 minutes. In some patients, small bowel overgrowth may increase H_2 exhalation even before lactulose reaches the colon (41). In some other patients, H_2 exhalation may not be observed because of absence of H_2-generating bacteria from the small intestine and colon (42).

THE BIOCHEMICAL FATE OF LACTULOSE IN THE COLON

Once in the cecum, lactulose is metabolized by colonic bacteria with the formation of volatile fatty acids, H_2 and, in some subjects, methane. Acetic acid, propionic acid, butyric acid and lactic acid presumably are important breakdown products (6, 11, 43-45), but other compounds may also be formed. The relative proportions of these metabolites are not adequately documented, yet acetic and lactic acid probably are the most prominent (6). These breakdown products probably are not specific for lactulose, but most likely result from the degradation of any carbohydrates that reach the cecum where they are metabolized by bacteria. Consequently, results of studies performed with analogous compounds or poorly digestible carbohydrate nutrients appear to represent direct analogies to the administration of lactulose. This situation has been well studied in ruminants, where the fermentation of carbohydrates was found to be associated with energy conservation and increased fecal nitrogen output (4, 46-49).

Evidence for the absorption of short-chain fatty acids by the human colonic mucosa is now quite good (50). With the dialysis bag technique, the rectal absorption of acetate, propionate and butyrate have been demonstrated (51). The mechanisms were investigated by a colon perfusion technique which showed that absorption of acetate, propionate and butyrate was proportional to the luminal concentration. Ionic diffusion was thought to account for about 40% of the acids and nonionic diffusion for 60%. The protons required for the latter process were thought to be derived from H_2CO_3 with the formation of HCO_3^- and alkalinization of the colonic contents (52). The situation may be different after lactulose administration when the pH of cecal contents becomes acid. Nevertheless, applicability of these data to the condition after lactulose administration has been documented in healthy subjects in whom oral doses of lactulose were followed by dose-dependent increments in peripheral venous acetate levels with peak concentrations of 99±23, 127±18, and 181±24 μmol per L after 5, 10, and 20 g of lactulose, respectively, the fasting concentrations being 54±4 μmol per L (11). In this study, propionate and butyrate were also looked for and not found in peripheral blood, presumably because of hepatic first-pass elimination.

Indirect evidence for absorption of sugar breakdown products can also be obtained from studies with uniformly ^{14}C-labelled glucose. When a dose of 12.5 g was placed into the cecum by intubation in four volunteers, exhalation of $^{14}CO_2$ was as rapid and as complete as when the same amount of the test substance was placed in the stomach (53). Since cecal contents are highly anaerobic, it is unlikely that $^{14}CO_2$ was formed *in situ*. Rather, the exhaled label must have resulted from intermediary metabolism of short-chain fatty acids. In these studies only 14% of the label could be recovered in feces of which only 17% was in a dialyzable form. The nondialyzable label was thought to be part of structural components of fecal bacteria. Similar results were obtained by Florent (6).

In view of the anaerobic conditions that exist within the colon, it is not surprising that molecular hydrogen is formed. In fact, this occurs whenever carbohydrates reach the cecum (32, 54-58) and has been used as a clinical tool to diagnose carbohydrate malabsorption. Depending on the prevailing colonic flora, it appears that in some subjects part of the H_2 formed is used for the synthesis of methane (44, 55-57). Presumably, these gases are responsible for the well-known bloating and flatulence after lactulose administration.

Breakdown of lactulose by colonic bacteria is also followed by a dramatic increase in hydrogen ion concentration. This seems to be most marked in the cecum (6, 59-61). Fecal pH falls only when lactulose is administered in doses large enough to induce diarrhea. In one study, lactulose was administered to healthy subjects in a dose of 30 to 40 g per day and the pH was measured with a telemetric capsule (60). After lactulose the pH significantly fell within the right colon from 6.0 (range 5.5

- 7.5) to 4.85 (3.5 - 6.1). Nonsignificant changes occurred within the left colon from 7.0 (6.0 - 7.6) to 6.7 (5.6 - 7.3) and within the rectum from 6.8 (6.2 - 7.6) to 6.55 (6.0 - 7.2). In another investigation 40 g of lactulose were given daily and fecal pH was measured by the dialysis bag technique. It decreased significantly in two of three subjects (61). Whether or not fecal pH is lowered by lactulose is probably only a matter of dose. Doses which are optimal for the treatment of PSE generally lower fecal pH.

It is likely that the colonic bacteria hydrolyze lactulose initially to galactose and fructose. If each of these sugars is further broken down to two fatty acids, the osmotic load in the colon is four times that of lactulose itself. On this basis it can be calculated that a lactulose dose of 20 g (30 ml of the commercial syrup) is equivalent to 193 ml of isotonic lactulose and in the colon to 770 ml of isotonic organic acids. In reality an osmotic load of this magnitude is unlikely, because formation and absorption of the fatty acids presumably occur simultaneously. Nevertheless, quadrupling of the osmotic load is a feature not shared by other osmotic laxatives and might in part explain the efficacy of lactulose as a laxative.

An important observation concerns the fact that with chronic administration of lactulose its colonic metabolism seems to change. This phenomenon is evident clinically as a decrease in symptoms such as bloating and flatulence. Its metabolic counterpart has been elucidated by Florent et al. (6) who showed that after eight days of continuous lactulose administration, cecal lactulose concentrations and H_2-exhalation rates decreased while cecal acetic and lactic acid concentrations and $^{14}CO_2$-exhalation from ^{14}C-lactulose increased. Cecal fluid pH dropped faster and to a greater degree on the eighth day. These data clearly show that chronic lactulose ingestion induces alterations in colonic bacterial metabolic pathways which enhance the degradation of lactulose. It is not clear, however, whether this is due to changes in the bacterial flora or to changes in enzyme activity of these bacteria.

INTERACTION OF LACTULOSE WITH THE BACTERIAL FLORA OF THE COLON

When lactulose was first used in the treatment of PSE, its benefits were presumed to be due to changes in the enteric flora (62-64). However, consistent changes in the relative proportions or in the absolute numbers of different bacterial species have been difficult to identify. Initially, microbiological studies focused on lactobacilli (65-68), but since then, bacteriologic methods have been remarkably improved.

In vitro, lactulose can be metabolized by a large number of strictly anaerobic bacteria, such as various bacteroides and lactobacilli species, *Streptococcus mutans*, *Clostridium perfringens* and *C. glycolyticum*. Among these species, only *C. perfringens* produces gas. Also, other facultative anaerobic bacteria such as enterobacter species, *E. coli*, Klebsiella, Citrobacter and enterococci can ferment lactulose. Gas has been formed by Enterobacter, Klebsiella, *E. coli* and Citrobacter (4, 7).

In view of the difficulties in performing strictly anaerobe cultures and of the many bacterial species that are capable of metabolizing lactulose *in vitro*, it is not surprising that the changes in bacterial composition observed after lactulose administration have not been clear cut. In four cirrhotic patients, Conn and Floch observed a slight decrease in total aerobic and a slight increase in total anaerobic counts (68). Bacteroides, lactobacilli, coliform, and streptococci also tended to increase, but none of these changes was statistically significant. Furthermore, fecal bacteria in six normal volunteers who took lactulose were not different from those of five others who took glucose. In a more extensive study, Vince et al. concluded that the observed changes could not be distinguished from dilutional effects (69). In other studies there was no correlation between the clinical response and the colonic bacterial changes induced by lactulose (70, 71).

EFFECTS OF LACTULOSE ON AMMONIA METABOLISM

Inasmuch as PSE was thought to be related to ammonia, it was logical to focus on the effects of lactulose on ammonia metabolism. In the initial studies of lactulose in PSE, it was noted that lactulose treatment was associated with decreased blood ammonia levels (72). These observations have been confirmed by more extensive clinical studies (73-78).

At first, the pharmacological effects of lactulose on blood ammonia were explained by the influence of colonic acidification on nonionic diffusion. Ammonia is a weak base with a pK of 9.3 that accumulates on the acid side of a lipid membrane. Studies in dogs showed that colonic luminal pH values above 6.0 were associated with movement of ammonia from the lumen to the blood (net absorption), whereas luminal pH values below 6.0 led to movement of ammonia from the blood to the lumen (79). On the basis of such considerations, the ammonia trapping theory was proposed. Further, it is the basis of the recommendation to measure stool pH of patients treated with lactulose and to titrate lactulose doses to pH levels <6.0 (80-84). The rapid clinical responses after lactulose enemas presumably are also explained primarily by the effects of the acid solution on nonionic diffusion, although metabolic mechanisms cannot be excluded (85).

If nonionic diffusion fully accounts for the lactulose-induced changes in ammonia metabolism, fecal ammonia content should be elevated during lactulose treatment. However, elevated fecal ammonia levels were not confirmed (61). Other mechanisms which may modify bacterial ammonia production were therefore investigated. *In vitro*, the largest amounts of ammonia were produced by gram-negative anaerobic rods, including bacteroides, clostridia, enterobacteria and bacillus species. Lactobacilli produce little ammonia. All groups of bacteria formed less ammonia at pH 5.0 than at pH 7.0 and the generation of ammonia was not inhibited when 30 mmol per L of ammonia were included in the medium. Most gram-negative bacteria produced only small amounts of ammonia when incubated with glucose, lactose or lactulose, but there were exceptions. Ammonia formation by gram-positive anaerobes (except clostridia) was not affected by carbohydrate fermentation (86). These results are consistent with the earlier finding that in the presence of lactulose fecal incubates utilize ammonia anabolically, rather than form it (87). Many bacteria seem to behave as though an unlimited energy supply as carbohydrates stimulates the incorporation of ammonia into bacterial protein. Instead of being a source of ammonia, these bacteria are a sink for ammonia.

The observations mentioned above are consistent with studies of the effects of lactulose on urea metabolism. It is well known that approximately one-fourth of the urea pool is eliminated by intestinal hydrolysis to ammonia rather than by renal excretion. Since under normal circumstances ammonia is easily absorbed, it reaches the liver where it is efficiently removed from blood and used for urea synthesis. Thus, in the form of ammonia, a large fraction of the urea pool undergoes enterohepatic cycling. If, in the presence of lactulose, ammonia is trapped in the colon by nonionic diffusion and by incorporation into bacterial proteins, fecal nitrogen excretion should increase at the expense of renal urea elimination. This is exactly what Weber et al. have shown (88-91) (Figure 1).

All the above observations may nicely be put together into a double hypothesis which combines the effect of lactulose on a bacterial ammonia metabolism with its effect on nonionic diffusion. It should be kept in mind, however, that recent observations in germfree rats are not explained by the above concepts and might necessitate yet another modification of the "lactulose theory" (92).

Within this context it has always been realized that hyperammonemia alone cannot explain the neuropsychiatric manifestations of PSE. It was thought, however, that ammonia might serve as model compound for other nitrogenous substances.

ADVERSE EFFECTS OF LACTULOSE

Laxative doses of lactulose are generally well tolerated. In the treatment of hepatic encephalopathy, lactulose doses should be titrated to achieve about two soft bowel movements per day and, if possible, to a pH <6.0. Consequently, the therapeutic margin, i.e., the difference between its therapeutic and its diarrhea-producing dose, is small. Excessive amounts may lead to watery stools, fluid loss and dehydration. In several patients, azotemia, hypernatremia, and hypokalemia have been reported (93). The spontaneous adverse drug reaction monitoring system of the drug committee of the "Deutsche Ärzteschaft" (German Society of Physicians) has received only 19 reports of adverse effects in the period from 1974 to 1987, 12 of them dealing with diarrhea, the others with minor nonspecific com-

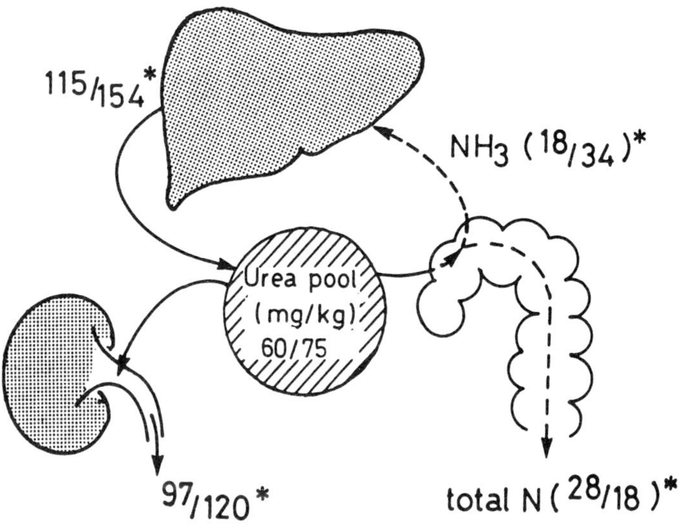

FIGURE 1. Effects of lactulose on urea metabolism. The numbers express nitrogen either in mg per kg (urea pool) or in mg per kg per day. The first number represents treatment with lactulose and the second stands for the control situation. * indicates significant changes at the 5% level. The data demonstrate that during lactulose treatment less ammonia is used for urea synthesis and more nitrogen is excreted in the feces. As a consequence, hepatic urea synthesis, the urea pool and renal urea elimination are all decreased during lactulose administration. The study consisted of cirrhotic patients consuming 1 g protein per kg per day (90).

plaints. Also the World Health Organization reporting system has no adverse effects of any serious nature on file (personal communications).

A minor adverse effect of lactulose is the aversion by some patients to its sweet taste. Although it appears to be trivial at first glance, it can contribute to noncompliance and to treatment failures. Nausea and vomiting have also been reported. They may result from the osmotic load to the upper gastrointestinal tract, which in the commercial syrup is increased by contaminating sugars such as lactose and galactose. Patients should be advised to camouflage the taste by diluting the syrup with orange juice or other beverages.

In view of the presence of galactose in lactulose syrup, it may not be appropriate to administer it to subjects on galactose-free diets.

A rare adverse reaction is the formation of pneumatosis coli (94).

If acidification of cecal contents is essential for the lactulose action, lactulose should not be combined with antacids which may reduce the effects of lactulose on nonionic diffusion of ammonia and other weak bases.

It is clear that the advantages of lactulose far outweigh its disadvantages.

CONCLUDING REMARKS

This brief review of the clinical pharmacology of lactulose deals almost exclusively with lactulose *per se*. The principles expressed, however, are applicable to crystalline lactulose, to lactitol and even to lactose when it is administered to lactase-deficient individuals. Obviously, there are differences in dosage, in the manner of ingestion, in clinical responsiveness to specific dosages, in side effects and subtle differences in the details of the metabolism of these related carbohydrates. Few comparative investigations of these differences have been performed or reported. Until such data are available, it is reasonable to practice the principles as they apply to lactulose and to extrapolate from these principles for these similar substances.

REFERENCES

1. ten Ham EJ. Biochemical experiments with lactulose. N.V. Philips-Duphar Research Laboratories. 1962: 1-16.

2. Täufel K, Krause W, Ruttloff H, et al. Zur intestinalen Spaltung von Oligosacchariden. Z Ges Exp Med, 1967; 144:54-66.

3. Dahlquist A, Gryboski JD. Inability of the human small intestinal lactase to hydrolyse lactulose. Biochim Biophys Acta 1965; 110:635-636.

4. Luginbühl M. Kulturelle Beeinflussung obligat und fakultativ anaerober Darmkeime durch Laktulose und Lactitol. Erklärungsversuch für die Wirksamkeit der Lactulose- oder Lactitoltherapie bei der portosystemischen Encephalopathie. Thesis 1985; Bern/Switzerland.

5. Flourie B, Florent C, Jouany JP, et al. Colonic metabolism of wheat starch in healthy humans. Gastroenterology 1986; 90:111-119.

6. Florent C, Flourie B, Leblond A, et al. Influence of chronic lactulose ingestion on the colonic metabolism of lactulose in man (an in vivo study). J Clin Invest 1985; 75:608-613.

7. Vince A, Killingley M, Wrong OM. Effect of lactulose on ammonia production in a fecal incubation system. Gastroenterology 1978; 74:544-549.

8. Vince A, Dawson AM, Park N, et al. Ammonia production by intestinal bacteria. Gut 1973; 14:171-177.

9. Edmiston CE, Avant GR, Wilson FA. Anaerobic bacterial populations on normal and diseased human biopsy tissue obtained at colonoscopy. Appl Environ Microbiol 1982; 43:1173-1181.

10. Pomare EW, Branch WJ, Cummings JH. Carbohydrate fermentation in the human colon and its relation to acetate concentrations in venous blood. J Clin Invest 1985; 75:1448-1454.

11. Aries V, Crowther JS, Drasar BS, et al. Bacteria and the aetiology of cancer of the large bowel. Gut 1969; 10:334-335.

12. Windholz, M, ed. The Merck Index, 10th ed. Rahway/USA: Merck and Co., Inc., 1983.

13. Loehry CA, Axon ATR, Hilton PJ, et al. Permeability of the small intestine to substances of different molecular weight. Gut 1970; 11:466-470.

14. Loehry CA, Kingham J, Baker J. Small intestinal permeability in animals and man. Gut 1973; 14:683-688.

15. Fordtran JS, Rector FC, Ewton MF, et al. Permeability characteristics of the human small intestine. J Clin Invest 1965; 44:1935-1944.

16. Chadwick VS, Phillips FC, Hofmann AF. Measurements of intestinal permeability using low molecular weight polyethylene glycols (PEG 400)—Chemical analysis and biological properties of PEG 400. Gastroenterology 1977; 73:241-246.

17. Chadwick VS, Phillips SF, Hofmann AF. Measurements of intestinal permeability using low molecular weight polyethylene glycols (PEG 400)—Chemical analysis and biological properties of PEG 400. Gastroenterology 1977; 73:247-251.

18. Carrulli N, Salvioli GF, Manenti F. Absorption of lactulose in man. Digestion 1972; 6:139-145.

19. Behrens RH, Docherty H, Elia M, et al. A simple enzymatic method for the assay of urinary lactulose. Clin Chim Acta 1984; 137:361-367.

20. Weaver LT, Laker MF, Nelson R. Enhanced intestinal permeability in preterm babies with blood stools. Arch Dis Child 1984; 59:280-281.

21. Beach RC, Menzies IS, Clayden GS, et al. Gastrointestinal permeability changes in the preterm neonate. Arch Dis Child 1982; 57:141-145.

23. Weaver LT, Laker MF, Nelson R. Intestinal permeability in the newborn. Arch Dis Child 1984; 59:236-241.

24. Cook GC, Menzies IS. Intestinal absorption and unmediated permeation of sugars in post-infective tropical malabsorption (tropical sprue). Digestion 1986; 33:109-116.

25. Ukabam SO, Cooper BT. Small intestinal permeability to mannitol, lactulose, and polyethylene glycol 400 in celiac disease. Dig Dis Sci 1984; 29:809-816.

26. Pearson AD, Eastham EJ, Laker MF, et al. Intestinal permeability in children with Crohn's disease and coeliac disease. Br Med J 1982; 85:20-21.

27. Ukabam SO, Clamp JR, Cooper BT. Abnormal small intestinal permeability to sugars in patients with Crohn's disease of the terminal ileum and colon. Digestion 1983; 27:70-74.

28. Ford RP, Menzies IS, Phillips AD, et al. Intestinal sugar permeability: relationship to diarrhoeal disease and small bowel morphology. J Pediatr Gastroenterol Nutr 1985; 4:568-574.

29. DuMont GC, Beach RC, Menzies IS. Gastrointestinal permeability in food-

allergic eczematous children. Clin Allergy 1984; 14:55-59.

30. Ukabam SO, Cooper BT. Small intestinal permeability as an indicator of jejunal mucosal recovery in patients with celiac sprue on a gluten-free diet. J Clin Gastroenterol 1985; 7:232-236.

31. Levitt MD. Production and excretion of hydrogen gas in man. N Engl J Med 1969; 281:122-127.

32. Levitt MD, Hirsh CA, Fetzer CA, et al. H_2 excretion after ingestion of complex carbohydrates. Gastroenterology 1987; 92:383-389.

33. Metz G, Drasar BS, Gassull MA, et al. Breath hydrogen test for small intestinal bacterial colonisation. Lancet 1976; 1:668-669.

34. Rhodes JM, Middleton P, Jewell DP. The lactulose H_2 breath test as a diagnostic test for small intestinal bacterial overgrowth. Scand J Gastroenterol 1979; 14:333-336.

35. Bond JH, Levitt MD. Investigations of small bowel transit time in man utilizing pulmonary hydrogen (H_2) measurements. J Lab Clin Med 1975; 85:546-555.

36. Corbett CL, Thomas S, Read NW, et al. Electrochemical detector for breath hydrogen determinations: measurement of small bowel transit in normal subjects and in patient with the irritable bowel syndrome. Gut 1981; 22:836-840.

37. Korth H, Müller I, Erckenbrecht JF, et al. Breath hydrogen as a test for gastrointestinal transit. Hepatogastroenterology 1984; 31:282-284.

38. Bond JH, Levitt MD. Use of breath hydrogen (H_2) to quantitate small bowel transit following partial gastrectomy. J Lab Clin Med 1977; 90:30-36.

39. Breuer N, Ptok A, Goetze H, et al. Methodische Aspekte zur Anwendung des Wasserstoff (H_2)-Atemtestes. Z Gastroenterol 1986; 24:80-84.

40. Wildgrube HL, Classen M. Wasserstoff (H_2-) Atemtests in der Diagnostik von Dünndarmerkrankungen. Z Gastroenterol 1983; 21:628-636.

41. King CE, Toskes PP. Comparison of the 1-gram [^{14}C]xylose, 10-gram lactulose H_2, and 80-gram glucose H_2 breath tests in patients with small intestine bacterial overgrowth. Gastroenterology 1986; 91:1447-1451.

42. Robb TA, Goodwin DA, Davidson GP. Faecal hydrogen production in vitro as an indicator for in vivo hydrogen producing capability in the breath hydrogen test. Acta Paediatr Scand 1965; 74:942-944.

43. Wrong O, Metcalfe-Gibson A, Morrison RBI, et al. In vivo dialysis of faeces as a method of stool analysis. I. Technique and results in normal subjects. Clin Sci (Oxf) 1965; 28:357-375.

44. Beaven J, Bjoerneklett A, Jenssen E, et al. Pulmonary hydrogen and methane and plasma ammonia after the administration of lactulose or sorbitol. Scand J Gastroenterol 1983; 18:343-347.

45. Cummings JH. Short chain fatty acids in the human colon. Gut 1981; 22:763-779.

46. Mason VC, Palmer R. The influence of bacterial activity in the alimentary canal of rats on faecal nitrogen excretion. Acta Agric Scand 1973; 23:142-150.

47. Thornton RF, Bird PR, Somer M, et al. Urea excretion in ruminants. III. The role of hind-gut (caecum and colon). Aust J Agric Res 1970; 21:345-354.

48. Bond JH, Currier BE, Buchwald H, et al. Colonic conservation of malabsorbed carbohydrate. Gastroenterology 1980; 78:444-447.

49. Oerskov ER, Fraser C, Mason VC, et al. Influence of starch digestion in the large intestine of sheep on caecal fermentation, caecal microflora and faecal nitrogen excretion. Br J Nutr 1970; 24:671-682.

50. Watson AJM, Kelly MJ, Wilks M, et al. Mechanism of acetate absorption in normal rat jejunum (Abstract). Gut 1985; 26:A1109.

51. McNeil NI, Cummings JH, James WPT. Short chain fatty acid absorption by the human large intestine. Gut 1978; 19:819-822.

52. Ruppin H, Bar-Meir S, Soergel KH, et al. Absorption of short-chain fatty acids by the colon. Gastroenterology 1980; 78:1500-1507.

53. Bond JH, Levitt MD. Fate of soluble carbohydrate in the colon of rats and man. J Clin Invest 1976; 57:1158-1164.

54. Perman JA, Modler S, Olson AC. Role of pH in production of hydrogen from carbohydrates by colonic bacterial flora. Studies in-vivo and in-vitro. J Clin Invest 1981; 67:643-650.

55. Pitt P, de Bruijn KM, Beeching MF, et al. Studies on breath methane: the effect of ethnic origins and lactulose. Gut 1980; 21:951-959.

56. Bond JH, Engel RR, Levitt M. Factors influencing pulmonary methane excretion in man. J Exp Med 1971; 133:572-588.

57. Bjoerneklett A, Jenssen E. Relationships between hydrogen (H_2) and methane (CH_4) production in man. Scand J Gastroenterol 1982; 17:985-992.

58. Anderson IH, Levine AS, Levitt MD. Incomplete absorption of the carbohydrate in all-purpose wheat flour. N Engl J Med 1981; 304:891-892.

59. Patil DH, Westaby D, Mahida YR, et al. Comparison of lactulose and lactitol on ileal and colonic pH (Abstract). Gut 1985; 26:P89.

60. Bown RL, Gibson JA, Sladen GE, et al. Effects of lactulose and other laxatives on ileal and colonic pH as measured by a radiotelemetry device. Gut 1974; 15: 999-1004.

61. Agostini L, Down PF, Murison J, et al. Faecal ammonia and pH during lactulose administration in man: comparison with other cathartics. Gut 1972; 13:859-866.

62. Ingelfinger FJ. Editorial comment. In: Beeson PB, et al., eds. Year Book of Medicine, 1964-1965 Year Book Series. Chicago: Year Book Medical Publishers, 1964: 591.

63. Phear EA, Ruebner B. The in vitro production of ammonium and amines by intestinal bacteria in relation to nitrogen toxicity as a factor in hepatic coma. Br J Exp Pathol 1956; 37:253-262.

64. Hoffmann K, Mossel DAA, Korus W, et al. Untersuchungen über die Wirkungsweise der Lactulose (B-galactosido-fructose) im Darm. Klin Wochenschr 1964; 42:126-130.

65. Petuely F. Bifidusflora bei Flaschenkindern durch bifidogene Substanzen (Bifidusfaktor). Z Kinderheilk 1957; 79:174-179.

66. Petuely F. Der Heutige Stand unseres Wissens über das Bifidusproblem in bakteriologischer, chemischer und klinischer Hinsicht. Arch Kinderheilk 1962; 165:209-218.

67. Petuely F. Der Bifidusfaktor. Dtsch Med Wochenschr 1957; 82:1957-1960.

68. Conn HO, Floch MH. Effects of lactulose and Lactobacillus acidophilus on the fecal flora. Am J Clin Nutr 1970; 23:1588-1594.

69. Vince A, Zeegen R, Drinkwater JE, et al. The effect of lactulose on the faecal flora of patients with hepatic encephalopathy. J Med Microbiol 1974; 7:163-168.

70. Bircher J, Haemmerli UP, Müller-Duysing W, et al. The mechanism of action of lactulose in portal systemic encephalopathy: colonic bacterial urease activity and bacterial flora in rats. Rev Eur Etudes Clin et Biol 1970; 15:1096-1100.

71. Bircher J, Haemmerli UP, Scollo-Lavizzari G, et al. Treatment of chronic portal-systemic encephalopathy with lactulose. Am J Med 1971; 51:148-159.

72. Bircher J, Müller J, Guggenheim P, et al. Treatment of chronic portal systemic encephalopathy with lactulose. Lancet 1966; 1:890-893.

73. Conn HO, Lieberthal MM. The Hepatic Coma Syndromes and Lactulose. Baltimore: Williams and Wilkins Company, 1979.

74. Fessel JM, Conn HO. Lactulose in the treatment of acute hepatic encephalopathy. Am J Med Sci 1973; 266:103-110.

75. Elkington SG, Floch MH, Conn HO. Lactulose in the treatment of chronic portalsystemic encephalopathy. N Engl J Med 1969; 281:408-412.

76. Zeegen R, Drinkwater JE, Fenton JCB, et al. Some observations on the effects of treatment with lactulose on patients with chronic hepatic encephalopathy. Q J Med 1970; 39:245-263.

77. Rorsman G, Sulg I. Lactulose treatment of chronic hepatoportal encephalopathy. Acta Med Scand 1970; 187:337-346.

78. Patil DH, Westaby D, Mahida YR, et al. Comparative modes of action of lactitol and lactulose in the treatment of hepatic encephalopathy. Gut 1987; 28:255-259.

79. Bircher J, Haemmerli UP, Trabert E, et al. The mechanism of action of lactulose in portal-systemic encephalopathy. Nonionic diffusion of ammonia in the canine colon. Rev Eur Etudes Clin et Biol 1971; 16:352-357.

80. Price JB, Sawada M, Voorhees AB. Clinical significance of intraluminal pH in intestinal ammonia transport. Am J Surg 1970; 119:595-598.

81. Wolpert E, Phillips SF, Summerskill WHJ. Transport of urea and ammonia production in the human colon. Lancet 1971; 2:1387-1390.

82. Castell DO, Moore EW. Ammonia absorption from the human colon. Gastroenterology 1971; 60:33-42.

83. Orloff J, Berliner RW. The mechanism of the excretion of ammonia in the

dog. J Clin Invest 1956; 35:223-235.

84. Down PF, Agostini L, Murison J, Wrong OM. The interrelations of faecal ammonia, pH and bicarbonate: evidence colonic absorption of ammonia by non-ionic diffusion. Clin Sci 1972; 43:101-114.

85. Kersh ES, Rifkind H. Lactulose enemas. Ann Intern Med 1973; 78:81-84.

86. Vince AJ, Burridge SM. Ammonia production by intestinal bacteria: the effects of lactose, lactulose and glucose. J Med Microbiol 1980; 13:177-191.

87. Vince A, Killingley M, Wrong OM. Effect of lactulose on ammonia production in a fecal incubation system. Gastroenterology 1978; 74:544-549.

88. Walser M, Bodenlos LJ. Urea metabolism in man. J Clin Invest 1959; 38:1617-1626.

89. Weber FL, Fresard KM, Lally BR. Effects of lactulose and neomycin on urea metabolism in cirrhotic subjects. Gastroenterology 1982; 82:213-217.

90. Weber FL, Fresard KM. Comparative effects of lactulose and magnesium sulfate on urea metabolism and nitrogen excretion in cirrhotic subjects. Gastroenterology 1981; 80:994-998.

91. Weber FL. The effect of lactulose on urea metabolism and nitrogen excretion in cirrhotic patients. Gastroenterology 1979; 77:518-523.

92. De Boers JE, Oostenbroek RJ, van Dongen JJ, et al. Sequential metabolic characteristics following portocaval shunt in rats. Eur Surg Res 1986; 18:96-106.

93. Kaupke C, Sprague T, Gitnick GL. Hypernatremia after the administration of lactulose (Letter). Ann Intern Med 1977; 86:745.

94. Zimmerman AL, Gupta JK, Ingegno AP. Pneumatosis coli following treatment with lactulose. NY State J Med; 1979:1896-1899.

13

CLINICAL TRIALS OF LACTULOSE THERAPY IN HEPATIC ENCEPHALOPATHY

Francesco Orlandi, M.D., Eugenio Brunelli, M.D., Antonio Benedetti, M.D., and Giampiero Macarri, M.D.

The introduction of lactulose as a therapeutic agent for the treatment of hepatic encephalopathy (HE) represents a major advance in the therapy of liver disease. At present, lactulose is the drug of choice in clinical practice in acute and chronic HE.

In revisiting the clinical experience on lactulose, we recall what Conn reminds us in his book on the hepatic coma syndromes (1): the drug was synthesized in 1930 (2) and evaluated by pediatricians in the following years. Franz Ingelfinger prophetically suggested in 1964 that it might prove helpful in hepatic disease (3), and in 1966 Bircher used it successfully in cirrhotic patients with hepatic encephalopathy (4). This "latency period" of the drug shows us how long the road can be for a molecule to become a valid drug for a specific clinical indication.

Since Bircher's paper, a number of clinical reports of orally administered lactulose have been published. We reviewed 30 of these trials, which represent a twenty-year cumulative clinical experience on the drug (5-33)(Table 1). Eight other trials on the efficacy of lactulose enemas in hepatic encephalopathy are not considered here. Sixteen of the 30 reviewed studies were controlled studies (8, 9, 12-17, 23, 24, 28-33). The three double-blind trials included a total number of 45 patients (8, 24, 29). Lactulose was compared with glucose or sorbitol in three studies published between 1969 and 1973 (8, 13, 24), with neomycin in eight other studies published between 1969 and 1981 (9, 15-17, 23, 28-30), and with branched-chain amino acid solutions or lactitol in three investigations published between 1982 and 1985 (31-33). Lactulose was therefore used in the 1970s as a potential, as-yet-unproved drug in a time dominated by neomycin, and in the 1980s as the first-choice conventional drug against newer agents. At present, the comparison of a new drug with placebo in hepatic encephalopathy is a procedure open to ethical criticism

TABLE 1. Results of Clinical Studies of Oral Administration of Lactulose in Cirrhotic Patients with Hepatic Encephalopathy

First author, date	Encephal-opathy	No. of patients treated with lactulose	Clinical improve-ment	Other therapy in controlled trials
Lande, 1968	Chronic	12	10	
Rottiers, 1968	Acute	11	8	
Demeulenaere, 1969	Chronic	7	7	
Elkington, 1969	Chronic	7	5	Sorbitol
Ma, 1969	Chronic	10	6	Neomycin
Gauthier, 1970	Chronic	30	24	
Geffroy, 1970	Chronic	20	18	
Siebner, 1970	Chronic	12	11	Antibiotics
Simmonds, 1970	Acute	11	10	Glucose
Zeegen, 1970	Chronic	7	3	$MgSO_4$
Bircher, 1971	Chronic	6	6	Neomycin, $MgS0_4$
Fung, 1971	Acute	10	6	
Fung, 1971	Chronic	5	5	Neomycin
Imler, 1971	Chronic	7	2	Neomycin
James, 1971	Chronic	6	5	
Cassi, 1972	Acute	6	5	
Kardel, 1972	Chronic	9	3	
Salvagnini, 1972	Chronic	12	6	
Almici, 1973	Chronic	19	16	
Fessel, 1973	Acute	24	20	Neomycin
Germain, 1973	Chronic	9	5	Sucrose
Eisenburg, 1974	Chronic	14	10	
Reikowski, 1974	Chronic	36	34	
Seidlova, 1974	Chronic	14	11	
Atterbury, 1977	Acute	22	18	Neomycin, sorbitol
Conn, 1977	Chronic	29	26	Neomycin, sorbitol
Orlandi, 1981	Chronic	91	28 *	Neomycin, $MgSO_4$
Rossi-Fanelli, 1982	Acute	17	8	Branched-chain amino acids
Fiaccadori, 1985	Acute	16	10	Branched-chain amino acids
Lanthier, 1985	Chronic	5	5	Lactitol

* Transition to a less severe grade of encephalopathy in two weeks of treatment, $p>0.05$ vs neomycin.

in view of the general acceptance of the efficacy and safety of lactulose.

The total number of patients treated with lactulose in the 30 studies was 484. The groups of patients treated with lactulose exceeded 20 individuals in only six investigations (10, 23, 26, 28-30)(Figure 1). Pilot studies based on few patients are common in clinical pharmacology, but difficulties peculiar to hepatic encephalopathy became evident to most investigators. For example, it took over four years to recruit homogeneous groups of patients in each of the two multicenter studies which are the largest randomized trials included in this review (29, 30).

The multifaceted pattern of the syndrome, which includes a number of clinical stigmata, has led also to the use of heterogeneous selection criteria in the 16 controlled studies. The course of acute forms of the syndrome has been evaluated in five of these investigations including 93 patients treated with lactulose (13, 23, 28, 31, 32). The other 11 studies were concerned with chronic hepatic encephalopathy. Requisites for admission ranged from coma in some studies to any grade of encephalopathy or only grades I and II in other studies. Some papers did not define clearly the outcomes observed in mild or severe forms of the syndrome. Acute nitrogenous encephalopathy was a requisite for admission in one study (23), and in other investigations the prevalence of nitrogenous forms was not indicated.

Five papers considered azotemia or renal insufficiency at the time of admission to be a reason for exclusion from the trial. Two other studies excluded

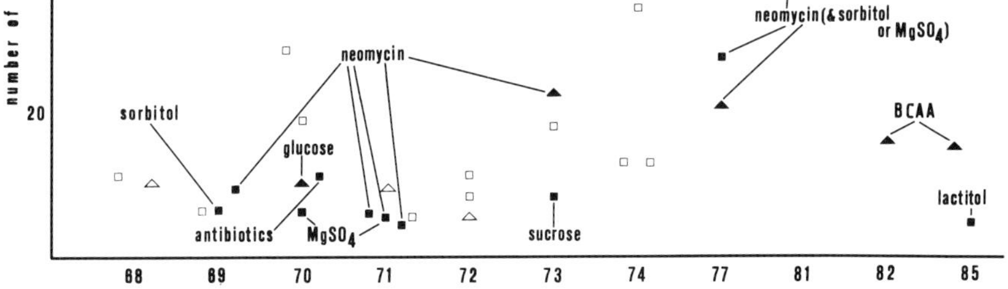

FIGURE 1. The clinical trials published between 1968 and 1985 on the treatment of hepatic encephalopathy with lactulose are represented. Each study concerning acute encephalopathy is indicated as a triangle and each investigation concerning chronic encephalopathy as a square. Controlled trials are indicated in black, and the drugs compared to lactulose are shown: neomycin or branched-chain amino acids i.v. (BCAA) or others. Note that 80% of the studies include less than 20 patients.

the hepatorenal syndrome, and three other papers identified a total of 12 patients with azotemia.

Ancillary therapy, which is another crucial point in evaluating the course of hepatic encephalopathy, has been clearly outlined in 6 out of 14 papers. Moreover, the effects of lactulose administration were evaluated in a wide range of durations of therapy, from 2 to 10 days in acute encephalopathy and from 5 to 90 days in chronic forms of the syndrome.

Such heterogeneous criteria for admission and for follow-up have been followed by heterogeneous rates of therapeutic success. The outcome was expressed in most studies as transition to a milder grade of HE (Figure 2).

The analysis of the 16 investigations, which resemble a series of dominoes, i.e., basically similar but different, with small numbers of patients, shows very heterogeneous criteria of inclusion, duration of therapy, dosage of the drug, ancillary regimens and other clinically relevant items. A cumulative statistical analysis seemed therefore open to a very real danger of bias.

The essential steps of knowledge, after Bircher's pilot study (4), were the evidence that in acute encephalopathy lactulose was more efficient than placebo, i.e., glucose (13), that restoration of mental state can be faster with lactulose than with neomycin if large doses of the disaccharide are administered on the first day of therapy (23), and that lactulose shows a better risk/benefit ratio than treatment with neomycin plus sorbitol (28). Similarly, evidence of the efficacy of the lactulose

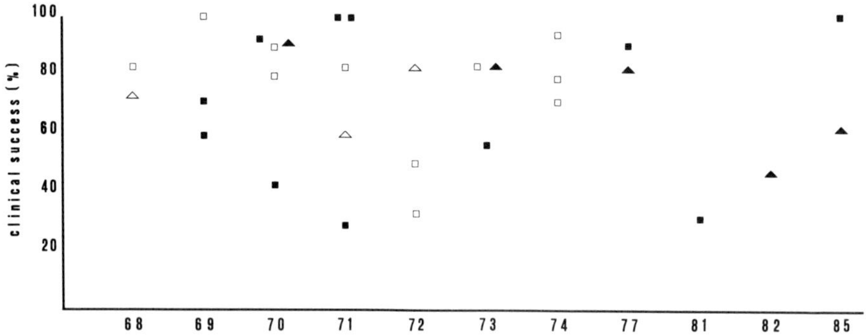

FIGURE 2. The therapeutic response rate observed in the 30 reviewed trials is shown here in terms of "clinical success," expressed in most studies as improvement to a less severe grade of encephalopathy. The meaning of the symbols is the same as in Figure 1. Criteria of admission to these studies, the duration of therapy, the dosage of the drugs administered and ancillary regimens were very heterogeneous in these studies. In the 16 controlled trials, lactulose showed a better risk/benefit ratio than the conventional or new drugs used in such investigations.

in chronic encephalopathy was obtained in 1969 and 1970 (8, 14), and a better risk/benefit ratio than for neomycin was demonstrated in 1978 to 1981 by two long-term multicenter randomized trials (29, 30).

These two independent studies are the largest investigations of hepatic encephalopathy, and their results can be considered to be examples of fortuitously complementary trials: one study was concerned with well-selected patients with stable cirrhosis and encephalopathy and excluded patients with encephalopathy induced by most extrinsic precipitating factors (29); the other study used more comprehensive criteria of selection (30). In spite of these different philosophies, the two trials reached substantially consistent results: lactulose was equally effective compared to neomycin-sorbitol (29) or neomycin-$MgSo_4$ (30), and it therefore became the drug of choice for the treatment of hepatic encephalopathy due to the potential toxicity of the antibiotic agent.

The semiquantitative assessment of mental state, expressed as clinical grades of encephalopathy, was the primary measure of the efficacy of lactulose in both trials. The efficacy of the drug is nevertheless underestimated when the clinical outcome is evaluated as transition from grade I to grade 0 (no abnormality detected) encephalopathy in a relatively short period of study.

The need for an objective and reliable evaluation of the drug efficacy was therefore a relevant methodological problem in such multicenter studies. Conn et al. devised the PSE Index (mental state, Number Connection Test, asterixis, electroencephalography and arterial ammonia) to grade the severity of the syndrome and to measure serially the effects of therapy (29). The index showed its excellent validity throughout a double-blind crossover investigation, and from then on it has been used in many other therapeutic trials. On the other hand, the serial assessment of disturbances of speech, behavior, memory, gait and writing showed 60% to 70% disappearance rates of these signs after two weeks of lactulose administration in grade I encephalopathy. The rate of improvement was 45% for asterixis, and 21% for Reitan A trailmaking test (30).

A number of measurements of the efficacy of treatment other than mental state have been evaluated in the reviewed studies, such as electroencephalographic changes, stool pH, arterial pH and blood ammonia levels and other biochemical tests. They are not considered here.

The side effects of lactulose administration have been clearly described in 18 studies concerning 298 patients. The pooled values are 18.3% for flatulence, 14.5% for diarrhea, 12.6% for abdominal pain, and 0.3% for vomiting. Such rates support the overall opinion that lactulose is well tolerated and practically free of toxicity.

In conclusion, a review of the published studies has shown that lactulose has been a "winner" in terms of risk/benefit ratio, simplicity, and cost when properly matched with other drugs.

All but two investigations were performed over one to three weeks of therapy, and the long-term acceptability of lactulose is therefore practically unknown. Lactitol has recently been shown to have a compliance rate better than lactulose in a three-month-long therapy of chronic encephalopathy (33).

Looking at the 30 investigations considered here, it is noteworthy that hepatologists did not coordinate their efforts, and spent most of their resources in a number of small, independent studies. Only a few multicenter randomized trials were performed and, not by chance, these few studies have been responsible for most of the information available. This is the main lesson of a twenty-year experience of lactulose in the treatment of hepatic encephalopathy.

SUMMARY

Thirty clinical trials on the treatment of acute or chronic hepatic encephalopathy in cirrhotic patients with lactulose were reviewed. The total number of lactulose-treated patients was 484. The clinical course of the syndrome in the groups of patients treated with lactulose was compared with the outcomes observed in patients treated with placebo, or neomycin or other drugs in 16 controlled investigations including a total number of 278 patients. A cumulative statistical analysis of the published data appears misleading due to heterogeneous selection criteria, durations of the therapy, dosages of drugs, and ancillary regimens used in most investigations. Multicenter randomized trials led to more clinical information than the independent small studies. In the 16 controlled studies, lactulose appeared superior to the therapies with which it was compared in terms of risk/benefit ratio, simplicity and cost.

REFERENCES

1. Conn HO, Lieberthal MM. The Hepatic Coma Syndromes and Lactulose. Baltimore: Williams & Wilkins, 1979: 248-250.

2. Montgomery EM, Hudson CS. Relations between rotatory power and structure in the sugar group XXVII. Synthesis of a new disaccharide ketose (lactulose) from lactose. J Am Chem Soc 1930; 52:2101-2106.

3. Ingelfinger F. Editorial comments. In: Beeson PB, et al., eds. Year Book of Medicine, 1964-1965 series. Chicago: Year Book Medical Publishers, 1964-1965: 591-592.

4. Bircher J, Müller J, Guggenheim P, et al. Treatment of chronic portasystemic encephalopathy with lactulose. Lancet 1966; 1:890-893.

5. Lande M, Clot-Paimboeuf C. Traitement des encephalopathies porto-caves par lactulose. Presse Med 1968; 76:1675-1676.

6. Rottiers R, Van Egmond J, Verbruggen R, et al. Cirrhosis, hyperammoniemia and lactulose. Overdruk Tydschrift Gastroenterol 1968; 11:123-139.

7. Demeulenaere L, Rottiers R, Van Egmond J, et al. Cirrhose,

hyperammoniémie et lactulose, traitement par lactulose de l'hyperammoniémie paroxystique spontanée ou provoquée et de l'hyperammoniémie chronique chez le cirrhotique. Probl Réanimation 1969; 5:855-868.

8. Elkington SG, Floch MH, Conn HO. Lactulose in the treatment of chronic portal-systemic encephalopathy. A double-blind clinical trial. N Engl J Med 1969; 281:408-412.

9. Ma MH, McLeod JG, Blackburn CRB. Long-term treatment of portal-systemic encephalopathy with lactulose. Aust Ann Med 1969; 18:117-123.

10. Gauthier A, Camatte R, Remacle J, et al. Traitement des encéphalopathies hépatiques chroniques par le lactulose. A propos de 30 observations. Thérapeutique 1970; 46:667-670.

11. Geffroy Y, Segrestin M, Geffroy PY. Intérét du lactulose dans le traitement de l'encéphalopathie portocave chronique, a propos de 20 observations. Thérapeutique 1970; 46:897-901.

12. Siebner H, Missmahl HP. The treatment of hepatoportal encephalopathy with lactulose. Dtsch Med Wochenschr 1970; 15:529-533.

13. Simmons F, Goldstein H, Boyle JD. A controlled clinical trial of lactulose in hepatic encephalopathy. Gastroenterology 1970; 59:827-832.

14. Zeegen R, Drinkwater JE, Fenton JCB, et al. Some observations on the effects of treatment with lactulose on patients with chronic hepatic encephalopathy. Q J Med 1970; 39:245-263.

15. Bircher J, Haemmerli UP, Scollo-Lavizzari G, et al. Treatment of chronic portal-systemic encephalopathy with lactulose. Report of six patients and review of the literature. Am J Med 1971; 51:148-159.

16. Fung WP, Khoo OT. Lactulose in the treatment of acute and chronic hepatic encephalopathy. Singapore Med J 1971; 12:176-180.

17. Imler M, Kurtz D, Bockel R, et al. Étude comparative du traitement de l'encéphalopathie porto-cave par le lactulose, les bacilles lactiques et les antibiotiques. Thérapeutique 1971; 47:237-248.

18. James IM, Garassini M. Effect of lactulose on cerebral metabolism in patients with chronic portosystemic encephalopathy. Gut 1971; 12:702-704.

19. Cassi E, Sala E, Beretta R, et al. Trattamento della encefalopatia porto-sistematica con il lattulosio. Clin Ter 1972; 63:531-556.

20. Kardel T, Olsen PZ, Stigsby B, et al. Hepatic encephalopathy evaluated by automatic period analysis of the electroencephalogram during lactulose treatment. Acta Med Scand 1972; 192:493-498.

21. Salvagnini M, Modena C, Naccarato R, et al. Rilievi preliminari intorno all'impiego del lattulosio nel trattamento protratto dell'encefalopatia porto-sistemica. Clin Ter 1972; 63:317-336.

22. Almici C, Inzoli MR, Poloni AE, et al. Il lattulosio nella terapia dell'encefalopatia porto-sistemica. Minerva Med 1973; 64:4596-4603.

23. Fessel JM, Conn HO. Lactulose in the treatment of acute hepatic encephalopathy. Am J Med Sci 1973; 266:103-110.

24. Germain L, Frexinos J, Louis A, et al. Étude en double aveugle du lactulose chez 18 malades atteints d'encéphalopathie hépatique chronique aprés shunt porto-cave. Arch Fr Mal App Dig 1973; 62:293-301.

25. Eisenburg J, Grunst HJ, Holl J. Effect of lactulose on blood ammonia levels in patients with chronic cirrhosis, encephalopathy and after portocaval shunt operation. In: Imler M, Szam I, eds. Recent Progress in Ammonia Metabolism. Baden-Baden, Brussels: Witzstrock G, 1974: 178-187.

26. Reikowski H, Reikowski J, Muting D. Effect of lactulose long-term treatment on increased ammonia levels in the blood and serum phenol values in 36 patients with cirrhosis of the liver. In: Imler M, Szam I, eds. Recent Progress in Ammonia Metabolism. Baden-Baden, Brussels: Witzstrock G, 1974: 174-177.

27. Seidlova V. Laktuloza v lecbe chronickych portosystemicych encefalopatti. Cesk Gastroenterol Vyz 1974; 28:201-207.

28. Atterbury CE, Maddrey WC, Conn HO, et al. Lactulose and neomycin-sorbitol in the treatment of acute portal-systemic encephalopathy: a double blind controlled clinical trial. Gastroenterology 1978; 23:389-406.

29. Conn HO, Leevy CM, Vlahcevic ZR, et al. Comparison of lactulose and neomycin in the treatment of chronic portal-systemic encephalopathy: a double-blind controlled trial. Gastroenterology 1977; 72:573-583.

30. Orlandi F, Freddara U, Candelaresi MT, et al. Comparison between neomycin and lactulose in 173 patients with hepatic encephalopathy. A randomized clinical study. Dig Dis Sci 1981; 26:498-506.

31. Rossi-Fanelli F, Riggio O, Cangiano C, et al. Branched-chain amino acids vs lactulose in the treatment of hepatic coma. A controlled study. Dig Dis Sci 1982; 27:929-935.

32. Fiaccadori F, Ginelli F, Pedretti G, et al. Branched-chain enriched amino acid solutions in the treatment of hepatic encephalopathy: a controlled trial. Ital J Gastroenterol 1985; 17:5-10.

33. Lanthier PL, Morgan MY. Lactitol in the treatment of chronic hepatic encephalopathy: an open comparison with lactulose. Gut 1985; 26:415-420.

14

ADVERSE REACTIONS AND SIDE EFFECTS OF LACTULOSE AND RELATED AGENTS

Harold O. Conn, M.D.

A chapter on the complications of lactulose and related disaccharides is destined to be a short chapter, indeed (Table 1). Although gastrointestinal side effects occur from the top to the bottom of the alimentary tract, the nature of the substance and its metabolic degradation does not lend itself to the production of hypersensitivity reactions or to the production of toxic intermediates.

GASTROINTESTINAL

At the apex of the alimentary tract, *aversion to the taste* of lactulose syrup and *anorexia* are common complaints. In our experience it is commented upon by one-third to one-half of the patients who receive lactulose for portal-systemic encephalopathy (PSE) that we have treated. However, it causes sufficient distress to be discontinued in less than 5% of patients. In half of them the aversion can be overcome by mixing the syrup with orange or lemon juice (it makes a tolerable lemonade) or applesauce. This suggests that part of the distaste may be the viscosity of the syrup as much as its excessive sweetness. Whatever the mechanism of the distaste, it sometimes interferes with appropriate treatment and, certainly, decreases compliance in outpatients. Compliance is a sufficient problem even with the ingestion of inert medications.

The use of lactulose as crystals or as tablets, neither of which are currently available in the United States, almost completely avoids this problem. However, converting crystalline lactulose to a solution for ease of administration may reconstitute the syrup and the distaste.

TABLE 1. Adverse Reactions and Side Effects of Lactulose and Related Agents.

- I. Gastrointestinal
  - A. Upper
    1. Anorexia
    2. Nausea
    3. Vomiting
  - B. Lower
    1. Flatulence
    2. Abdominal pain
    3. Diarrhea
    4. Rectal burning
    5. Pneumatosis intestinalis
- II. Metabolic
  - A. Metabolic acidosis
  - B. Lactase deficiency
  - C. Galactosemia
- III. Drug interactions
  - A. Antibiotic agents
  - B. Cathartic agents
  - C. Constipating agents
  - D. Analgesic, sedative, tranquilizing agents

Lactitol, which is less sweet than lactulose, is better tolerated as a syrup than lactulose.

Lactose, which is much less sweet than lactulose, is well tolerated.

Nausea is not uncommon. It was reported to occur about 25% more frequently in normal subjects receiving lactulose (30 ml per day) than in those receiving a glucose placebo (1). However, this study was performed in volunteers at a prison and nausea was reported frequently in both groups. It is possible that the frequent nausea (16% and 42% in the two groups, respectively) was artifactually exaggerated in the prison setting. In controlled studies of "normal" individuals being treated for constipation, nausea is rare (2-5), but the usual dosage administered is only one-fourth that used in PSE.

Vomiting has not been reported in studies of lactulose as a cathartic. However, it was noted in about 15% of a total of >400 patients treated for PSE (6-9).

Mild nausea occurred in about 5% of patients treated for PSE with lactitol (10-12) or lactose (10) and vomiting was not mentioned at all (10).

Flatulence is apparently the normal status of prisoners, but occurred more commonly in those taking lactulose (1). It appears occasionally in those being treated for constipation (2-5). Flatulence and abdominal cramps are frequently found in patients receiving treatment for acute PSE with large doses of lactulose (6-9). These symptoms are often seen when lactulose is first started and disappears after several days of continued administration.

Flatulence, and/or abdominal discomfort, was observed in 20% to 25% of patients treated for PSE with lactitol or lactulose (10-12) and abdominal pain in 15% and 5%, respectively (10).

Diarrhea can be a major side effect of lactulose treatment. One can quibble about whether or not diarrhea is truly a complication of lactulose. After all, lactulose is used as a cathartic agent, and diarrhea may be considered *evidence of its efficacy*. Indeed, it is our recommendation in acute PSE that lactulose be administered in large (30 to 50 ml), hourly doses until two watery bowel movements occur (8). In that situation diarrhea is an endpoint of therapy, in effect, an effect, rather than a side effect.

In normal subjects, diarrhea may be precipitated in about one-fourth of patients getting 30 ml per day (1). In constipated patients, small doses of lactulose do not induce diarrhea (2-5). In the treatment of PSE, diarrhea may occur in 15% (6), but in most controlled series, notable diarrhea was only an occasional event (7, 8) and required discontinuation in less than 3% (9).

A significant fraction of patients have lactase deficiency to some degree. It is common in blacks, Orientals, Jews, and Indians from India and from America. Conceivably, many patients who exhibit diarrhea while receiving lactulose may have it from the 7 g per 100 ml of lactose that are present in lactulose syrup.

Three reports have been published in which *hypernatremia* has been thought to be a complication of lactulose administration (13-15). Kaupke et al. described a cirrhotic patient who had been treated with 200 ml of lactulose per day (13). It had been continued for four days, *despite the passage of five or six watery stools each day*. On the fifth day he was found comatose, hypotensive, without measurable central venous pressure, and with a BUN of 92 mg per dl and a serum sodium level of 164 mEq per L. These findings were undoubtedly a consequence of excessive administration of lactulose rather than a complication of the agent *per se*.

Warren et al. described hypernatremia (serum sodium >145 mEq per L) in 60% of 25 patients with cirrhosis and PSE (14). The mean serum sodium in these patients was 153 mEq per L. Two-thirds of them had been treated with lactulose, usually 120 ml daily. Nelson et al. retrospectively reviewed the course of 75 hospitalized patients to whom lactulose had been administered (15). In 20 patients, hypernatremia (serum sodium >145 mEq per L) developed (22%). The hypernatremic patients had received a mean daily dose of 118 ml of lactulose. The hypernatremia was not related to renal failure as determined by serum creatinine levels nor to diuretic drugs. It was associated with increased BUN concentration. Unfortunately, the authors do not present the mean duration nor mean total dose of lactulose. Furthermore, data were insufficient to evaluate body weight, fluid intake or output, stool frequency, or stool volume. The authors state, however, that "diarrhea was specifically mentioned in five of the nine patients who died with hypernatremia, but in no instance in those who died with normal serum sodium levels." Diarrhea had also been noted in 8 of 11 survivors with hypernatremia (73%). Thus, diarrhea had been specifically noted in 13 of the 20 patients with hypernatremia (65%). The authors conclude, but are unable to prove, that lactulose-induced diarrhea was probably responsible for the hypernatremia.

In both reports, the mortality was significantly higher in the hypernatremic patients than in those with normal serum sodium levels.

It seems clear that "hypernatremia" is a misnomer. Rather, it seems to me that dehydration and prerenal azotemia are more appropriate terms. The hypernatremia merely represents one component of the dehydration syndrome. In my opinion, the hypernatremia is not a complication of the use of lactulose; it is a complication of the *abuse* of lactulose.

Many physicians believe that lactulose exerts its anticoma effects by its cathartic action, i.e., by the reduction of substrate and product (see Chapter 7). This is an erroneous impression. Lactulose acts via its own degradation by bacteria which produce short-chain fatty acids which acidify the intestinal contents, suppress ammonia production, trap ammonia in the acidified lumen, incorporate ammonia into bacterial protein and speed the elimination of these nitrogenous substances. Diarrhea is not a prerequisite for effective lactulose action. Ideally, the dosage of lactulose should be adjusted to induce two or three soft, acidic bowel movements each day. The induction of diarrhea is a warning sign; when it occurs, the dosage should be reduced since its persistence is potentially dangerous.

Lactulose, which is present in small amounts in commercial baby milks, may occasionally induce diarrhea (16). These formulae contain enough lactulose to induce diarrhea in adults on a gram per kilogram body weight basis. It seems clear that lactitol or lactose in lactase-deficient patients when administered in excessive dosage can cause diarrhea as does lactulose.

Another unusual presumed complication of lactulose administration is pneumatosis intestinalis (Figure 1). The mechanism of this rare lesion is not known. Conceivably, it may be associated with the production of molecular hydrogen from lactulose, which may somehow penetrate the colonic mucosa. The patient complained of abdominal distention and crampy pain. The gas and symptoms disappeared after the lactulose had been discontinued. Conceivably, the pneumatosis was unrelated to the lactulose.

METABOLIC

No metabolic complications have been reported. There is no increase in serum glucose levels in diabetic subjects.

It has been suggested that the large amount of acid in the intestinal tract may induce systemic acidosis. Surprisingly, this phenomenon is rare, if it occurs at all. In a letter to the editor, Mann et al. reported severe lactic acidosis in a patient

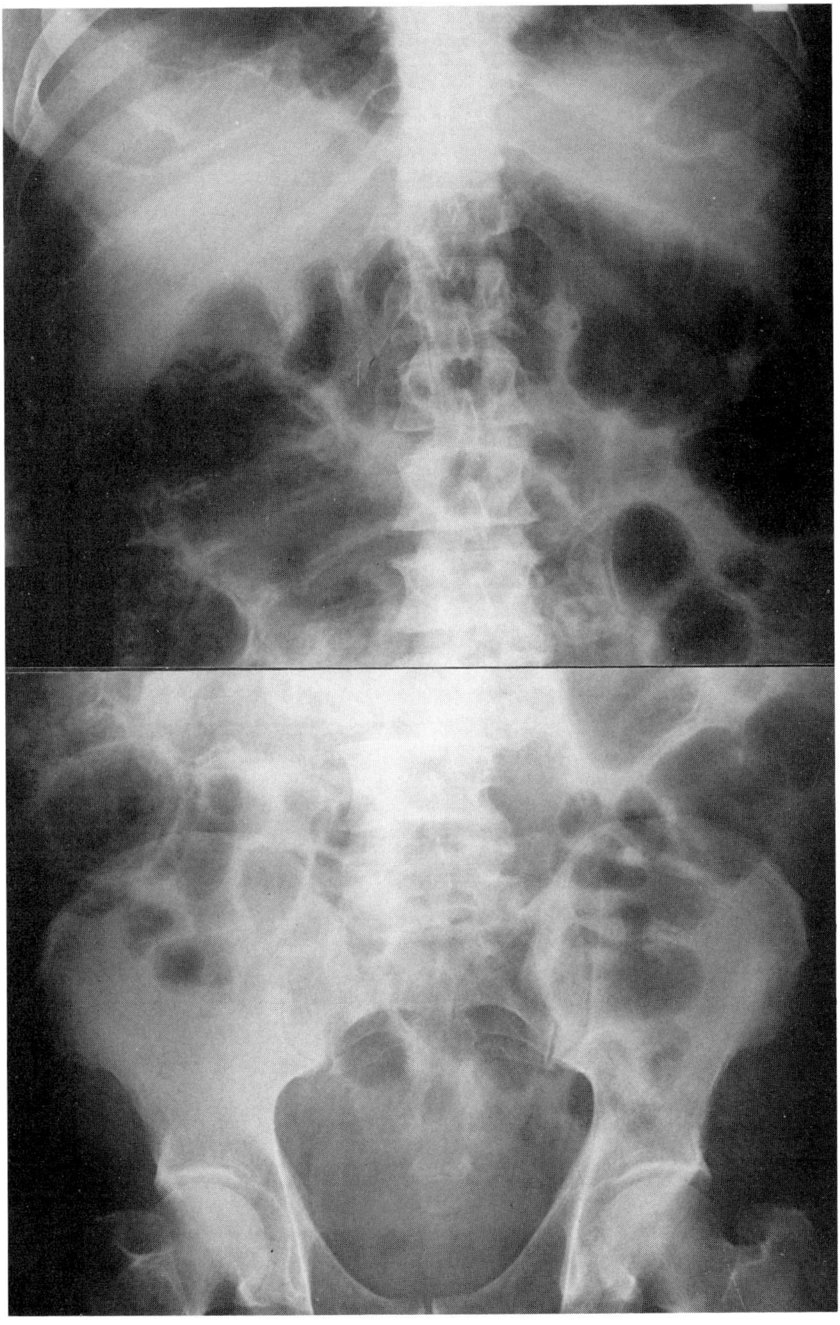

FIGURE 1. Pneumatosis intestinalis in a patient receiving lactulose. Gas outlines the bowel wall.

with congenital hepatic fibrosis and a portacaval shunt who was receiving lactulose (17). This patient had severe azotemia (BUN >90 mg per dl) and acidosis on admission (arterial pH 7.24, serum lactate level 10 mEq per L). Certainly, the lactulose-induced intestinal acidosis may have worsened the preexisting metabolic acidosis in this patient. However, the lactic acidosis, which may occur in fulminant hepatic failure (18), predisposes to systemic acidosis and may exaggerate it in patients receiving lactulose.

No evidence of acidosis developing *de novo* as a consequence of the intracolonic accumulation of acid has been reported. Indeed, the total amount of hydrogen ion produced by therapeutic amounts of lactulose is probably insufficient to cause a systemic metabolic acidosis of significance.

In the rare patient with galactosemia or who otherwise requires a galactose-deficient diet, the administration of lactulose syrup, which contains about 1 g per dl of galactose, is contraindicated. This situation will not come up in clinical conversation very often.

Conceivably, other contaminating carbohydrates such as tagatose, which is present in lactulose syrup (0.4 g per dl), may induce side effects in susceptible patients.

No side effects of lactulose or lactitol enemas have yet been reported (18-21). Occasionally, side effects associated with lactose enemas have been reported (21). These include hyponatremia, hyperglycemia and rectal bleeding. It seems clear that the same kinds of complications can occur with any of these disaccharides, but these probably reflect the dosage administered and the duration of retention of the enema rather than the biochemical structure of the individual sugars.

INTERACTIONS BETWEEN LACTULOSE AND OTHER MEDICATIONS

Theoretically, lactulose, lactitol and lactose, all of which require bacterial degradation, may be inactive in patients who are receiving *antibiotic* agents that inhibit the metabolism of lactulose. In practice this is an uncommon, rarely significant problem. When both lactulose and antibiotics are required, one may attempt to select the antibiotic agents accordingly. Alternatively, one may monitor stool pH to determine whether the carbohydrate is being degraded by bacteria despite the antibiotic coverage (22).

Cathartic agents may have an additive effect with lactulose or related substances on intestinal transit; therefore, the combination of cathartic agents and these carbohydrates should be avoided. Magnesium-containing antacids may act as cathartic agents and may require changing the antacid or increasing the dose of lactulose.

Constipating agents may diminish the efficacy of the carbohydrate by preventing the excretion of nitrogenous wastes. Antacids containing aluminum hydroxide may have obstipating properties.

Antacids may buffer acidification of the colonic contents by lactulose and related sugars and may, thereby, reduce the beneficial effects. The combination should be avoided. Some substances like antacids may adsorb and prevent degradation of the carbohydrate and/or may neutralize the acidification of the carbohydrate.

Analgesic, sedative, tranquilizing agents used simultaneously may obscure the beneficial effects of carbohydrate therapy.

It seems clear that the benefits of disaccharide therapy for hepatic encephalopathy far outweigh its complications.

REFERENCES

1. Bodi T. A safety evaluation of lactulose in normal subjects. Unpublished data on file, Merrell-National Laboratories, Cincinnati, OH 45215.

2. Wesselius-De Casparis A, Braadbaart S, Bergh-Bohlken GE, et al. Treatment of chronic constipation with lactulose syrup. Results of a double-blind study. Gut 1968; 9:84-86.

3. Connoly P, Hughes IW, Ryan G. Comparison of 'Duphalac' and 'Irritant' laxatives during and after treatment of chronic constipation. A preliminary study. Curr Med Res Opin 1975; 2:620-625.

4. Sanders JF. Lactulose syrup assessed in a double-blind study of elderly constipated patients. J Am Geriatr Soc 1978; 26:236-239.

5. Bocklehurst JC, Kirckland JL, Martin J, et al. Constipation in long-stay elderly patients. Its treatment and prevention by lactulose, poloxalkol-dihydroxyanthroquinolone and phosphate enemas. Gerontology 1983; 29:181-184.

6. Conn HO, Lieberthal MM. Formulation and pharmacology of lactulose. In: The Hepatic Coma Syndromes and Lactulose. Baltimore, Maryland: Williams & Wilkins, 1978: 248-277.

7. Conn HO, Leevy CM, Vlahcevic ZR, et al. Comparison of lactulose and neomycin in the treatment of chronic portal-systemic encephalopathy. A double-blind controlled trial. Gastroenterology 1977; 72:573-583.

8. Atterbury CE, Maddrey WC, Conn HO. Neomycin-sorbitol and lactulose in the treatment of acute portal-systemic encephalopathy. A controlled, double-blind clinical trial. Am J Dig Dis 1978; 23:398-406.

9. Orlandi F, Feddara U, Candelaresi MT, et al. Comparison between neomycin and lactulose in 173 patients with hepatic encephalopathy. A randomized clinical study. Dig Dis Sci 1981; 26:498-506.

10. Uribe M, Toledo H, Perez F, et al. Lactitol, a second-generation disaccharide for treatment of chronic portal-systemic encephalopathy. A double-blind, crossover, randomized clinical trial. Dig Dis Sci 1987; 32:1345-1353.

11. Morgan MY, Hawley KE. Lactitol vs lactulose in the treatment of acute

hepatic encephalopathy in cirrhotic patients: a double-blind randomized trial. Hepatology 1987; 7:1278-1284.

12. Heredia D, Teres J, Orteu N, et al. Lactitol vs lactulose in the treatment of chronic recurrent portal-systemic encephalopathy (PSE) (Abstract). J Hepatol 1987; 5, suppl 1:S143.

13. Kaupke C, Sprague T, Gitnick GL. Hypernatremia after the administration of lactulose (Correspondence). Ann Intern Med 1977; 86:745.

14. Warren SE, Mitas JA, Swerdlin AHR. Hypernatremia in hepatic failure. JAMA 1980; 243:1257-1260.

15. Nelson DC. McGrew WRG Jr, Hoyumpa AM Jr. Hypernatremia and lactulose therapy. JAMA 1983; 249:1295-1298.

16. Hendrickse RG, Wooldridge MAW, Russell A. Lactulose in baby milks causing diarrhoea simulating lactose intolerance. Br Med J 1977; 1:1194-1195.

17. Mann NS, Russman HB, Mann SK, et al. Lactulose and severe lactic acidosis (Correspondence). Ann Intern Med 1985; 102:637.

18. Kersh ES, Rifkin H. Lactulose enemas. Ann Intern Med 1973; 78:81-84.

19. Ratnaike RN, Hicks EP, Hislop IG. The rectal administration of lactulose. Aust NZ J Med 1975; 5:137-140.

20. Uribe M, Berthier JM, Lewis H, et al. Lactose enemas plus placebo tablets vs neomycin tablets plus starch enemas in acute portal-systemic encephalopathy. A double-blind randomized controlled study. Gastroenterology 1981; 81:101-106.

21. Uribe M, Campollo O, Vargas F, et al. Acidifying enemas (lactitol and lactose) vs nonacidifying enemas (tap water) to treat acute portal-systemic encephalopathy: a double blind, randomized clinical trial. Hepatology 1987; 7:639-643.

22. Conn HO, Lieberthal MM. Lactulose and neomycin: combined therapy. In: The Hepatic Coma Syndromes and Lactulose. Baltimore, Maryland: Williams & Wilkins, 1978: 340-345.

15

COMBINATION THERAPY WITH LACTULOSE AND ANTIBIOTICS

FREDRICK L. WEBER, JR., M.D.

Clinical trials have amply demonstrated that both lactulose and antibiotics are effective in the treatment of acute and chronic portal-systemic encephalopathy (PSE) (1-7). A question of considerable practical importance is whether combining lactulose with an antibiotic such as neomycin or metranidazole can give a better therapeutic effect than single-agent therapy alone. In spite of the frequent need for information to answer this clinical dilemma, firm evidence to support either approach is limited.

In considering a rationale for combination therapy it must be emphasized that the beneficial effects of lactulose depend on its metabolism by the colonic flora (3). The question then becomes whether lactulose can be metabolized by a subset of intestinal bacteria which is resistant to neomycin or some other antibiotic of choice. In fact, because of the variability of the colonic flora between individuals, probably no two patients will have the same response to combination therapy. This review will, however, tentatively conclude that some, but not all, patients respond better to a combined regimen than to single agent therapy alone. In approaching this topic, four general areas will be reviewed: a) evidence that antibiotic treatment alone is effective; b) theoretical problems concerning the addition of antibiotics to lactulose treatment; c) metabolic data indicating additive effects of lactulose and antibiotics; and d) a review of the scant clinical data that exists on the therapeutic effect of combination therapy in patients.

ANTIBIOTIC TREATMENT

Early observations indicated that neomycin was particularly effective in the treatment of PSE (8-10). Although these early studies did not meet rigorous modern standards of being double-blind and controlled, the initial evidence was compelling and subsequent clinical efficacy so apparent that antibiotics assumed a major role in the treatment of PSE. One rationale for antibiotic therapy was that it would inhibit urease-containing bacteria and hence reduce the amount of ammonia produced in the large intestine. Evidence obtained by Macbeth et al. indicated that neomycin treatment significantly reduced fecal urease activity when enzyme activity was expressed in terms of concentration or as the total amount excreted per day (11). Proteolytic enzyme activity, which might also contribute to the production of ammonia or other cerebral toxins, was also substantially inhibited (11). Early evidence also indicated that the effectiveness of antibiotics was not solely due to reducing ammonia production and that other bacterial metabolites could precipitate PSE. The administration of the amino acid methionine was shown by Phear et al. to cause hepatic encephalopathy without increasing blood ammonia whereas pretreatment with chlortetracycline reversed this effect of methionine (12).

More recently antibiotics have been evaluated in the treatment of both acute and chronic PSE in double-blind, controlled studies where protein intake was sufficiently controlled to permit comparisons (Table 1). Conn et al. evaluated both neomycin and lactulose in patients with chronic PSE. They found that neomycin and lactulose were equally effective when compared to control periods when treatment was omitted (3). Morgan et al. evaluated neomycin and metronidazole in patients with chronic PSE and found that both antibiotics were approximately equally effective when compared to a control period without treatment (5). In acute PSE, treatment trials using control periods are not available; however, neomycin

TABLE 1. Double-blind, Controlled Studies Demonstrating the Efficacy of

Antibiotic Regimen	Comparison Treatment(s)	Patients
Neomycin 6 g per day (+ sorbitol)	Control period and placebo tabs plus lactulose	Chronic PSE (n=29)
Neomycin 4 g per day vs metronidizole 0.8 g per day	Control period	Chronic PSE (n=18)
Neomycin 6 g per day (+ sorbitol)	Lactulose plus placebo tablets	Acute PSE (neomycin Rx, n=23; lactulose Rx, n=22)
Neomycin 3 g per day (+ starch enemas)	Lactose enemas plus placebo tablets	Acute PSE (neomycin Rx, n=10; lactulose enemas, n=8)

has been compared to other regimens and found to be at least equally effective. Atterbury et al. compared a regimen of neomycin (6 g per day) plus sorbitol to lactulose and placebo tablets and found equal treatment effects with both regimens (1). Uribe et al. compared neomycin (3 g per day) plus starch enemas to placebo tablets and lactulose enemas and also found that both treatments were equally effective (13). A further controlled study, although not double-blinded, found that the response to neomycin and lactulose was similar in a large group (n=173) of patients with both acute and chronic PSE (14). Although neomycin therapy has been considered the standard against which other therapies were to be compared, it has finally been established in double-blind, controlled trials that neomycin is indeed effective (as we thought all along).

THEORETICAL PROBLEMS CONCERNING COMBINATION THERAPY WITH LACTULOSE AND ANTIBIOTICS

The beneficial effects of antibiotic treatment clearly depend upon inhibiting bacterial activity within the bowel lumen while the effectiveness of lactulose therapy depends upon the metabolism of this disaccharide by intestinal bacteria. When determining whether to add an antibiotic to lactulose therapy, one must consider whether or not organisms that can metabolize lactulose are likely to be resistant to the antibiotic. Antibiotics that inhibit the growth of lactulose-metabolizing bacteria might be effective in their own right, but at the expense of abolishing

Antibiotics in Acute and Chronic PSE

Study characteristics	Author(s)
Neomycin and lactulose both effective compared to control	Conn et al., 1977
Neomycin and metronidazole both effective compared to control	Morgan et al., 1982
Neomycin and lactose of equal efficacy	Atterbury et al., 1978
Oral neomycin and lactose enemas of equal efficacy	Uribe et al., 1981

the effects of lactulose. Alternatively, the effectiveness of neomycin could be reduced by the metabolism of lactulose since an acid environment reduces the activity of the aminoglycoside antibiotics (15).

Previous studies have indicated that lactulose can be metabolized by a wide variety of bacterial species which include obligate anaerobes, microaerophilic organisms such as lactobacillus species, and facultative anaerobes (16). Table 2 lists some of the bacterial organisms known to metabolize lactulose along with data obtained *in vitro* concerning their resistance to neomycin and metronidazole (17-19). A number of bacterial species capable of metabolizing lactulose are likely to be resistant to neomycin. Although the facultative anaerobes are almost uniformly sensitive to neomycin (17), anaerobic organisms outnumber aerobes by a factor of 100 to 10,000 (20), and anaerobes are uniformly resistant to neomycin (21) because transport of the aminoglycosides into bacteria is an energy-dependent process which requires molecular oxygen (22). Anaerobes would thus be likely to survive and metabolize lactulose in the presence of neomycin. Furthermore, a study by Read et al. has shown that lactobacilli isolated from the stool of cirrhotic patients are frequently resistant to oral neomycin (23). Metronidazole, on the other hand, might be expected to inhibit a larger proportion of the lactulose-metabolizing bacteria because of its effectiveness against anaerobes.

These speculations, however, taken from *in vitro* data may have little practical importance when one is actually concerned with the sum of certain metabolic processes contributed to by a vast array of individual bacterial species present in the large bowel. The proportion of individual species present in different patients undoubtedly varies as does their resistance to antibiotics and their ability to metabolize lactulose. Conn has postulated several different effects of combination therapy with lactulose and antibiotics on the enteric flora (24), and the test of whether these two agents can act additively needs to be conducted in human patients.

METABOLIC DATA INDICATING ADDITIVE EFFECTS OF LACTULOSE AND NEOMYCIN

Thus far, studies focusing on metabolic effects have suggested that lactulose and neomycin can act additively when administered to patients with cirrhosis. One way of assessing the interaction of these drugs is to monitor stool pH. Lactulose is known to acidify the stool because bacteria produce organic acids as they metabolize lactulose. If the stool remains acidic after an antibiotic is introduced, one would conclude that lactulose-metabolizing bacteria have survived and that one might see an additional effect of the antibiotic. On the other hand, if the stool becomes neutral, one would conclude that lactulose-metabolizing bacteria have been eliminated by the antibiotic.

A third possible outcome after the addition of an antibiotic is that the stool

TABLE 2. Colonic Bacteria Capable of Metabolizing Lactulose and Their Antibiotic Resistance

	Neomycin	Metronidazole
Obligate anaerobes:		
Bacteroides sp	R	
Bifidobacteria sp.	R?	R±
Clostridium perfringens	R	
Microaerophilic		
Lactobacillus sp.	R?	
Facultative anaerobes		
Enterobacterial sp.		R
Enterococcal sp. (*E. coli*)		R
Staphylococcal sp. (*S. aureus*)		R

R indicates *in vitro* resistance to the antibiotic listed.

pH will rise, although not to neutrality, indicating that the total capacity of the colonic flora to metabolize the disaccharide has been partially, but not totally, impaired. Conn et al. studied 22 patients who either received lactulose or neomycin followed by combination treatment with lactulose and neomycin (25). Approximately one-third of the group demonstrated each of the three postulated outcomes on combination therapy: that is, a) the stool pH remained acidic on combination therapy; b) the pH rose to neutrality; or c) the pH rose, but remained within the acidic range. These patients would be considered to have received full therapeutic doses of each agent, that is, 60 to 80 g per day of lactulose which is usually found to produce two to four bowel movements per day and 6 g per day of neomycin.

Our laboratory reported six patients whose stool pH was acidic during lactulose therapy and showed no change after the addition of 4 g per day of neomycin (26). Hence, based on observations of stool pH the data indicate that lactulose-metabolizing bacteria will survive in a substantial majority of patients when neomycin is given in doses ranging from 4 to 6 g per day.

Two other observations suggest that neomycin will not totally abolish bacteria which are active in the metabolism of carbohydrates. Gilat et al. found that neomycin caused no inhibition of lactulose metabolism by bacteria as assessed by breath hydrogen production (27). Furthermore, Murphy and Calloway found that neomycin had no consistent effect on intestinal gas production after bean ingestion, indicating that neomycin permitted ongoing bacterial metabolism of another carbohydrate (28).

Contradictory findings have been reported by Patil et al. (29). Using a radiotelemetry device to monitor colonic pH, they found that in three normal subjects neomycin (2 to 4 g per day) abolished the fall in right colonic pH caused by lactulose. In higher concentrations, neomycin also appeared to inhibit lactulose in a fecal incubation system. One singular aspect of these studies was that lactulose alone failed to reduce significantly the fecal pH of these subjects indicating that they received a low dose of lactulose in relation to its usual therapeutic effect. An additional study in rats also found that neomycin administration abolished the fall in colonic pH normally caused by lactulose (30).

Although most of these data indicate that lactulose may continue to be metabolized after the administration of neomycin, they do not establish whether the two agents act additively to cause beneficial alterations in nitrogen metabolism in patients with PSE. We have used urea production and degradation rates to assess the effects of lactulose alone and the combination of lactulose and neomycin in reducing the production of urea precursor nitrogen, presumably ammonia nitrogen, within the intestinal lumen (31, 32).

With stable cirrhotic patients, lactulose alone caused a fall in stool pH to a mean value of 5.5 and a 25% reduction in the urea production rate. This drop in the urea production rate was mainly accounted for by a large increase in fecal nitrogen excretion and a corresponding reduction in urinary urea excretion. An additional component of the reduction in the urea production rate was a modest fall in the urea degradation rate. A fall in the serum urea concentration primarily accounted for the reduction in urea degradation, and only an occasional patient showed a significant drop in intestinal urea clearance which was more likely to reflect directly a change in bacterial ureolysis than the urea degradation rate. Therefore, this study did not confirm the findings of Vince et al. *in vitro* which indicated that an acidic pH similar to that obtained with lactulose would predictably inhibit bacterial urease activity (33).

In further studies we assessed the effects of combination therapy with lactulose and neomycin on urea and nitrogen metabolism in cirrhotic patients (26). Six stable cirrhotic patients were studied during treatment periods lasting eight to nine days. Lactulose was given in doses to produce two to four bowel movements per day (mean dose 55±5 g per day; mean±SEM); then neomycin in a dose of 4 g per day was added to lactulose. After the addition of neomycin, the urea degradation rate fell by 70% which entirely accounted for a 14% reduction in the urea production rate. The intestinal urea clearance rate also fell by 68%. Therefore, neomycin clearly inhibited urea breakdown, but there was no evidence that neomycin reversed the effects of lactulose since stool nitrogen excretion remained high and urinary urea excretion remained low. As previously mentioned, stool pH was acidic during the administration of lactulose and showed no rise when neomycin was added.

In this study we have further analyzed the output of fecal solids and their distribution in the fiber, bacterial, and soluble fractions of stool (34). Nitrogen in the bacterial fraction was significantly reduced by 28% after the addition of neomycin from 1.41±0.2 to 1.01±0.1 g per day. This relatively small reduction indicated that a significant portion of the colonic bacterial flora probably remained viable after the administration of neomycin.

Pirotte et al. obtained further evidence suggesting that lactulose and neomycin may act additively to reduce ammonia production (35). In their study, nine cirrhotic subjects were maintained on a constant protein intake and evaluated during a control period and during periods when they received lactulose alone in a fixed dose of 45 g per day, neomycin alone (1 g per day), and a combination of lactulose and neomycin given in the same dosages. Arterial blood ammonia was determined during fasting and after administration of an oral ammonia load. Both lactulose and neomycin decreased the fasting ammonia concentration when compared to control. Ammonia was further reduced during combination therapy with lactulose and neomycin when compared to either lactulose or neomycin alone. Combination therapy also caused lower peak ammonia concentrations after an ammonia load than single agent therapy with either lactulose or neomycin.

One criticism of this study is that both agents were given in doses which would generally be considered substandard. Lactulose in a dose of 45 g may not produce two to four bowel movements in all patients and 1 g per day of neomycin is certainly less than has been used in most other studies. Nevertheless, in defense of the study it should be noted that lactulose alone caused a reduction in stool pH to below 5 in all patients, and neomycin alone caused a significant reduction in fasting blood ammonia, indicating that there were demonstrable metabolic effects with both agents.

Hence, the available evidence does suggest that the combination of lactulose with an antibiotic such as neomycin can cause additive metabolic effects on nitrogen metabolism that one would expect to be beneficial. A reduction in blood ammonia does not necessarily mean that the encephalopathy has improved, but many studies in patients with chronic PSE have found a good correlation between the blood ammonia concentration and the course of encephalopathy (3, 36-38), including studies where the treatment might be expected to reduce blood ammonia selectively (39, 40).

THERAPEUTIC EFFECTS OF COMBINATION THERAPY WITH LACTULOSE AND NEOMYCIN

There is little clinical information on the efficacy of combination therapy in the treatment of PSE itself. Imler et al. found that neither lactulose (45 g per day) nor neomycin (2 g per day) individually normalized the mental state of two patients with hepatic encephalopathy, but a combination of lactulose and neomycin did cause further improvement in mental status, blood ammonia and EEGs (41).

Over the course of several years we have studied eight patients with stable cirrhosis and mild (no greater than grade I) encephalopathy who had an inadequate response to lactulose alone when given in doses to produce two to four acidic bowel movements a day. Patients were then systematically evaluated during a control period, a lactulose period, and a period when neomycin (4 g per day) was added to lactulose; each period lasted at least seven days.

All of these patients were closely monitored on a metabolic ward and received a constant protein intake of either 1 g per kg or 0.6 g per kg body weight depending on individual tolerance. Liver tests, blood electrolytes and renal function were stable throughout the study, and patients were free of infection, gastrointestinal bleeding, renal failure and electrolyte abnormalities. Blood ammonia levels (42), Number Connection Tests (43) and electroencephalograms (44) were all performed and evaluated by blinded observers on two separate occasions at the end of each period.

Lactulose alone had no significant effect on any parameter except stool pH when compared to the control period (Table 3). After neomycin was added to lactulose, two of the eight patients showed no further improvement in encephalopathy or in blood ammonia concentration, and both of these patients developed less acid stools. The other six patients whose stools remained acidic had significant improvement in blood ammonia levels and Number Connection Tests when compared to the control period. In four of these six patients, EEGs also showed substantial improvement on combination therapy when compared to the lactulose or control period.

It should be acknowledged that this study does not strictly meet the standards of a double-blind, controlled trial, nor was there a control period at the end of the study to insure that steady state conditions were present throughout the study period. Nevertheless, we believe the study does establish that combination therapy may be more effective than lactulose therapy alone. In particular, when lactulose alone has failed to restore normal mental status, the results suggest that a majority of patients will have a better response to combination therapy.

Although one would certainly like more data concerning the effects of combination therapy with lactulose and antibiotics in patients with PSE, a rationale does exist for the use of combination therapy when there has been an incomplete

TABLE 3. Additive Effect of Lactulose and Neomycin in PSE (n=6)

	Control	Lactulose	Lactulose + neomycin
Blood ammonia (mg nitrogen per dl)	175±13	161±19	129±11*
Number Connection Tests (seconds)	56±3	51±4	45±4*
Stool pH	7.0±0.2	5.3±0.3*	5.3±0.3*

* Significantly different from control by analysis of variance and multiple comparison procedures.

response to single agent therapy alone. In this regard, there is the most experience with neomycin among the antibiotics and there is a theoretical rationale to suggest that this relatively narrow spectrum antibiotic is more likely to permit lactulose-metabolizing bacteria to survive than metronidazole. If patients are treated with combination therapy, it is most appropriate to monitor stool pH, and if one observes a significant rise after the antibiotic is added, combination therapy should probably not be continued. In this situation, one would most likely be left with neomycin as the sole effective therapeutic agent. Depending on the assessment of clinical response, one may stop the antibiotic and restart lactulose or continue neomycin alone since individual patients may have a better response to one or the other agent.

REFERENCES

1. Atterbury CE, Maddrey WC, Conn HO. Neomycin-sorbitol and lactulose in the treatment of acute portal-systemic encephalopathy. Am J Dig Dis 1978; 23:398-406.
2. Bircher J, Haemmerli UP, Scollo-Lavizzari G. Treatment of chronic portal-systemic encephalopathy with lactulose. Am J Med 1971; 51:148-159.
3. Conn HO, Leevy CM, Vlahcevic ZR, et al. Comparison of lactulose and neomycin in the treatment of portal systemic encephalopathy. Gastroenterology 1977; 72:573-583.
4. Elkington SG, Floch MH, Conn HO. Lactulose in the treatment of chronic portal-systemic encephalopathy. A double-blind clinical trial. N Engl J Med 1969; 281:408-412.
5. Morgan MH, Read AE, Speller PCE. Treatment of hepatic encephalopathy with metronidazole. Gut 1982; 23:1-7.
6. Simmons F, Goldstein H, Boyle JD. A controlled clinical trial of lactulose in hepatic encephalopathy. Gastroenterology 1970; 59:827-832.
7. Zeegen R, Drinkwater J, Fenton J, et al. Some observations on the effects of treatment with lactulose on patients with chronic hepatic encephalopathy. Q J Med 1970; 39:245-263.
8. Dawson AM, McLaren J, Sherlock S. Neomycin in the treatment of hepatic coma. Lancet 1957; 2:1262-1268.
9. Fisher CJ, Faloon WW. Blood ammonia levels in hepatic cirrhosis. Their control by the oral administration of neomycin. N Engl J Med 1957; 256:1030-1035.
10. Najarian JS, Jew J, Dakin RL, et al. Control of ammonia production in the colon with neomycin enemas. Arch Surg 1959; 78:844-850.
11. Macbeth WAAG, Kass E, McDermott WV Jr. Treatment of hepatic encephalopathy by alteration of intestinal flora with lactobacillus acidophilus.

Lancet 1965; 1:399-403.

12. Phear EA, Ruebner B, Sherlock S, et al. Methionine toxicity in liver disease and its prevention with chlortetracycline. Clin Sci 1956; 15:93-117.

13. Uribe M, Berthier JM, Lewis H, et al. Lactose enemas plus placebo tablets vs. neomycin tablets plus starch enemas in acute portal systemic encephalopathy. A double-blind randomized controlled study. Gastroenterology 1981; 81:101-106.

14. Orlandi F, Freddara U, Candelaresi MT. Comparison between neomycin and lactulose in 173 patients with hepatic encephalopathy. Dig Dis Sci 1981; 26:498-506.

15. Sabath LD, Tuftegard I. Rapid microassays for clindamycin and gentamycin when present together and the effect of pH and of each other on the antibacterial activity of the other. Antimicrob Agents Chemother 1974; 6:54-59.

16. Hoffman K, Mossel DA, Korus W. Untersuchungen uber de wirkungsweise der lactulose (ß-galactosido-fructose in darm). Klin Wochenschr 1964; 42:126-130.

17. Lorian V. Antibiotics in Laboratory Medicine, 2nd ed. Baltimore: Williams and Wilkins Co, 1986.

18. Sutter VL. Antimicrobial agents and chemotherapy. American Society for Microbiology 1976; 10:736-752.

19. Lechevalier HA, Bryson V. Antimicrobial activity of neomycin. In: Waisbren SA, Waisbren BA, eds. Neomycin. Baltimore: Williams and Wilkins Co, 1958: 87-100.

20. Simon GL, Gorbach SL. Intestinal flora in health and disease. Gastroenterology 1984; 86:174-193.

21. Ristuccia AM. Aminoglycosides. In: Ristuccia AM, Cunha BA, eds. Antimicrobial Therapy. New York: Raven Press, 1984: 305-328.

22. Hancock REW. Aminoglycoside uptake and mode of action with special reference to streptomycin and gentamycin. I. Antagonists and mutants. J Antimicrob Chemother 1981; 8:249-276.

23. Read AE, McCarthy CF, Heaton KW, et al. Lactobacillus acidophilus ((Enpac) in treatment of hepatic encephalopathy. Br Med J 1966; 1:1267-1269.

24. Conn HO. Complications of portal hypertension. In: Gitnick G, ed. Current Hepatology. New York: John Wiley and Sons, 1984: 224-226.

25. Conn HO, Lieberthal MM. Lactulose and neomycin: combined therapy. In: The Hepatic Coma Syndromes and Lactulose. Baltimore: Williams and Wilkins Co, 1979: 340-345.

26. Weber FL Jr, Fresard KM, Lally BR. Effects of lactulose and neomycin on urea metabolism in cirrhotic subjects. Gastroenterology 1982; 82:213-217.

27. Gilat T, Ben Hur H, Gelman-Malachi E, et al. Alterations of the colonic flora and their effect on the hydrogen breath test. Gut 1978; 19:602-605.

28. Murphy EL, Calloway DH. The effect of antibiotic drugs on the volume and composition of intestinal gas from beans. Am J Dig Dis 1972; 17:639-642.

29. Patil DH, Westaby D, Mahida YR. Comparative modes of action of lactitol

and lactulose in the treatment of hepatic encephalopathy. Gut 1987; 28:255-259.

30. Mann NS, Borkar BB, Narenderan KP. Effect of lactulose, neomycin, and antacid on colonic pH recorded continuously with an implanted electrode. Am J Gastroenterol 1979; 72:141-145.

31. Weber FL Jr. The effect of lactulose on urea metabolism and nitrogen excretion in cirrhotic patients. Gastroenterology 1979; 77:518-523.

32. Weber FL Jr, Fresard KS. Comparative effects of lactulose and magnesium sulfate on urea metabolism and nitrogen balance in cirrhotic subjects. Gastroenterology 1981; 80:994-998.

33. Vince A, Dawson AM, Park N. Ammonia production by intestinal bacteria. Gut 1973; 14:171-177.

34. Weber FL Jr, Banwell JG, Fresard KM. Nitrogen in fecal bacterial, fiber and soluble fractions of cirrhotic patients; effects of lactulose and lactulose plus neomycin. J Lab Clin Med 1988; 110:259-263.

35. Pirotte J, Guffens JM, Devos J. Comparative study of basal arterial ammonemia and of orally-induced hyperammonemia in chronic portal systemic encephalopathy, treated with neomycin, lactulose and an association of neomycin and lactulose. Digestion 1974; 10:435-444.

36. McDermott WV Jr, Adams RD, Riddell AG. Ammonia metabolism in man. Ann Surg 1954; 140:539-556.

37. Stahl J. Studies of the blood ammonia in liver disease. Its diagnostic, prognostic, and therapeutic significance. Ann Intern Med 1963; 58:1-24.

38. Weber FL Jr, Reiser BJ. Relationship of plasma aminoacids to nitrogen balance and portal-systemic encephalopathy in alcoholic liver disease. Dig Dis Sci 1982; 27:103-110.

39. Hirayama C, Ichida F, Takahashi Y. A controlled clinical trial of nicotinohydroxamic acid and neomycin in advanced chronic liver disease. Digestion 1982; 25:115-123.

40. Mendenhall CL, Rouster S, Marshall L. A new therapy for portal systemic encephalopathy. Am J Gastroenterol 1986; 81:540-543.

41. Imler M, Kurtz D, Bockel R. Étude comparative du traitment de l'encephalopathie porto-cave par le lactulose, les bacilles lactiques et les antibiotiques. Thérapeutique 1971; 47:237-248.

42. Seligson P, and Hirahara K. Measurement of ammonia in whole blood, erythrocytes, and plasma. J Lab Clin Med 1957; 49:962-974.

43. Conn HO. Trailmaking and number connection tests in the assessment of mental state in portal-systemic encephalopathy. Dig Dis Sci 1977; 22:541-550.

44. Parsons-Smith BG, Summerskill WHJ, Dawson AM, et al. The electroencephalograph in liver disease. Lancet 1967; 2:867-871.

SECOND GENERATION "LACTULOSES"

16

LACTITOL: CHEMICAL AND BIOLOGICAL PROPERTIES

JOHN A. VAN VELTHUIJSEN, PH.D.

Lactitol is a sweet-tasting sugar alcohol derived from lactose (milk sugar) by reduction of the glucose part of this disaccharide; it has not been found in nature. It was described in the literature for the first time by Senderens (1) in 1920; the first useful preparation was made by Karrer and Büchi in 1937 (2).

Lactitol is also named lactit in German, lactositol and lactobiosit. The CAS registry number is 585-86-4. The molecular weight of anhydrous lactitol ($C_{12}H_{24}O_{11}$) is 344.32 (Figure 1).

Lactitol:
4-0-(β-D-Galactopyranosyl)-D-Glucitol

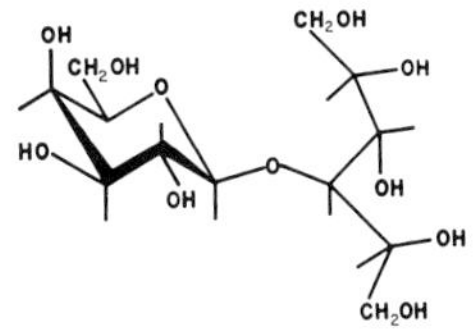

Lactulose:
4-0-(β-D-Galactopyranosyl)-D-Fructose

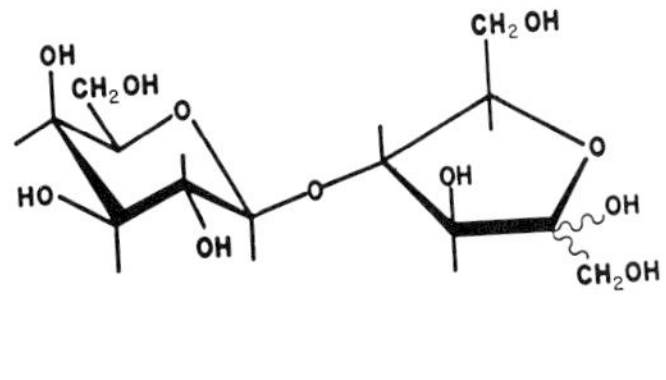

FIGURE 1. The chemical structure of lactitol compared to that of lactulose.

PREPARATION

The principles of the preparation of lactitol are of general knowledge. The industrial process is a hydrogenation of a 30% to 40% lactose solution at about 100°C with a Raney Nickel catalyst (3). The reaction is carried out in an autoclave under a hydrogen pressure of 40 bar or more. Upon sedimentation of the catalyst the hydrogenated solution is filtered and purified by means of ion-exchange resins and activated carbon. The purified lactitol solution is then concentrated and crystallized.

The monohydrate as well as the dihydrate can be prepared depending on the conditions of crystallization (4).

Hydrogenation under more severe conditions (130°C, 90 bar) results in partial epimerization to lactulose and partial hydrolyzation to galactose and glucose and hydrogenation to the corresponding sugar alcohols lactitol, lactulitol, sorbitol and galactitol (dulcitol) (5).

PHYSICAL PROPERTIES

Lactitol is very soluble; crystalline anhydrous lactitol can be obtained from ethanol solutions, having a melting point of 146°C. This substance is very hygroscopic and not for practical use. Crystallization from aqueous solutions results in nonhygroscopic white monohydrate or dihydrate crystals. The dihydrate has a melting point of 76 to 78°C and the monohydrate has a more complicated melting behavior: under the melting microscope, most of the crystals melt at 121 to 123°C, but part of the crystalbound water evaporates below 100°C, converting this monohydrate into the anhydrous form. The melting point determination of the monohydrate by differential scanning calorimetry shows the main endothermal peak in the range of 96 to 107°C (water evaporation). X-ray diffraction analysis has been performed with the monohydrate and dihydrate. The crystal and molecular structures of both hydrates have been fully elucidated (6). The relative density of the orthorhombic monohydrate is 1.523 g per cm^3 and for the tetragonal dihydrate it is 1.445 g per cm^3.

The specific rotation, calculated as anhydrous lactitol, is:

$$[\alpha]^{25}_{D} = +14.2^\circ$$

The relative sweetness of lactitol, compared with an 8% sucrose solution is 0.39. Although lactitol is not as sweet as sucrose, it has a clean, sweet taste that closely resembles sucrose in character.

For pharmaceutical use, the monohydrate is preferred because of its lower water content and the higher melting point. In this chapter, only the physical properties of the monohydrate will be mentioned since only the lactitol monohy-

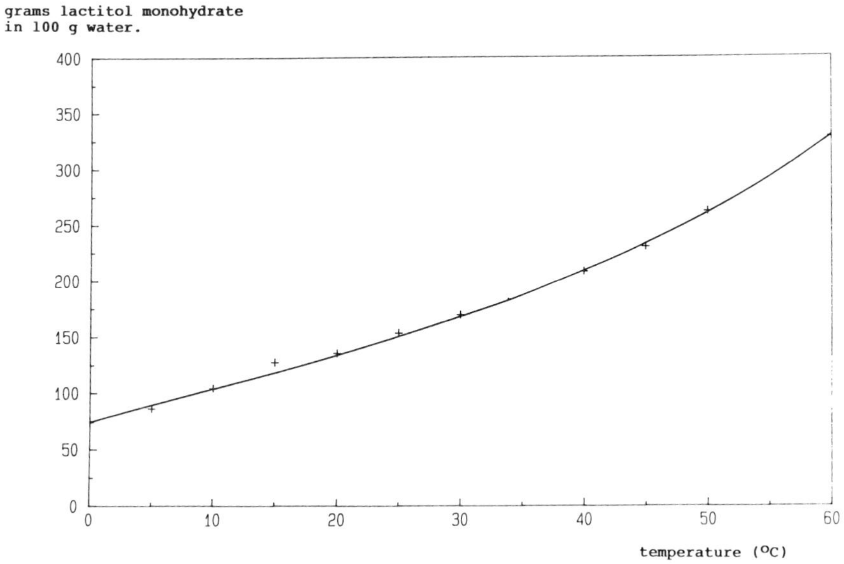

FIGURE 2. Solubility of lactitol monohydrate in water at different temperatures. + = monohydrate.

drate is prepared for medical use.

Solubility. Lactitol is highly soluble in water. At 25°C, 150 g of lactitol monohydrate dissolve in 100 ml water, resulting in a solution with 60% d.s. Solubility increases with increasing temperature, as shown in Figure 2.

It is only soluble in polar organic solvents (Table 1).

Heat of solution: when lactitol is dissolved in water, the crystals require energy to dissolve, the so-called cooling effect. The heat of solution is -52.1 J per g for lactitol monohydrate.

Viscosity. The viscosity of lactitol at different concentrations is shown in Figure 3. The viscosity of aqueous lactitol solutions is similar to the viscosity of sucrose solutions at equal concentrations (Table 2).

Hygroscopicity and water activity. Lactitol monohydrate is essentially nonhygroscopic. It is far less hygroscopic than sorbitol and xylitol and is approximately equal to mannitol (Figure 4).

TABLE 1. Solubility in 100 g of Solvent

Dimethylsulfoxide	25°C	233	g monohydrate
Dimethylformamide	25°C	39	g monohydrate
Ethanol	25°C	0.75	g monohydrate
	50°C	0.88	g monohydrate
Ether	25°C	0.40	g monohydrate

TABLE 2. Viscosities of Lactitol and Sucrose Solution at Equal Concentrations

	Lactitol 60% d.s.	Sucrose 60% d.s.
30°C	47 cP	45 cP
50°C	21 cP	19 cP

The hygroscopicity of the solid material is related to the water activity of the aqueous solution and the relative humidity at equilibrium (ERH).

$$A_w = \frac{P}{Po} = \frac{\text{vapor pressure of solution}}{\text{vapor pressure of water}} = \frac{ERH}{100}$$

Water activity is important in regulating the attraction or release of moisture. It also influences microbial activity, enzymatic activity and fat oxidation.

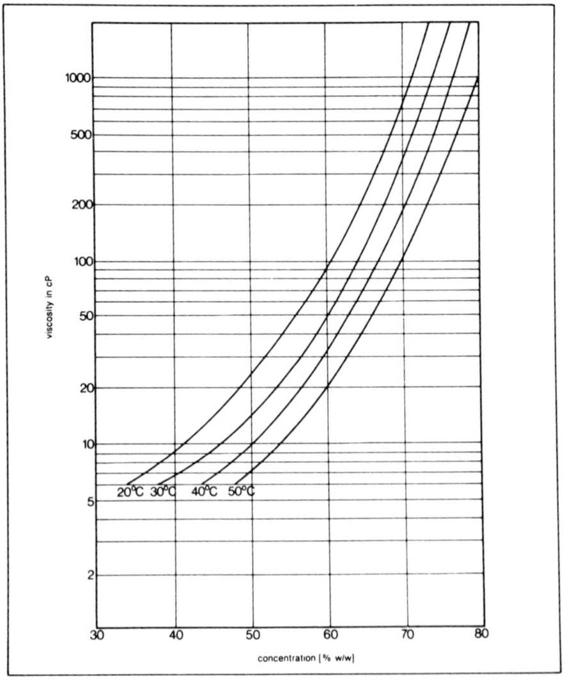

FIGURE 3. Viscosities of lactitol solutions.

As water activity is related to molar concentration, it is not surprising that the water activities of lactitol solutions are similar to those of sucrose solutions (Figure 5).

CHEMICAL PROPERTIES

Lactitol is a polyol with nine OH-groups, which can be esterified with fatty acids resulting in emulsifiers (3), or which can react with propylene oxide (to produce polyurethanes). Due to the absence of a carbonyl group, lactitol is chemically more stable than related disaccharides like lactose. The stability in the presence of alkali is much higher than that of lactose. The stability of lactitol in the

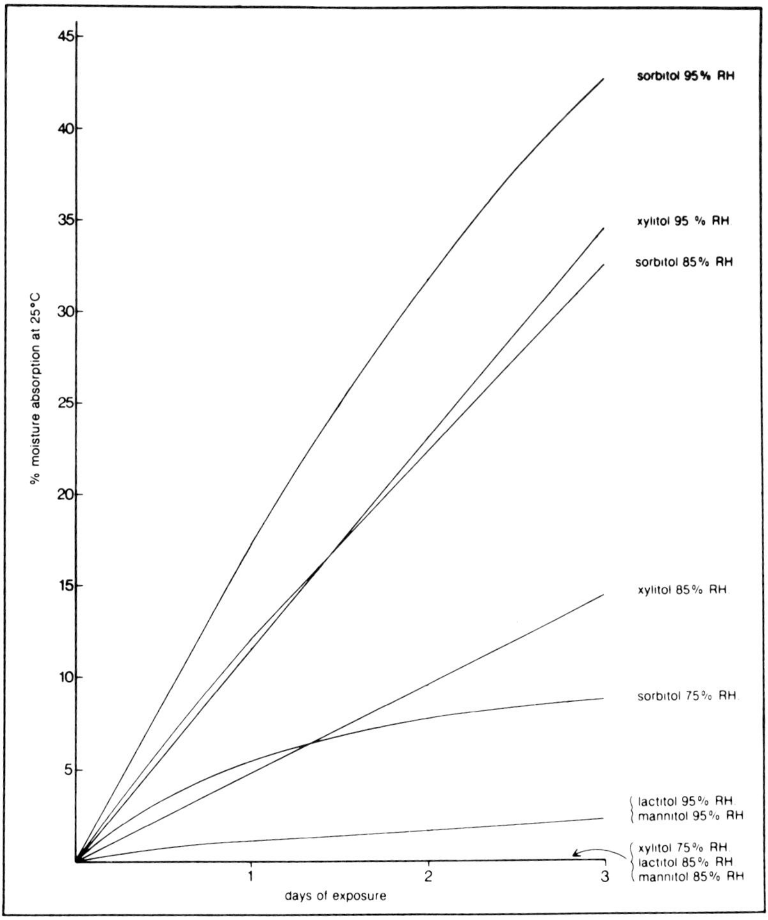

FIGURE 4. Moisture absorption of crystalline polyols at different relative humidities.

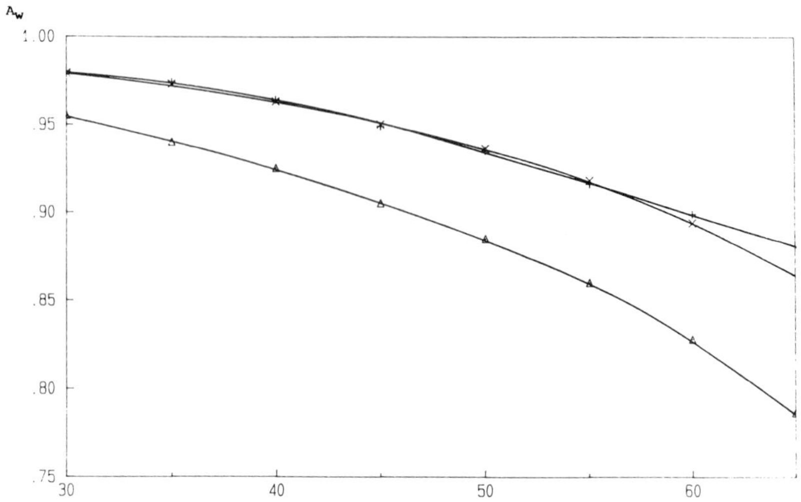

FIGURE 5. Water activity (A_w) of sucrose, sorbitol and lactitol solutions at different concentrations. x = sucrose; + = lactitol; Δ = sorbitol.

presence of acid is similar to that of lactose. The absence of a carbonyl group also means that lactitol does not take part in nonenzymatic browning (Maillard) reactions.

Lactitol solutions have an excellent storage stability in the pH range 3.0 to 7.5 at temperatures up to 60°C. Ten percent lactitol solutions in the range of pH 3.0 to 7.5 at 60°C show no decomposition after one month. After two months at pH 3.0 some decomposition (15%) is detected but not at higher pH. With increasing temperature and especially with increasing acidity, hydrolytic decomposition of lactitol is observed. Sorbitol and galactose are the main decomposition products. At high pH lactitol is stable even at 105°C (Table 3).

TABLE 3. Decomposition of a 10% Lactitol Solution under Extreme Conditions of pH and Temperature

	% weight recovery at 24 h at 105°C			
	Lactitol	Galactose	Sorbitol	Not identified
pH 2.0	42.9	28.1	21.4	7.6
pH 10.0	98.0	-	-	2.0 (acids)
pH 12.0	98.3	-	-	1.7 (acids)

When heated to temperatures of 179° to 240°C, lactitol is partly converted into anhydrous derivatives (lactitan), sorbitol and lower polyols.

Analytical methods for the determination of lactitol. There are several methods for determining polyalcohols in general. The best specific analytical method is the modern high performance liquid chromatography (HPLC) using an ion-exchange column. Aminex HPX-87, manufactured by Biorad, New York, with dimensions of 300 x 7.8 mm, are useful columns.

The working procedure is as follows: make a lactitol solution in water, filter it through a 0.45 μm membrane filter and inject a small volume on the HPLC column that is maintained at 85 °C. The eluent is water and the detector a differential refractometer at 40°C. The typical elution times for polyols are shown in Table 4.

USE AND PURPOSE OF LACTITOL BASED ON BIOLOGICAL PROPERTIES

Lactitol is a sweet-tasting sugar alcohol with interesting nutritional, physiological and pharmaceutical properties. It is not metabolized in animals and man as a carbohydrate since it is neither hydrolyzed nor absorbed in the small intestine. It is metabolized by bacteria in the large intestine where it is converted into biomass, organic acids, CO_2 and a small amount of H_2.

Lactitol consumption does not induce an increase of blood glucose or insulin levels, making it a desirable sugar substitute for diabetic patients.

Furthermore, it has been demonstrated that its nutritional caloric utilization is half that of carbohydrates, with a metabolic energy value of maximum 2 kcal per g or maximum 8.4 kJ per g.

TABLE 4. HPLC Elution Times in Minutes

	HPX 87 C (Ca-form)	HPX 87 P (Pb-form)
Lactose	9.19 min.	12.25 min
Galactose	12.03	15.73
Lactulitol	10.72	17.71
Glucose	10.75	13.40
Lactitol	**12.13**	**23.60**
Maltitol	12.31	21.50
Fructose	13.37	18.00
Ribitol	15.19	22.51
Erythritol	15.92	22.50
Glycerol	16.49	21.70
Mannitol	17.54	28.63
Dulcitol	20.50	36.81
Sorbitol	21.15	39.55

It is very slowly converted to organic acids (lactic acid) by tooth-plaque bacteria, so that lactitol does not cause dental caries and satisfies the Swiss regulations as safe for teeth. These properties already suggest dietary applications, e.g., products for diabetic patients, noncariogenic confections and low calorie foods.

Medically applied, lactitol is useful in the same circumstances as lactulose, such as the treatment of portal-systemic encephalopathy (7) and as a laxative. Medical applications and clinical studies are discussed elsewhere.

TOXICOLOGY

All the required toxicity studies for a food additive have been carried out. There are no deleterious effects of feeding lactitol at levels up to 10% of the diet. There are no toxicological effects at 2%. The Joint Expert Committee of Food Additives FAO/WHO approved lactitol in April 1983. The committee allocated an ADI (Acceptable Daily Intake) "not specified" to lactitol (8).

The Scientific Committee on Food of the EEC evaluated lactitol and consider it to be a safe product; they stated that "consumption of the order of 20 g per person per day of polyols is unlikely to cause undesirable laxative symptoms" (9).

Safety studies in experimental animals included long-term feeding studies at high dietary levels for two and a half years in rats and for two years in mice.

The safety data are summarized here. Full data are described in CIVO-TNO (Zeist, Holland) reports, which are not published. These reports have been evaluated by WHO, SCF-EEC and FDA.

Short-term studies. In acute oral toxicity studies the LD_{50} exceeds 10 g per kg body weight. At this dose, considered to be the highest tolerable amount given as a single oral dose, no deaths or toxicity occurred. With dermal or occular application, there were no adverse effects of lactitol. Acute aqueous toxicity was tested at the maximum concentration 1% in water. No toxicity was found for *Poecilia reticulata* (guppy) or for daphnia (waterflea).

In a biodegradability test, lactitol showed a COD of 955 mg per g of lactitol and a BOD 20 value of 550 mg per g.

Biodegradation was complete within five days, whereas only 50% of the theoretically required oxygen was used. This implies that it is mainly used for growth of microorganisms.

Mutagenicity. Lactitol does not show any mutagenic activity in the Salmonella/microsome mutagenicity tests. In a chromosome analysis of cultured human lymphocytes treated *in vitro* with lactitol or lactose, it was demonstrated that neither substance showed any clastogenic activity.

Subchronic toxicity in rats/liver pathology. A 90-day feeding study with lactitol and lactose showed a resemblance in the various effects caused by either substance. Although more pronounced in the 20% lactitol group than in the 25% lactose group, the similarity suggests a common cause. The most obvious effect is an increase in the weights of the cecum in all lactitol- and lactose-treated rats. Because no histological changes were detected in the cecum and because this is a well-known phenomenon with incompletely digestible carbohydrates, this effect is considered to be an adaptive, rather than a pathological, condition.

There were microscopic liver changes seen (swollen hepatocytes, together with excessively homogeneous cytoplasm) in the 10% and 20% lactitol groups, but not in the 5% lactitol group. The hepatic changes resemble those found in the 25% lactose group.

Similar microscopical abnormalities were found later in F_{3b} young of the multigeneration study, when lactitol diets were fed up to four weeks after weaning, in all test diets (2%, 5% and 10% lactitol). These liver changes were not found in rats on a one-year feeding study.

Consultant pathologists regard the homogeniety change as trivial and of no pathological significance.

In order to find out whether the slight microscopical changes in hepatocytes occur in adult rats, a study was conducted in three-month-old rats (20 males and 20 females per group) with diets containing 0% (control), 10% or 20% lactitol and 20% lactose. After feeding periods of 4, 8 and 12 weeks, the livers of rats/sex/group were examined microscopically. These examinations did not show the homogenous cytoplasm. These negative findings in adult rats suggest that the adult rat is less sensitive to these minor hepatic effects of lactitol than the very young rat.

Multigeneration study in rats. The purpose of this study is to provide data concerning the effect of lactitol-feeding on the reproductive performance, embryotoxicity and litter data of rats for three generations (Figure 6).

Growth rate and survival of the offspring were decreased in the groups fed 10% lactitol or 20% lactose. No unfavorable effect of lactitol on pup survival was seen, however, in the F_3-litters. The results did not reveal any deleterious effect of feeding lactitol on the reproduction parameters, namely, fertility, gestation index, duration of gestation period, resorption quotient and litter size.

Embryotoxicity/teratogenicity study. Lactitol was fed to female rats which had been pretreated *in utero* and subsequently after birth for 15 weeks prior to mating. This study was done with the F_{2a}-young, the second generation rats. Pregnant females continued to be fed the test diets until day 21 of pregnancy at levels of 0% (control), 2%, 5% and 10% in the diet. It was concluded that lactitol at concentrations of 2%, 5% and 10% in the diet does not induce any embryotoxic or teratogenic effect in rat fetuses.

One-year feeding study with rats. In this study with lactitol and lactose in the F_{1a} rats, body weights in all groups fed lactitol or lactose were lower than those of the controls. There was a dose-related increase in feces production (g dry matter per 100 g dry feed) in the groups fed on lactitol. The fecal output with 20% lactose was about the same as with 10% lactitol.

The moisture content of the feces tended to be increased in both lactitol- and lactose-fed groups. The pH of the feces did not show any differences among the groups. From the data of feces production, calculations of digestibility were made. For each 10 g lactitol or 20 g lactose, the amount of fecal dry matter excreted was 3.4 g more than the amount excreted from 10 g sucrose or 20 g sucrose plus starch in 100 g of the control diet. The differences suggest that lactitol has a caloric value 66% that of sucrose, and lactose of 83% of sucrose.

Gross and microscopic examination did not reveal pathological changes which could be ascribed to the ingestion of the test substance.

Life span oral toxicity and carcinogenicity study in rats, pretreated in utero. F_{1a} rats of the five diet groups are fed during a lifetime period of 130 weeks.

Mortality rate was not found unfavorably affected in any of the treated groups. The overall mortality after 130 weeks amounted to 66% for males and 55% for females.

There were no noticeable changes in the composition of the fecal microflora or in the levels of lactic acid and volatile fatty acids in the cecal content and in feces. The levels of lactitol and lactose in the cecum and in the feces were very low, indicating almost complete degradation in the gastrointestinal tract.

The relative weight of the cecum was increased in rats fed lactitol or lactose. Non-neoplastic and hyperplastic histophatological changes observed in kidneys, adrenals and testes consisted of pelvic nephrocalcinosis, mainly in females, and adrenal medullary hyperplasia in males fed lactitol. Similar changes occurred in rats fed lactose. Moreover, male animals fed lactose or lactitol showed increased interstitial cell proliferation in the testes.

The incidence of pheochromocytomas in the adrenals of males was relatively high in the 2% and 10% lactitol groups and the 20% lactose group. The number of testicular Leydig cell tumors was considerably higher in males fed 10% lactitol or 20% lactose than in controls.

The conclusion is that feeding of lactitol may result in changes similar to those obtained upon feeding lactose.

Life span oral carcinogenicity study with lactitol in mice. Lactitol was examined for possible carcinogenicity in mice by feeding the material at levels of 0% (control), 2%, 5% or 10%, incorporated in the basal diet at the expense of sucrose, to groups of 50 male and 50 female mice for two years. From the results of this study it was concluded that feeding of lactitol at dietary levels up to 10% to mice throughout the major part of their lifetime failed to show carcinogenic properties or any other effects of obvious toxicological significance.

Evaluation of carcinogenicity data in rats. An independent expert, Dr. Francis J. C. Roe, who is advisor in experimental pathology and cancer research, has reviewed all data of the long-term feeding study in rats. Further, he has carried out his own examination of the relevant slides of histological sections. In addition, an age- standardized statistical analysis in tumor data for males is done by Mr. Peter Lee. Based on these data and knowledge of the toxicity of lactose and various sugar alcohols, such as sorbitol, xylitol and mannitol, an explanation for these common phenomena has been developed.

The nongenotoxic mechanism(s) by which the administration of lactitol to laboratory rats increases the incidence of some endocrine tumors (adrenal medulla and testis) and decreases the incidence of others (pancreatic islet cell, pituitary) are yet not known, but almost certainly they are the same as those by which lactose produces similar effects. High dietary concentrations of lactose fed to rats cause enlargement of the cecum, increased absorption of calcium from the gut, increased urinary excretion of calcium, pelvic and corticomedullary nephrocalcinosis, acute tubular nephropathy, urinary calculus formation and both hyperplasia and neoplasia of the adrenal medulla.

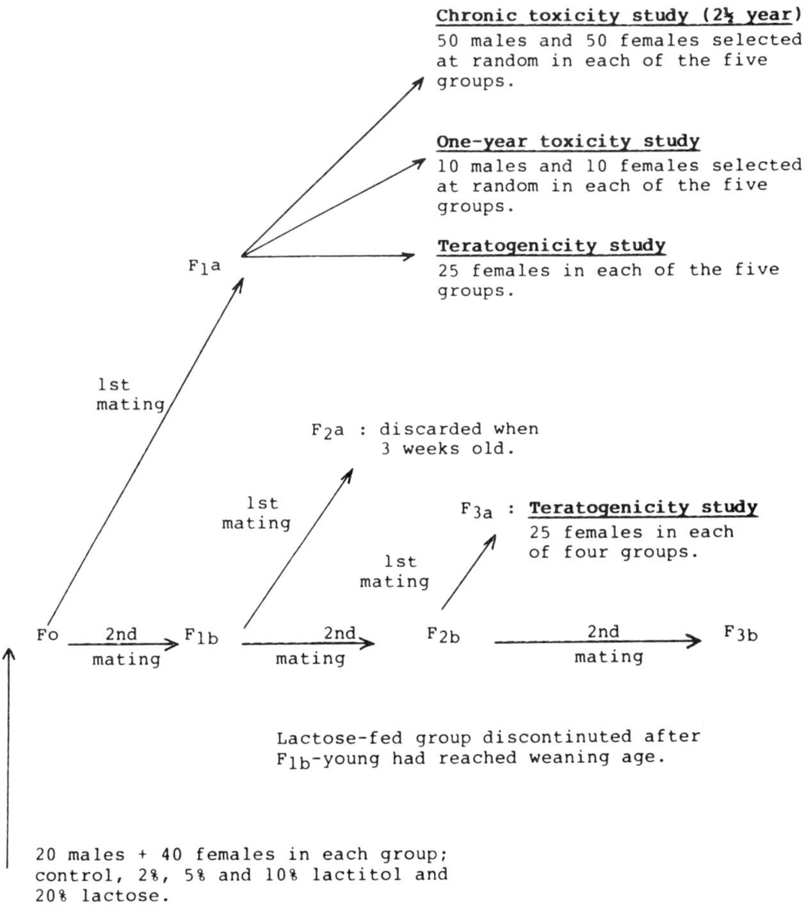

FIGURE 6. Multigeneration study with rats.

Other polyols, such as sorbitol, xylitol and lactitol, exhibit similar effects. Recent evidence suggests that in rats, but not in mice or humans, excessive calcium absorption stimulates the adrenal medulla. The fact that humans do not develop chromaffin-negative nonfunctional tumors of the adrenal medulla even in circumstances where there is hypercalcemia, suggest that there are no real risks of adrenal medullary hyperplasia or neoplasia in man. Finally, the fact that neither lactose nor polyols such as xylitol materially increase calcium absorption in humans in the same way or to the same extent as they do in rats, provides reassurance that these substances will not give rise to nephrocalcinosis in man.

By analogy one may predict that lactitol will not predispose to any form of endocrine tumor by either genotoxic or nongenotoxic mechanisms in man.

FDA/FASEB evaluation of tumor data. In September 1985, FDA requested the Federation of American Societies for Experimental Biology (FASEB) to review the health aspects of sugar alcohols and lactose. All reports and data on lactitol, lactose and other sugar alcohols were studied by an Ad Hoc Experts Panel. Their evaluation is published in a report (10) in September 1986.

Six-month feeding study with lactitol in beagle dogs. Subchronic oral toxicity was examined by feeding lactitol at dietary levels of 0% (control), 5%, 10% or 15% to groups of six male and six female dogs for 26 weeks. An extra group of six male and six female dogs, fed a diet containing 15% lactose, was used for comparison.

The most marked treatment-related effect was an increase in the weight of the cecum, colon and small intestine in males of all lactitol groups and an increase in cecal weight in females of the 10% and 15% lactitol groups (small intestines and colon were not weighed in females). Gross and microscopic examination did not reveal any pathologic changes that could be attributed to the feeding of lactitol or lactose.

BIOCHEMICAL ASPECTS

Absorption, distribution and excretion. Three male rats (150 to 200 g, six to eight weeks of age, one not pretreated and two habituated to a diet containing 7% lactitol) were orally intubated with approximately 2 mg D-(sorbitol-1-^{14}C) lactitol. In the studies with the rats habituated to lactitol, 9% to 15% of the radioactivity was recovered from the air exhaled in the period 0-5 hours and 48% from the air exhaled in the period 0-24 hours.

The urine and the feces contained a minor proportion of the administered radioactivity (urine, 2.3% after five hours and 6.8% after 24 hours; feces, 11.7% after 24 hours). The gastrointestinal tract contained 33% of the radioactivity after five hours and 5% after 24 hours; the remainder of the body contained 20% after five hours and 9% after 24 hours. It was concluded that lactitol is extensively degraded in the rat after oral administration primarily by the intestinal microflora and that habituation of the rats to unlabelled lactitol did not essentially affect the rate and extent of degradation. It was shown that the microbial degradation of lactitol yields products like volatile fatty acids, which are readily absorbed from the gut and are normal intermediates in several metabolic processes.

In another study, the metabolic fate of intravenously administered ^{14}C-lactitol in rat has been examined. It was found that 87% of the lactitol is excreted unchanged in the urine within eight hours.

In a patent application (11), it was demonstrated in rats that lactitol inhibits the absorption of sucrose and the formation of cholesterol. The increase of the blood glucose, after consumption of a 1:1 mixture of sucrose and lactitol, was about half of the increase after consumption of sucrose alone. However, the formation of liver glycogen with the 1:1 mixture was only one-fifth of that with only sucrose. When added to diets containing cholesterol, it was shown that lactitol reduces the hepatic and serum cholesterol levels in rats by as much as 50%.

Enzymatic hydrolysis and absorption. Karrer and Büchi (2) have studied the action of galactosidase-containing enzyme preparations on the splitting of lactitol into galactose and sorbitol. They found that lactitol is only hydrolyzed very slowly by these enzyme preparations.

Later studies reported in a German patent (12) have confirmed that lactitol is only slowly split by enzymes with about a tenth of the speed at which lactose is split. Based on both these *in vitro* studies, a reduced caloric value of lactitol can be expected.

In patients of Hayashibara (13,14), it is claimed that lactitol has no caloric value because it is not digested or absorbed. The intestines of test rabbits not fed for 24 hours beforehand were closed at both ends and were injected with a 20% aqueous solution of lactitol or with an equimolar amount of a sucrose solution. After a lapse of several hours, the lactitol or sucrose left in the intestines was determined. While 85% of the sucrose intake had been lost due to absorption and digestion, all of the lactitol was still present.

Metabolic energy and metabolism in the small intestine. From studies in Lund (15) based on human intestinal biopsies, it was demonstrated that human intestinal mucosa do not show any significant disaccharidase activity towards lactitol as substrate (1% to 2% of that for lactose).

Further reports concerning the same kind of analysis on small intestinal pieces from minipigs towards lactitol, maltitol and isomalt (Palatinit®), have demonstrated that 5% of lactitol is split in germfree pigs and approximately 10% in conventional animals (in man 1%) compared to lactose; 20% to 25% of maltitol is split (in man 13%) compared to 4% of maltose and isomalt (in man 4%) compared to sucrose (invertase).

The activity in human biopsies towards maltitol was about as high as the activity towards threhalose and lactose. This means that significant amounts of ingested maltitol can be digested by man. From these results it can be concluded that the caloric utilization in conventional pigs will be higher than in man in case of lactitol and maltitol, but not with Palatinit®.

A metabolic energy study with human volunteers at the Agricultural University in Wageningen (16) was carried out. In this study 11 volunteers were kept for four days in a respiration room twice. Once they had a diet of 49 g sucrose per day, and once the sugar was replaced by 50 g lactitol monohydrate per day. Extrapolated to 100% lactitol versus 100% saccharose, this would mean considerably lower energy value of metabolic energy of lactitol versus saccharose, showing for lactitol a 60% lower value.

In fact, lactitol monohydrate (containing 5% water) is meant by "lactitol." Further, with regard to the inaccuracy (SE 10%) of the determination, the conclusion that the metabolic energy value of lactitol does not exceed 50% of sucrose is justified.

The caloric value of lactitol (dry substance) is thus established in man as 2 kcal per g. These volunteers had little discomfort during the days of taking 50 g lactitol monohydrate per day, divided in four to six portions during the day. There was no diarrhea. Only in the lactitol period was there more feces per day and the content of the dry matter in feces was lower (13.7% relative). Tolerance is dependent on the manner of consumption and adaptation.

The laxative properties of lactitol and other polyols. It is well known that polyols (hydrogenated sugars) have a laxative effect when consumed in large amounts. When addressing the subject of the laxative effect of polyols, it should be stressed that this effect can not be considered to be toxic. The laxative effect is based on the slow absorption rate of pentitols (xylitol) and hexitols (sorbitol, mannitol) due to the passive absorption mechanism and/or partly incomplete resorption of disaccharide alcohols (isomalt [Palatinit®], lactitol and maltitol) and polydextrose in the small intestine in which case these substances reach lower bowel areas where microbial degradation takes place.

These characteristics can lead to diarrhea caused by an osmotic effect, which limits the use of these substances. The osmotic activity of low-molecular compounds causes a higher water content in the gastrointestinal tract. The colon is endowed with an extraordinary capacity to save fluid and electrolytes for the human body in order to maintain homeostasis.

Polyols have an influence on osmoregulation. The monosaccharide alcohols (xylitol, sorbitol, mannitol) have the strongest osmotic effect, followed by disaccharide alcohols (maltitol, lactitol) and polydextrose according to their molecular weight. Sugars like glucose and sucrose also result initially in water transport into the gastrointestinal tract, but these sugars are rapidly absorbed by an active mechanism. The osmotic effect depends on the dosage given and the osmoregulation (a hormonal regulation) which can be improved by adaptation.

The laxative threshold of lactitol has been determined and compared to that of sorbitol in a double-blind, randomized cross-over study on 21 normal subjects. This study was carried out in the Central Middlesex Hospital, London (17). Laxative threshold in this study was defined as the dose at which the test substance produced unacceptable levels of side effects or the maximum dose of the study (130 g per 24 h) was reached. The administration of test substances was discontinued if the subjects developed more than four bowel movements per 24 h.

The mean "laxative" threshold dose of lactitol was 74 (SE 6) g and for sorbitol 71 (SE 5) g per 24 h. Only two subjects reached the maximum predetermined dose of 130 g lactitol per 24 h. The "laxative" threshold in this study is the limit on account of diarrhea or severe gastrointestinal symptoms. The findings suggest that it would be quite acceptable to administer up to 40 g lactitol per day.

Different from the above "laxative" (diarrhea) dose level is the laxative effect as a favorable effect for treatment in constipation. The laxative effect is defined as the dose at which one normal stool per day is achieved. Many laxative studies have been carried out in patients with constipation.

When given as a single dose, the average daily dose for adults was about 20 g, corresponding to 350 mg per kg body weight for a 65 kg woman (18). In some cases, such as in the study of pregnant constipated women or in elderly patients (19, 20), the average daily dosage was lower, 13 to 16 g per day.

When given in a divided dose in the morning and in the evening, the applied dosage (21, 22) was either similar as in the studies carried out in the UK, 20 or 22 g (23), or markedly higher at 26 g and 29 g (24, 25). Whatever the applied dose, when given twice a day, lactitol appeared to increase the occurrence of abdominal complaints voiced by the patients. In conclusion, a single daily dose is to be preferred in constipation.

Children (26, 27) need comparatively somewhat lower doses than adults, i.e., around 250 mg per kg body weight (range: 150 to 350 mg per kg).

Lactitol was constantly found to be an efficacious laxative, especially when it was given in a single daily dose. Only a tiny minority of patients failed to respond. Lactitol's laxative action was also found to be more predictable (28, 29) and more regular than that of lactulose; the dosage (30), once individually determined, did not need to be changed as did that of lactulose.

During the study of Professor van Es in Wageningen (16) on the metabolic energy of lactitol, the volunteers had very little discomfort from eating 50 g per day of lactitol monohydrate, divided in four to six portions during the day, after a four-day adaptation period. There was no diarrhea; in the lactitol period, the feces had a lower dry matter content and more feces was expressed as dry substance (in the publication in Table 1, the dry substance was not mentioned). As a mean value, 6.77 g additional dry feces is produced per day with consumption of 47.5 g per day dry lactitol compared to 49 g of sucrose.

The type of a laxative effect of sorbitol is different compared to that of lactitol. Sorbitol has an osmotic laxative effect, whereas lactitol induces more feces and gas formation resulting in a laxative effect of more feces-biomass.

The effect of lactitol of inducing more frequent stools in a predictable way is very useful; the side effects of gas formation (CO_2, H_2) can be inconvenient. The same effects are induced by a number of natural food ingredients, such as dietary fiber.

The effect of lactitol on the metabolic activity of the colonic flora of the pig and the human. The metabolic activity of the gut bacterial flora has been recognized for many years. Among the products of importance are ammonia (by amino acid deamination and urea hydrolysis), organic acids (by carbohydrate fermentation and amino acid deamination), bile acid metabolites (by deconjugation and dehydroxylation of the biliary bile acids), indole (by metabolism to tryptophan), volatile phenols (by metabolism of tyrosine) and cholesterol metabolites (by reduction of the 5-6 double bond of cholesterol). The roles of such metabolites are of importance in the causation of gallstones (31), colorectal cancer (32) and hepatic coma (33). A decreased rate of formation of such metabolites might therefore be of importance in improving public health.

The metabolic energy study with lactitol in Wageningen with human volunteers (16) was also used to study the effects on metabolic activity of colonic flora comparing this with the effect of lactitol in pigs (34). The metabolites studied were the products of bile acid and cholesterol metabolism (analyzed in feces) and the urinary volatile phenols produced by the colonic bacterial metabolism of tyrosine. In addition, the effect of lactitol on the composition of the flora of the proximal colon was assessed in pigs. Lactitol feeding inhibited both 7-dehydroxylation of bile acids and reduction of the 5-6 double bond of cholesterol in the minipigs. In the fecal flora, the most notable effect was the decrease in numbers of the aerobic organisms (70-fold for the enterobacteria, principally *E. coli.*)

In all eight human subjects, lactitol feeding resulted in a major decrease in the fecal concentration of cholesterol and its metabolites. In all eight volunteers, lactitol feeding resulted in a massive decrease in fecal bile acid concentration, but there was no decrease in the extent of bile acid dehydroxylation and no consistent effect on the ratio of lithocholic to deoxycholic acid.

In contrast to the human, in the pig lactitol produced a massive increase in urinary volatile phenol production. It is known that such an increase can be achieved by small-bowel overgrowth (where the tyrosine concentration is very much higher than in the large bowel). In contrast to the human, the pig has profuse bacterial flora in the ileum and significant flora in the upper small bowel.

CONVERSIONS OF LACTITOL BY MICROORGANISMS

Tooth-protective properties. Sugars are a major factor in the pathogenesis of dental caries. Oral bacteria convert sugars into polysaccharides that are deposited on the teeth; these plaque sugars are then fermented into acids. The acid demineralizes the enamel and causes cavities.

At the University of Zürich, a special method has been developed for the *in vivo* determination of the plaque pH in humans. After consumption of chocolate or confections in which sucrose is replaced by lactitol, changes in plaque acidification are detected by the electrodes and transmitted electronically to a graph recorder.

The term "Zahnschonend" (safe for teeth/friendly to teeth) is used officially in Switzerland when the pH of a dental plaque does not decrease below 5.7 during a 30-minute period. Professor Mühlemann demonstrated in chocolates that lactitol is "safe for teeth" (35).

In Figure 7, it is shown that during and after eating 13 g Lacty®-chocolate (plain lactitol-containing chocolate), the plaque-pH is not affected, whereas with a 15 ml 10% sucrose solution, the plaque-pH is reduced to about 4.5, which indicates that sucrose is being fermented into acids by the oral bacteria. In another study, it was demonstrated that *Streptococcus mutans* and other bacteria like Lactobacillus and Bifidobacterium isolated from the dental plaque form acids from lactitol, but that acid formation is slow, comparable to that of sorbitol. Moreover, no dental plaque is formed from lactitol (36).

The cariogenicity of lactitol was also tested in rats (37). For this purpose, lactitol was incorporated in a powdered diet, consisting of 50% of a basal diet (SPP, Trouw & Co., Putten, The Netherlands), 25% wheat flour and 25% of test substance.

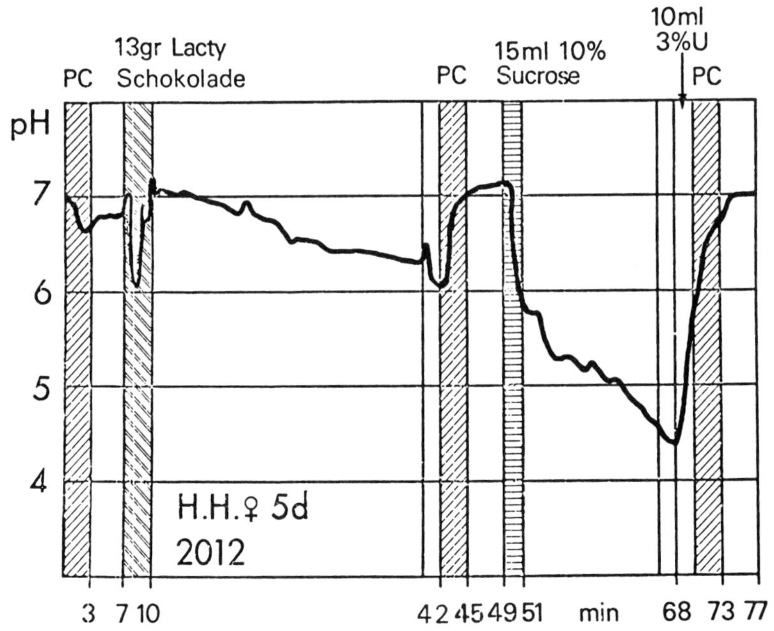

FIGURE 7. Telemetrically recorded pH of 5-day interdental plaque in subject H. H. during and after consumption of 13 g Lacty® plain chocolate. A 10% sucrose solution was used as a positive control. PC = 3 min. paraffin chewing. U = rinsing with 3% Carbamid, 10 ml.

Lactitol was compared with sorbitol, xylitol, sucrose and a control consisting of 50% wheat flour and 50% basal diet. The rats were program-fed. None of the animals suffered from diarrhea. Especially, in the lactitol group no significant adverse effects on general health were observed. The results are shown in Table 5. Obviously, substitution of sucrose by lactitol significantly reduced caries. The caries results for sorbitol and xylitol were in accord with other studies in which these polyols were used.

General fermentability of lactitol. Many bacteria which are able to ferment lactose (e.g., Enterobacteriaceae) are not able to ferment lactitol, e.g., *E. coli*.

LACTITOL AND DIABETES

In a study at the Medical College of the University of Groningen (38) on the effect of lactitol on blood glucose and insulin content in human diabetic subjects and "normal subjects," it has been shown that lactitol is potentially a useful sweetener for diabetic patients. Consumption of lactitol, 24 g per day, does not influence the blood glucose nor insulin concentrations of either group.

Influence of lactitol on blood carbohydrate levels. This test has been described in a CIVO-TNO report (39). Loading tests have been carried out in eight healthy persons, by the intake of 50 g sucrose, 50 g lactose, 50 g lactitol and 50 g lactitol plus 50 g sucrose, respectively.

Increase of galactose or lactitol in the blood was negligible. Consumption of lactitol does not increase the blood glucose content; consumption of lactitol plus

TABLE 5. Average of Carious Fissure Lesions and Weight Gains in Five Dietary Groups of 12 Rats

Diet	Number of fissure lesions[1] B		C		Weight gain g	
Sucrose	5.75		2.58		82.0	
Sorbitol	1.33	*	0.42	*	46.0	**
Lactitol	1.17	*	0.33	*	72.2	
Wheat flour	0.67	*	0.25	*	80.8	
Xylitol	0.42	*	0	*	48.6	**
Pooled standard error	0.56		0.43		5.4	

[1] 12 fissure at risk.

* $p<0.01$, ** $p<0.001$: significantly different from the sucrose group (Tukey's test).

sucrose clearly gives a lower increase in the blood glucose content than does sucrose alone. Increase of blood glucose after the intake of 50 g lactitol plus 50 g sucrose was at the same level as after intake of 50 g lactose.

Lactitol as a bulk sweetener for diabetic patients. As lactitol does not have any effect on blood glucose or insulin levels, it is suitable for insulin-dependent diabetic patients (type I). It can also be consumed by noninsulin-dependent diabetic patients (type II). This group can limit its diabetic status by taking dietetic measures. Lactitol fits in their diets because of its reduced calorie value in comparison to sucrose and sorbitol, and its similar metabolism to dietary fiber.

Study on effect of lactitol on the alloxan diabetic rat. In view of the intended application of lactitol as a sugar substitute for diabetic patients, it is of interest to study the effects on the physiology and pathology of diabetic experimental animals. In particular, the effects on eyes, kidneys and arteries are known to be affected in diabetes. A well-established technique for inducing diabetes mellitus in laboratory animals is the administration of alloxan, which results in destruction of beta cells in the pancreas and, thus, in decreased insulin production.

In a CIVO-TNO report (40), "Effects of different carbohydrates and polyols in the alloxan diabetic rat," the results of a three-month study in 12 groups of rats, each diet group consisting of ten rats of each sex, is cited. The diabetic rats were fed on a diet containing starch or on diets in which part of the starch has been replaced by either lactitol, lactose, sorbitol, sucrose or by fructose, at levels of 15% and 30%. The experimental animals were made diabetic by a single, intravenously administered dose of 40 mg alloxan per kg body weight. Only animals with blood glucose levels between 20 and 30 mmol per L were used. The various groups consisted of ten males and ten females each.

A group of ten males and ten females, not treated with alloxan, served as a nondiabetic control.

Body weight, food intake, water intake, blood glucose level, urine excretion, and urine glucose concentration were measured and opthalmoscopic observations were made throughout the study.

Ceca (both filled and empty), kidneys, and liver were weighed at autopsy. These organs and, in addition, eyes, pancreas and aorta, were microscopically examined. The mean body weights of the male and female diabetic rats were 20% to 30% and 10% to 20%, respectively, lower than those of the nondiabetic controls.

Food and water intake were increased in all diabetic groups, when compared on a g per kg body weight basis with the nondiabetic controls. In the lactitol and sorbitol groups they were dose-relatedly lower than in the other diabetic groups.

The blood glucose levels were higher in the diabetic groups than in the nondiabetic controls. They were dose-relatedly lower in the lactitol and sorbitol groups than in the other diabetic groups.

The mean urine excretion was considerably greater in the diabetic groups (particularly the wheat starch, sucrose, and fructose groups) than in the nondiabetic controls. In the 30% lactitol and 30% sorbitol groups the excretion was at most twice as large. The mean urinary glucose concentrations in the diabetic groups were, with only a few exceptions, in the range of 400 to 500 mmol per L.

A high incidence of cataracts (25% to 70% for both sexes combined) occurred in the rats in the wheat starch, sucrose, and fructose groups. Only isolated cases were observed in the other groups.

It was concluded that lactitol and sorbitol had a marked, ameliorating effect on several typical symptoms of diabetes mellitus: hyperglycemia, hyperphagia, polydipsia, glycosuria, polyuria and appearance of cataracts. The same applied to lactose, although to a lesser extent.

Evaluation of histological changes in the kidneys by means of factor analysis. In the above mentioned report (40), microscopic examination revealed changes in the kidneys which were obviously due to the diabetic condition. However, there was no consistent relationship between the type of carbohydrate or polyol in the diet and the nature or incidence of the lesions.

In a further CIVO-TNO report, a more detailed examination of the data of the individual animals is given.

Histopathological kidney data, obtained in a study on the effects of different carbohydrates and polyols in alloxan diabetic rats, have been subjected to factor analysis. The results point to a primary and a secondary effect of the diabetic state on the kidney of the rat. The primary effect, labelled "diabetes factor," is responsible for dilation of cortical tubules and the formation of dilated distal tubules with coarsely vacuolated, glycogen-containing epithelial cells. It is associated with typical signs of diabetes, e.g., hyperglycemia. The secondary effect is complex in nature and is associated with inflammatory processes. Both in males and females it includes a "degeneration factor" which manifests itself in an increased number of basophilic tubules and a thickening of basal lamina in Bowman's capsule. In males it involves, moreover, a "protein factor" which gives rise to expansion of the mesangial matrix and the appearance of proximal tubules with vacuolated epithelial cells, filled with eosiniphilic material. The analysis showed that incorporation of polyols has an ameliorating effect on the renal changes induced by the diabetes factor (41).

Lactitol as a sugar substitute for diabetics. Diet has been recognized as a cornerstone of therapy for diabetes mellitus since the disease was first described. After the discovery of insulin, controversy continued as to whether the carbohydrate content of diet should be relatively high or low, but low carbohydrate diets were used for many years. After 1971 the trend reversed and the American Diabetes Association recommended that the carbohydrate content of diabetic patients be liberalized (42). This position was supported by observations that high carbohydrate intakes led to improvement in glucose tolerance and insulin sensitivity and the desire to reduce total and saturated fat content. Currently, most experts suggest that carbohydrate should comprise 50% to 60% of total calories; however, the more important issue is related to the type of carbohydrate used.

The recommendation of limiting simple sugars (mono- and disaccharides) and of using complex carbohydrates or starches was based on the assumption that complex carbohydrates are more slowly digested and absorbed. However, recent studies have demonstrated different glycemic responses to different starches. A flattened glycemic response compared to glucose or sucrose is now desired.

It has been suggested that dietary recommendations concerning blood glucose control be based on the measured physiologic response to food. Jenkins and his colleagues suggest the use of a glycemic index to classify carbohydrate-containing foods (43). The glycemic index is the area under the blood glucose response curve for each food expressed as a percentage of the area after taking the same amount of carbohydrate as glucose. Cooked starches demonstrated high glycemic indexes, like cornflakes, carrots and potatoes (80% to 90%), bread (70%) comparing with lower glycemic indexes for milk (30% to 39%) and fructose (20% to 29%). The effect of dietary fibers are different: water-insoluble fibers (cereals) do not have a significant impact on postprandial glycemic responses, whereas water-soluble fibers, such as guar and pectins have greater influence on the rate of glucose absorption *in vivo* with low glycemic responses.

As lactitol itself does not have an effect on blood glucose nor blood insulin, it is suitable for insulin-dependent diabetic patients (type I). Since individuals with type I diabetes are usually young and lean, they should consume the calories necessary for normal growth and development.

Metabolically, lactitol is a water-soluble fiber and it is mentioned earlier that the increase of blood glucose after intake of 50 g lactitol plus 50 g sucrose was significantly less than after intake of 50 g sucrose only (39). So in order to have intake of enough calories from carbohydrates, with a flattened glycemic response, combinations of carbohydrates plus lactitol mixed in the diet of type I diabetic patients can be recommended.

Lactitol is also suitable for the noninsulin-dependent diabetic patients (type II). Between 80% to 90% of individuals with type II diabetes are overweight and the usual first principle of therapy is the restriction of calories to induce weight loss. Lactitol fits in their diets because of its reduced calorie utilization (50% of starch and sugar) and its similar metabolism to dietary fiber.

CONCLUSIONS

Lactitol is toxicologically a safe product with the same metabolism as water-soluble dietary fibers, which are not digested in the small intestine but fully fermented by the microflora of the large intestine. This metabolism not only gives lactitol interesting nutritional properties, but also provides for lactitol's therapeutic applications based on its behavior in the gut.

REFERENCES

1. Senderens JB. Catalytic hydrogenation of lactose. CR Acad Sci (III) 1920; 170:47-50.

2. Karrer P, Büchi J. Reduktionsprodukte von Disacchariden: Maltit, Lactit, Cellobit. Helvetica Chim Acta 1937; 20:86-90.

3. van Velthuijsen JA. Food additives derived from lactose: lactitol and lactitolpalmitate. J Agric Food Chem 1979; 27:680-686.

4. Wijnman CF, van Velthuijsen JA, van den Berg H. Lactitol monohydrate and a method for the production of crystalline lactitol. European Patent 1983; 39981.

5. Saijonmaa T, Heikonen M, Kreula M, et al. Preparation and characterization of milk sugar alcohol, lactitol. Milchwissenschaft 1978; 33:733-736.

6. van Bommel M, Kanters JA. The crystal and molecular structures of lactitol monohydrate and lactitol dihydrate (Abstract). Sixth European Chrystallograph Meeting, Barcelona 1980: 26.

7. Bircher J, Bührer M, Franz K, et al. Erstmalige anwendung von lactitol in der behandlung der portosystemischen Enzephalopathie. Schweiz Med Woschenschr 1982; 112:1306-1307.

8. Joint FAO/WHO Expert Committee on Food Additives. IPCS Toxicological evaluation of certain food additives and contaminants: lactitol. 27th report Geneva, WHO Food Additives Series 1983; 18:82-94.

9. The Scientific Committee for Food. Report on sweeteners. EC-Document III/1316/84/CS/EDUL/27 rev. (1984)

10. Life Sciences Research Office Federation of American Societies for Experimental Biology, Bethesda, MD 20814, USA. Health aspects of sugar alcohols and lactose. September 1986.

11. Hayashibara K. Preparation of sucrose containing sweeteners or sucrose/sweeteners containing foods. Netherlands Patent Appl. 1974: 7313151.

12. Maizena GmbH. Verwendung von Lactit als Zuckeraustauschstoff. German Patent BRD 1974: 2, 133, 428.

13. Hayashibara K. Improvements in and relating to the preparation of foodstuffs. UK Patent 1971: 1, 253, 300.

14. Hayashibara K, Sugimoto K. Containing lactitol as a sweetener. US Patent 1975: 3, 973, 050.

15. Nilsson U, Jägerstad M. Hydrolysis of lactitol, maltitol and Palatinit® by human intestinal biopsies. Br J Nutr 1987; 58:199-206.

16. Van Es AJH, de Groot L, Vogt JE. Energy balances of eight volunteers fed on diets supplemented with either lactitol or saccharose. Br J Nutr 1986; 56:545-554.

17. Patil DH, Grimble GK, Silk DBA. Lactitol, a new hydrogenated lactose

derivative; intestinal absorption and laxative threshold in normal human subjects. Br J Nutr 1987; 57:195-199.

18. Heitland W, Mauersberger H, Claas H, et al. Clinical study on lactitol as a once-a-day laxative in adult chronically constipated patients. Unpublished report from Eberhard-Karls-Universität Tübingen. October 1986.

19. De Cecco L. Studio clinico di lattitolo in pazienti con stipsi cronica nel corso della gravidanza. Unpublished report from Instituto di Clinica Ostetrica e Ginecologica, Genova (Italy). 1986.

20. Bockel R, Doffoel M. Etude de tolerance sur 6 mois ches 14 sujets ages, constipes chroniques traites par lactitol. Unpublished report from Hospices Civils de Strasbourg, Centre Hospitalier Regional, Dept Med Interne. May 1986.

21. Harries EHL. An open randomised comparison of two weeks treatment with lactitol or lactulose in patients with functional constipation. Unpublished report. May 1986.

22. Murphy D. An open randomized comparison of two weeks treatment with lactitol or lactulose in two hundred patients with functional constipation. Unpublished report. March 1986.

23. Hodkinson HM, Exton-Smith AN, Barnes KE, et al. A controlled study comparing lactitol with lactulose in the treatment of chronic constipation in the elderly. Unpublished report. February 1985.

24. Heitland W, Wiedmann KH. Untersuchung der laxierenden Wirkung von lactitol bei bettlägerigen Patienten. Unpublished report from Eberhard-Karls-Universität Tübingen, Chirurgische Klinik, Tübingen (D). August 1986.

25. Endres M, Feller J, Maier M, et al. Untersuchung der laxativen Wirkung von lactitol an über 65-jährigen Patienten. Unpublished report. May 1986.

26. D'Apuzzo V. Open study on the effect of lactitol administered as a laxative to chronically constipated children. Unpublished report from Ospedale Beata Vergine, Mendrisio (Switzerland). August 1986.

27. Giambonini S. Lactitol as a laxative in chronically constipated children - an open clinical trial. Unpublished report from Malattie dei bambini, Lugano (Italy). September 1986.

28. Verga L, Zanolla W. Studio clinico comparative sull impiego del lattitolo nel trattamento della stasi intestinale di pazienti ospedalizzati. Unpublished report from Ospedale Mellini, Divisione di Medicina, Chiari (Italy). April 1986.

29. Verga L, Zanolla W. Relazione clinica sull'impiego del preparato lattitolo in compresse nel trattamento della stasi intestinale di pazienti ospedalizzati. Unpublished report from Ospedale Mellini, Divisione di Medicina, Chiari (Italy). April 1986.

30. Durand P, Martino AM. Relazione sugli effetti del lattitolo nel trattamento della stasi intestinale in eta'pediatrica studio clinico comparativo. Unpublished report from Instituto Giannina Gaslini, Genovo (Italy). April 1986.

31. Low-beer TS, Butter S. Colonic bacterial activity, biliary cholesterol saturation and pathogenesis of gallstones. Lancet 1978; 2:1063-1065.

32. Hill MJ. Microbes and Human Cancer. London: Edward Arnold, 1986.

33. Vince A. Microbial Metabolism in the Digestive Tract. Hill MJ, ed. Boca Raton: CRC Press, 1986: 83-106.

34. Hill MJ. The effect of lactitol on the metabolic activity of the colonic flora of the pig and the human. Unpublished report from Bacterial Metabolism Laboratory of Public Health Laboratory Services, Porton Down (UK). February 1987.

35. Mühlemann HR. Gutachten über die zahnschonenden Eigenschaften von Lacty Schokolade und Lacty milch-schokolade der Firma CCA, Holland. Unpublished report from Zahnärztliches Institut der Universität Zürich. July 1977.

36. Havenaar R. Microbial investigations on the cariogenicity of the sugar substitute lactitol. Unpublished report from the University of Utrect (Netherlands), Department of Preventive Dentistry and Oral Microbiology. June 1976.

37. van der Hoeven JS. Cariogenicity of lactitol in program-fed rats. Caries Res 1986; 20:441-443.

38. Doorenbos H. Metabolism of lactitol. Unpublished report from Rijksuniversiteit Groningen, Kliniek voor Inwendige Geneeskunde (Netherlands). July 1977.

39. Zaal J, Ottenhof A. Influence of lactitol in blood sugar levels after sucrose intake. Unpublished report from CIVO-TNO, Zeist (Netherlands). August 1977.

40. Leegwater DC, Spanjers MT, Kuper CF. Effects of different carbohydrates and polyols in the Alloxan diabetic rat. Unpublished report from CIVO-TNO, Zeist (Netherlands). March 1982.

41. Leegwater DC, Kuper CF. Evaluation of histological changes in the kidneys of the Alloxan diabetic rat by means of factor analysis. Food Chem Toxicol 1984; 22:551-557.

42. Bierman EL, Albrink MK, Arky R, et al. Principal of nutrition and dietary recommendations for patients wih diabetes mellitus: 1978. Diabetes 1987; 20:633-634.

43. Jenkins DJA, Wolever TMS, Taylor RH, et al. Glycemic index of foods: a physiological basis for carbohydrate exchange. Am J Clin Nutr 1981; 34:362-366.

17

LACTITOL FOR THE TREATMENT OF HEPATIC ENCEPHALOPATHY

MARSHA Y. MORGAN, MB. ChB. FRCP.

CHEMISTRY AND METABOLISM

Lactitol (β-galactosido-sorbitol) is a disaccharide analogue of lactose (1). Lactitol monohydrate is a white, odorless, nonhygroscopic crystalline solid with a pleasant, sweet taste. Its solubility in water at 25°C is 149 g per 100 ml and the pH of a 10% solution lies between 6 and 7. Solutions are extremely stable at neutral pH and can be boiled without denaturing the sugar; hydrolysis occurs at a pH of 2. The monohydrate has a melting point of 115 to 120 C.

Animal experiments and low dose oral tolerance tests in normal subjects suggest that lactitol is not absorbed from the mammalian small intestine (1) and this has been confirmed in a jejunal perfusion study in healthy volunteers (2). In this study, six individuals aged between 20 and 30 years were intubated with a double-lumen perfusion tube and a 30 cm perfusion segment of upper jejunum isolated by use of a proximal occlusion balloon. Test solutions of 10, 30, 60 and 100 mmol per L of lactitol labelled with 1 μCi of 1-^{14}C-lactitol per L containing 4 g per L polyethylene glycol (PEG) labelled with 1 μCi of ^{3}HPEG per L, were made isotonic with plasma by adding sodium chloride. The solutions were maintained at 37°C and infused in random order at a rate of 15 ml per min. After equilibration, three 10-minute samples of the jejunal contents were collected and stored at 4°C together with samples of the infusates, until assayed for galactose content. The amounts of labelled PEG and of labelled lactitol in the samples were measured by liquid scintillation counting.

Galactose was not detected in aliquots of either the infused solutions or the intestinal aspirates obtained during perfusion. Thus, it is highly unlikely that lactitol is hydrolyzed by brush border hydrolases. Similarly there was no significant disappearance of the ^{14}C label during the perfusion experiments indicating that lactitol is not absorbed intact in the unhydrolyzed form. Lactitol is not, therefore, assimilated by the human small intestine.

Evidence suggests, however, that lactitol is extensively metabolized in the human colon (3). In a recent study, six healthy volunteers were given 20 g of lactitol in water daily for 15 days and received 10 µCi of universally labelled ^{14}C-lactitol (D-[U-^{14}C] lactitol, 14 µCi $mmol^{-1}$) on the eighth day. ^{14}C excretion in breath, feces and urine was subsequently monitored. Total recoveries of ^{14}C averaged 71%; nearly 90% of this was in expired carbon dioxide, while less than 10% was excreted in stools. The label was very rapidly cleared, mainly during the first 24 hours.

Recently, the colonic metabolism of lactitol has been further characterized. Stools from healthy human volunteers were incubated in an *in vitro* culture system developed to simulate the anaerobic metabolism of human colonic bacteria *in vivo* (4). The system contained either lactitol or lactulose in a concentration of 20 g per L. Aliquots of samples were collected at 0 and 24 hours and kept at -20 °C until analyzed for their volatile fatty acid content by modified gas liquid chromatography. Both sugars were readily metabolized by fecal bacteria as evidenced by the amount of sodium hydroxide required to maintain the reaction mixture at pH 7. During the 24-hour incubation period, acetic, propionic, butyric and lactic acids were liberated from media containing lactitol and lactulose, in similar amounts.

The effects of lactitol and lactulose on terminal ileal and colonic pH have been compared in six healthy volunteers by use of a pH-sensitive radiotelemeter (4). Subjects were treated for three to four days with increasing amounts of both sugars to final daily doses of 40 to 180 g of lactitol or 30 to 80 g of lactulose given in two to four divided doses. Subjects passed two to three semiformed stools per day. The mean (1SD) basal right-sided colonic pH was 6.51 0.48 and this fell significantly during treatment with both lactulose, 5.18 0.82 ($p<0.01$) and lactitol, 5.63 0.54 ($p<0.05$). The pH in the ileum and in the rest of the colon remained unchanged during disaccharide ingestion.

Thus, lactitol shares many properties with lactulose and should be equally as effective in the treatment of hepatic encephalopathy. However, as lactitol is available as a pure crystalline powder which is highly soluble in water and, as it has a low relative sweetness, its use might be associated with fewer side effects.

CLINICAL STUDIES IN HEPATIC ENCEPHALOPATHY

In 1982, Bircher and coworkers (5) described the use of lactitol in the treatment of hepatic encephalopathy for the first time. Their patient, a 61-year-old man with alcoholic cirrhosis, developed hepatic encephalopathy following portal-systemic shunt surgery for relief of portal hypertension. His response to protein restriction and lactulose in doses of up to 90 ml daily was unsatisfactory. The patient was therefore hospitalized and his neuropsychiatric state stabilized on a regime of protein restriction and 150 ml of lactulose daily. He was, however, intolerant of this regime. In consequence, he was started on treatment with lactitol to a maximum of 75 g daily. Although no significant further improvement was observed in his clinical state or neuropsychiatric performance, he tolerated the lactitol much better than the lactulose, as it was less sweet in taste and did not produce nausea.

Since this initial report, a number of controlled comparisons of lactitol with lactulose have been undertaken in cirrhotic patients with both acute and chronic hepatic encephalopathy.

CONTROLLED STUDIES IN CHRONIC HEPATIC ENCEPHALOPATHY

In the first published study (6), a small number of patients with chronic hepatic encephalopathy, previously on long-term maintenance therapy with lactulose, were treated with lactitol for three months under carefully monitored conditions. As close monitoring is known to have a beneficial effect on this condition, possibly because of better compliance with therapy, a monitored three-month treatment period on lactulose was included for comparison.

The study group comprised five patients with cirrhosis and chronic hepatic encephalopathy maintained in stable condition by use of protein restriction and oral lactulose (Table 1). All five patients experienced worsening of their clinical condition, psychometric performance and electroencephalogram (EEG) mean cycle frequency if inadvertently allowed to become constipated or to discontinue protein restriction or lactulose. None of the alcoholic patients had abused alcohol for at least two years.

After an initial, baseline, inpatient assessment, patients were discharged from hospital with no change in their dietary regime or their lactulose dosage. They were then monitored carefully for three months on an outpatient basis, adjusting their lactulose dosage to achieve two semisoft stools per day. After reassessment, lactitol was substituted for lactulose in the treatment regime in a dose of 0.5 g per kg body weight daily to be increased to 0.75 g per kg, if necessary, to ensure passage of two semisoft stools per day. The patients were reassessed in hospital after three months' treatment with lactitol. Throughout the trial, the patients kept a diary in which they recorded their daily disaccharide dosage, stool frequency and consistency and an assessment of symptoms and side effects, if any. Each month, they were asked to score treatment efficacy and acceptability on a scale of 1 (poor) to 4 (excellent).

The patients showed few, if any, clinical abnormalities while on maintenance lactulose although all five showed substantial deficits on psychometric testing. Very little change was observed in their clinical condition during the trial and no changes were observed in mean psychometric test scores after monitored treatment over three months with either lactulose or lactitol. Mean venous blood

TABLE 1. Details of Five Cirrhotic Patients on Maintenance Lactulose for Treatment of Chronic Hepatic Encephalopathy

Patient	Age (yr)	Sex	Etiology of cirrhosis	Serum bilirubin (μmol/L) *(5-17)	Serum AST[+] (U/L) (5-40)	Plasma albumin (g/L) (35-50)	PT[**] (s) (control =13)	Portal systemic shunt	Duration of encephalopathy	Daily treatment regime
RG	63	M	Alcoholic	29	78	32	17	Spontaneous	4 mo	40 g protein 20 ml lactulose
JB	61	M	Alcoholic	20	37	33	17	Spontaneous	5 mo	40 g protein 20 ml lactulose
LC	53	M	Alcoholic	5	46	34	13	Spontaneous	4 yr	30 g protein 40 ml lactulose 7.5 mg bromocriptine
EH	54	M	Cryptogenic	38	27	38	21	Mesocaval shunt 1975	7 yr	60 g protein 30 ml lactulose
NT	41	M	Cryptogenic	57	41	32	15	Portacaval shunt 1967	11 yr	30 g protein 20 ml lactulose 10 mg bromocriptine

* Reference range; [+] Aspartate transaminase; ** Prothrombin time.

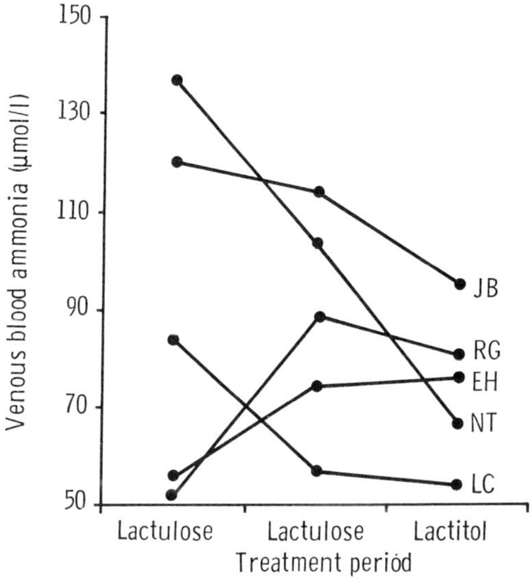

FIGURE 1. Changes in venous blood ammonia concentrations in five patients with chronic hepatic encephalopathy while on maintenance lactulose, after three months of monitoring on lactulose and after three months of monitoring on lactitol. Reference range 15 to 60 μmol per L.

ammonia concentrations (Figure 1), EEG mean cycle frequencies (Figure 2) and cerebral blood flow measurements (Figure 3) were abnormal throughout the trial, although consistent improvements were observed in a few patients.

Three patients considered lactitol to be as efficacious as lactulose while

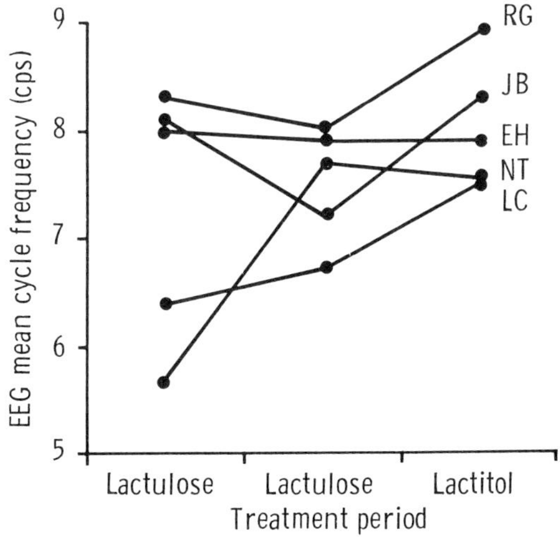

FIGURE 2. Changes in electroencephalogram (EEG) mean cycle frequency in five patients with chronic hepatic encephalopathy while on maintenance lactulose, after three months of monitoring on lactulose and three after months of monitoring on lactitol. Each value is the mean of three measurements of mean cycle frequency taken at daily intervals. Mean cycle frequency in an alert adult >8.9 cps.

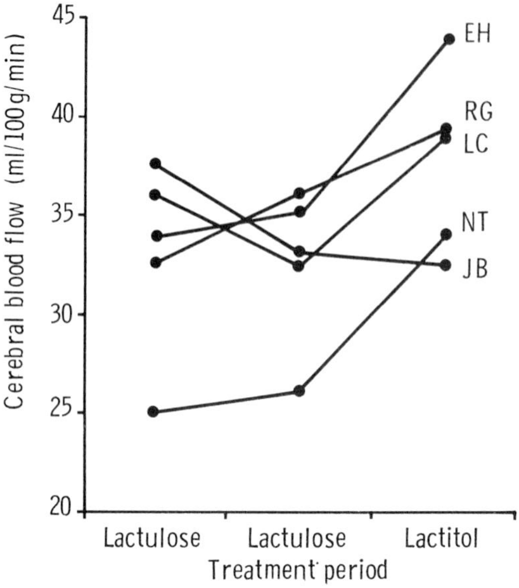

FIGURE 3. Changes in cerebral blood flow measured by inhalation of radioactive (^{133}Xe) in five patients with chronic hepatic encephalopathy while on maintenance lactulose, after three months of monitoring on lactulose and after three months of monitoring on lactitol. Reference range 45±5 ml per 100 g brain per min.

two patients considered its effects to be superior. All five patients felt that treatment with lactitol was more acceptable, because its cathartic effect was more predictable (Figure 4), its less sweet taste was preferred and its powder form was more convenient to use. Two patients experienced abdominal discomfort, flatulence and some urgency of defecation while taking lactulose but were symptom-free on

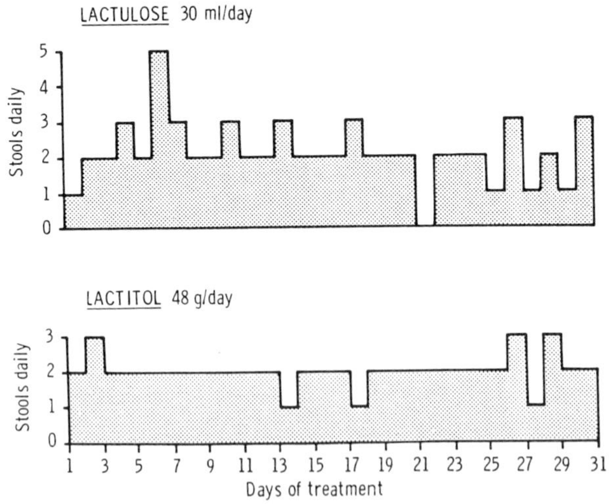

FIGURE 4. Daily stool frequency in one patient during the second month of monitored treatment with either lactulose or lactitol for chronic hepatic encephalopathy. Throughout, the patient took a 60 g protein diet.

lactitol. No other side effects were noted. In order to achieve two semisoft stools per day, patients required a mean of 44 ml (range 20 to100 ml) of lactulose or 64 g (48 to 84 g) of lactitol. No convenient formula of equivalent dosage could be derived; 1 ml of lactulose appeared equivalent in effect to between 0.84 to 2.67 g of lactitol.

Because the patient acceptability of lactitol was so high in this study, it might be argued that despite the close monitoring, patient compliance with treatment was better, thus making it difficult to assess the true efficacy of the compound. In consequence, solutions of lactitol and lactulose, identical in appearance and taste and sharing a number of important physico-chemical properties were prepared which contained either 66.7 g per 100 ml of lactitol or 66.7 ml (44.5 g) per 100 ml of lactulose syrup (Table 2). These solutions were then used to compare the efficacy of lactitol and lactulose in the treatment of 12 patients with chronic hepatic encephalopathy requiring long-term maintenance therapy (7).

All patients were assessed initially in hospital and were then randomized blindly to treatment with either lactitol or lactulose solutions dispensed in an initial dose of 0.75 ml per kg body weight daily in four divided doses which provided0.5 g per kg of lactitol or 0.5 ml (0.3 g) per kg of lactulose. The dosage was adjusted subsequently, as necessary, to achieve two semisoft stools per day.

The patients were assessed at regular intervals in the outpatient department for three months and were then admitted to hospital for a full reassessment. On discharge from hospital, treatment was crossed-over to the alternative sugar

TABLE 2. Formulation and Physio-chemical Properties of the Lactitol and Lactulose Solutions Prepared to Treat Patients with Hepatic Encephalopathy

	Lactitol	Lactulose
Formulation	Lactitol 40 g Distilled water 60 ml	Lactulose syrup 40 ml (66.7 g/100 ml) Distilled water to 60 ml
	Blackcurrant syrup dropwise to colour	Blackcurrant syrup dropwise to colour
Concentration (g/100 ml)	66.7	44.5 (66.7 ml/100 ml)
Weight/ml (g)	1.2053	1.2167
Refractive Index	1.422	1.422
Viscosity (cps)	78.85	79.50
Osmolarity (mOsm/L)	2947	2911
pH	4.6	4.6
Optical rotation (°)	147.2	147.3

solution and the monitoring procedure repeated (Figure 5). No wash-out period was possible between treatments because these patients had all experienced worsening of their clinical condition, psychometric performance and EEG mean cycle frequency if inadvertently allowed to become constipated or to discontinue their long-term treatment regime. No changes were made in dietary protein restriction nor in essential medications during the trial. Clinical complications such as gastrointestinal bleeding or infections were treated appropriately, if and when they arose. Throughout the trial, patients kept a diary in which they recorded their daily solution requirements, stool frequency and consistency and an assessment of symptoms or side effects, if any.

Treatment efficacy and acceptability were assessed at each outpatient and inpatient visit by use of the PSE Sum and Index as described by Conn (8). The PSE Sum is an arbitrary index of the severity of hepatic encephalopathy derived by adding scores for the degree of abnormality in mental status, the severity of asterixis, the reduction in Number Connection Test time (NCT), the increase in blood ammonia concentration and the reduction in electroencephalogram (EEG) mean cycle frequency, all expressed on a scale of 0 (absent) to 4 (severe).

Each of these five components is arbitrarily weighted in proportion to its importance. Thus, mental state is weighted by a factor of three, while the other variables are assigned a factor of one. The PSE Sum is the total of the weighted scores; its maximum possible value is 28. If information on one or more of the

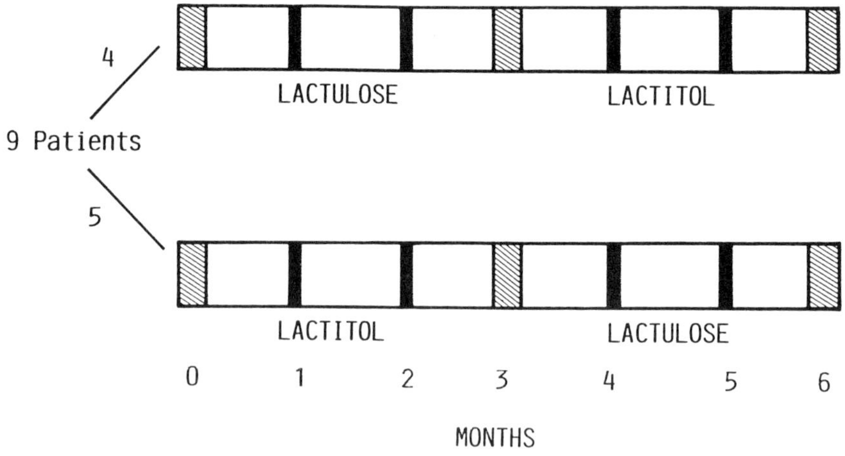

FIGURE 5. Overall study design for the double-blind, randomized, cross-over study of lactulose versus lactitol in the treatment of chronic hepatic encephalopathy. ▨ Comprehensive inpatient assessment; ■ Outpatient assessment

components of the PSE Sum is not available then PSE Sums calculated at different time points may not be directly comparable. The PSE Index was devised to take account of this eventuality; this index is the ratio of the assessed PSE Sum to the maximum possible PSE Sum. Use of the PSE Index permits a comparison of the severity of hepatic encephalopathy to be made at differing times or on different treatments, even if all the data are not available.

During this double-blind comparison of the efficacy and acceptability of lactitol and lactulose, one patient died and two repeatedly defaulted from treatment during the first month of the trial and were thus excluded from further analyses; the remaining nine patients completed the trial. Four patients (JB, EH, LC, DA) were initially randomized to lactulose, while the remaining five (JD, NT, DC, HM, SP) were randomized to lactitol (Table 3). There were no treatment failures. Overall, no significant differences were observed in clinical status, NCT test times, venous blood ammonia concentrations, EEG mean cycle frequencies or in the PSE Indices during treatment with either of the two sugars. However, during the last month of treatment with lactitol, clinical events likely to cause decompensation arose in five of the nine trial patients, whereas only one patient suffered an episode likely to cause decompensation during the last month of treatment with lactulose.

Patients required a mean equivalent (±ISD) of 31.9±11.2 g of lactitol or 32.9 16.7 ml (21.9 11.1 g) of reconstituted lactulose to produce two semisoft stools per day. Four of the nine (44.4%) patients developed dose-related flatulence during treatment with both sugars. However, dose-independent flatulence occurred in five patients during treatment with lactulose (55.6%) but in only two during treatment with lactitol (22.2%). Diarrhea, defined as the passage of four or more stools per day, occurred in eight patients during treatment with lactulose (88.9%) but in only four during treatment with lactitol (44.4%); the development of diarrhea was invariably dose-related. The difference in the incidence of side effects during treatment with the two sugars was not, however, statistically significant.

In this study, lactitol appeared as efficacious as lactulose in the treatment of chronic hepatic encephalopathy. In addition, lactitol was effective in preventing severe deterioration in clinical, psychometric and EEG performance in five of the patients when events otherwise likely to precipitate encephalopathy supervened. Overall, patients experienced fewer side effects with lactitol despite the fact that lactulose was diluted in preparation of the solution and was therefore not taken in its usual concentration.

Similar observations were made by Heredia and coworkers (9) in their comparison of the efficacy and patient acceptability of lactitol and lactulose in the treatment of chronic hepatic encephalopathy. These workers undertook a randomized, controlled, cross-over study of lactitol powder and lactulose syrup in 25 cirrhotic patients who had been maintained on protein restriction to 40 to 60 g daily and long-term lactulose. These patients were randomized, after an initial, detailed assessment, to three months' treatment with either 40 g of lactitol or 60 g of lactulose daily, in divided doses, and were then crossed over to the alternative treatment for

TABLE 3. Characteristics of Nine Patients Completing the Double-blind Trial of Lactitol versus Lactulose in Chronic Hepatic Encephalopathy

Patient	Age (yr)	Sex	Etiology of cirrhosis	Portal-systemic shunt	Total serum bilirubin (µmol/L) *(5-17)	PT** (s) (12-14)	Serum AST⁺ (U/L) (5-40)	Plasma albumin (g/L) (30-50)	Duration of treatment (mo)	Daily regime before entry to trial
JB	64	M	Alcoholic	Spontaneous	13	15	39	40	24	Lactitol 64-80 g
EH	67	M	Cryptogenic	Surgical	25	18	22	36	100	Protein 40 g Lactitol 40 g
LC	55	M	Alcoholic	Spontaneous	10	13	54	35	41	Protein 50 g Lactitol 60 g Bromocriptine 7.5 mg
JD	60	F	Alcoholic	Surgical	16	16	35	40	22	Protein 50 g Lactitol 48 g
NT	44	M	Cryptogenic	Surgical	50	16	44	32	156	Lactitol 40 g Bromocriptine 5 mg
DC	35	F	Cryptogenic	Spontaneous	33	17	63	39	12	Lactitol 16 g
DA	75	F	Cryptogenic	Spontaneous	18	15	42	41	15	Lactitol 24 g
HM	63	F	Cryptogenic	Spontaneous	26	14	36	44	41	Lactitol 12 g
SP	53	M	Alcoholic	Spontaneous	42	22	54	32	12	Lactulose 40 ml

* Reference range; ** Prothrombin time; ⁺ Aspartate transaminase

a further three-month period. The disaccharide dosage was adjusted, as necessary, to produce two bowel movements daily. The patients were reviewed monthly as outpatients and kept a daily diary of their drug dosage, stool frequency and consistency, treatment acceptability and treatment side effects, if any.

Twenty patients completed this study. Both treatments were equally efficacious when assessed by clinical status, NCT times, EEG mean cycle frequencies, blood ammonia concentrations and PSE Indexes. However, the patients showed a significant preference for lactitol because it was less sweet and produced less nausea. These authors suggest, therefore, that lactitol is a good alternative to lactulose for the treatment of chronic hepatic encephalopathy.

Balducci and coworkers (10) compared the efficacy of lactitol and lactulose in preventing the development of hepatic encephalopathy in cirrhotic patients who had undergone portal-systemic shunt surgery. They studied 31 patients who had been operated upon a mean (±ISD) of 49±12 months previously and who had been maintained on protein restriction and lactulose up to the time of their inclusion in the study. The patients were then allocated randomly to treatment with either lactitol powder or lactulose syrup in doses adjusted to produce two bowel motions daily, for a period of six months. Twenty-nine patients completed the study.

In the 12 months preceding the study, 42% of the patients had experienced one or more episodes of hepatic encephalopathy. During the study period, 4 of the 14 patients treated with lactitol (28.6%) and 6 of the 15 patients treated with lactulose (40.0%) experienced one or more such episodes. Over the six-month study period, the PSE Index improved in 8 of the 14 patients treated with lactitol (57%) and in 6 of the 15 patients treated with lactulose (40%). These results suggest that lactitol is at least as efficacious as lactulose in preventing the development of recurrent hepatic encephalopathy in cirrhotic patients after portal-systemic shunt surgery. No details were provided, however, of the acceptability of treatment or of the incidence of side effects.

No other comparisons of the efficacy and acceptability of lactitol and lactulose in the treatment of chronic hepatic encephalopathy are available. However, Uribe and coworkers (11) undertook a double-blind comparison of lactitol and lactose in the treatment of chronic hepatic encephalopathy in a group of cirrhotic patients who were lactase-deficient. The study included four treatment periods. During the first and third periods of two weeks each, patients received 3 g of neomycin and 70 ml of magnesium hydroxide daily. During the second and fourth periods, each of one month duration, patients received either lactitol or lactose in random order. The dose of both sugars was adjusted to achieve two to four stools per day. An adequate catharsis was achieved with a mean of 39 13 g of lactitol or 65 12 g of lactose daily. Lactitol and lactose were equally effective in the treatment of chronic hepatic encephalopathy, but, in general, lactitol was better tolerated and was preferred by the majority of patients.

CONTROLLED STUDIES IN ACUTE HEPATIC ENCEPHALOPATHY IN CIRRHOTIC PATIENTS

A small number of controlled studies have been undertaken to assess the efficacy and patient acceptability of lactitol in the treatment of acute hepatic encephalopathy in cirrhotic patients.

Morgan and Hawley (12) undertook a double-blind comparison of these two sugars in 25 cirrhotic patients who among them experienced 28 episodes of acute hepatic encephalopathy. These patients were randomized as soon as possible after admission to hospital to treatment with either lactitol (n=15) or lactulose (n=13) in solutions identical in appearance and taste and with similar physico-chemical properties (Table 2). These solutions were dispensed in an initial dose of 0.75 ml per kg body weight which was then adjusted every 12 hours to achieve two soft or semisoft stools per day. On entry to the trial and at 12 hours, the bowel was cleansed by use of neutral phosphate enemata. Dietary protein was restricted to 10 g daily for the five days of the trial. However, once patients showed a sustained improvement in their mental state, protein intake was increased by increments of 20 g every third day. Other medications were prescribed as necessary to treat the underlying liver disease or to ameliorate the events which had precipitated the episode of encephalopathy. Neurological observations were made hourly and full reassessments were made at 12-hour intervals throughout the trial. A detailed stool chart was kept and probable or definite side effects of treatment noted. The severity of the encephalopathy on entry to the trial and every 12 hours thereafter was assessed by calculating the PSE Sum and Index (8).

The patients in the two treatment groups were comparable on entry to the trial (Table 4). Treatment was discontinued in three patients taking lactitol for reasons unconnected with treatment; one patient developed paralytic ileus eight hours after entry into the trial and was therefore unable to take oral medication; a second patient had a profound gastrointestinal hemorrhage after 96 hours and required esophageal transection, while a third patient developed nausea unrelated to the medication at 72 hours. All three patients were treated with cleansing enemata and the 12-hour assessments continued so that their results could be included in the trial analysis.

During the trial, significant improvement occurred in clinical status, psychometric performance, EEG mean cycle frequency and the PSE Sum and Index in the majority of patients in both treatment groups (Table 5). A mean (±ISD) improvement in PSE Sum of 54 43% was observed in the patients in the lactitol group and of 52 23% in the lactulose group by day 5; by this time ten patients treated with lactitol (67%) and nine patients treated with lactulose (69%) were clinically normal. However, recovery occurred significantly more rapidly in patients treated with lactitol (Figure 6). Thus, after 24, 36, 48 and 72 hours of treatment, significantly greater mean percentage improvements were observed in PSE Indexes in patients

TABLE 4. Details of Cirrhotic Patients Studied and Treated for Acute Hepatic Encephalopathy with Lactitol and Lactulose

	Lactitol (n=15)	Lactulose (n=13)
Mean (±ISD) age (yr)	48.4 12.5 (range 32-77)	48.3 15.8 (range 23-74)
Sex ratio	7M : 8F	8M : 5F
Etiology of liver disease		
Alcoholic	8 (53.3%)	7 (54.6%)
Chronic active hepatitis	2 (13.3%)	3 (23.1%)
Others	5 (33.4%)	3 (23.1%)
Mean Pugh's Score*	10.8 1.9	10.2 2.9
(Range) (5 - 15)	(7.0 - 13.0)	(7.0 - 15.0)
Child's Grade** B (n)	4	6
Child's Grade C (n)	11	7
Mean weight (kg)	64 13	68 15
Mean PSE Sum on entry (0-28)	13.3 3.9	12.2 5.2
Mean PSE Index on entry (0-1)	0.48 0.14	0.46 0.19
Mean duration of pre-coma before study (hr)	36.5 25.9	28.3 9.6
Precipitant of hepatic encephalopathy		
Gastrointestinal bleeding	6 (40.0%)	8 (61.5%)
Infection	11 (73.3%)	8 (61.5%)
Hypokalemia	6 (40.4%)	5 (38.5%)
Multiple	11 (73.3%)	8 (61.5%)
Drugs within 48 hours of entry		
Diazemuls	7 (53.8%)	6 (46.1%)
General anesthesia	2 (13.3%)	1 (7.7%)
Antibiotics	11 (73.3%)	10 (76.9%)
Potassium	8 (53.3%)	6 (40.0%)

* Reference 13; ** Reference 14.

treated with lactitol than in patients treated with lactulose (Table 5).

There were no deaths during the trial. The three individuals in whom treatment with lactitol was discontinued died 6, 9 and 13 days after the trial, the first of bowel infarction and septicemia and the other two of uncontrollable gastrointestinal hemorrhage. One further patient treated with lactitol developed hepato-renal syndrome and died 13 days after the trial. One patient treated with lactulose died eight days after the trial as a result of uncontrollable gastrointestinal hemorrhage and sepsis. All five patients had severely decompensated liver disease.

Patients required a mean (±1SD) of 39±7 ml (range 24-48 ml) of lactitol solution or 46±11 ml (28-64 ml) of lactulose solution to achieve two semisoft stools per day. This is equivalent to a dose of 26±5 g (16 to 32 g) of lactitol or 31±7 ml (19 to 43 ml) of lactulose syrup or 21±5 g (13 to 29 g) of lactulose. Six patients treated with lactitol and four patients treated with lactulose developed diarrhea which was defined as the passage of four or more stools per day. In general, the diarrhea abated when the disaccharide dosage was reduced except in one patient

TABLE 5. Summary of Changes in Encephalopathy throughout the Double-blind, Randomized Trial of Lactitol versus Lactulose in Acute Hepatic Encephalopathy in Cirrhotic Patients

	Lactitol (n=15)		Lactulose (n=13)	
	Day 0	Day 5	Day 0	Day 5
Mean clinical assessment	1.7±0.7	0.2±0.5	1.4±0.9	0.2±0.4
(0-4)	*p<0.005		*p<0.005	
Mean blood ammonia	66±38	82±36	80±31	68±29
(<60 μmol/L)	ns		ns	
Mean NCT	104±53	52±23	97±34	58±23
(<30 s)	p<0.005		p<0.001	
Mean EEG	5.7±1.3	7.0±1.5	5.8±1.3	7.6±1.6
(>8.9 cps)	p<0.05		p<0.01	
Mean PSE Sum	13.3±3.9	5.3±4.0	12.2±5.2	5.2±2.5
(0 - 28)	p<0.002		p<0.001	
Mean PSE Index	0.48±0.14	0.19±0.14	0.46±0.19	0.19±0.09
(0 - 1)	p<0.001		p<0.001	
Mean % improvement in PSE Index by:				
12 hr	15±40		10±18	NS
24 hr	30±45		12±27	** p<0.05
36 hr	41±52		23±33	p<0.05
48 hr	41±58		28±26	p<0.02
72 hr	46±55		34±15	p<0.01
96 hr	46±46		46±17	NS
120 hr	54±43		52±23	NS

* Significance of the difference between values at the beginning and the end of the trial in each treatment group;

** Significance of the differences between values during treatment with lactitol and lactulose;

NS Not significant.

treated with lactulose in whom the diarrhea persisted to the end of the trial. In another patient treated with lactulose, the diarrhea was associated with the development of hypernatremia after 96 hours of treatment. He responded to treatment with intravenous fluids and a reduction in the lactulose dosage.

Thus, acute hepatic encephalopathy in patients with cirrhosis can be effectively treated with both lactitol and lactulose. However, in this study, resolution of the symptoms and signs of hepatic encephalopathy was significantly more rapid in the lactitol-treated group. This suggests that lactitol might be the treatment of choice for this condition.

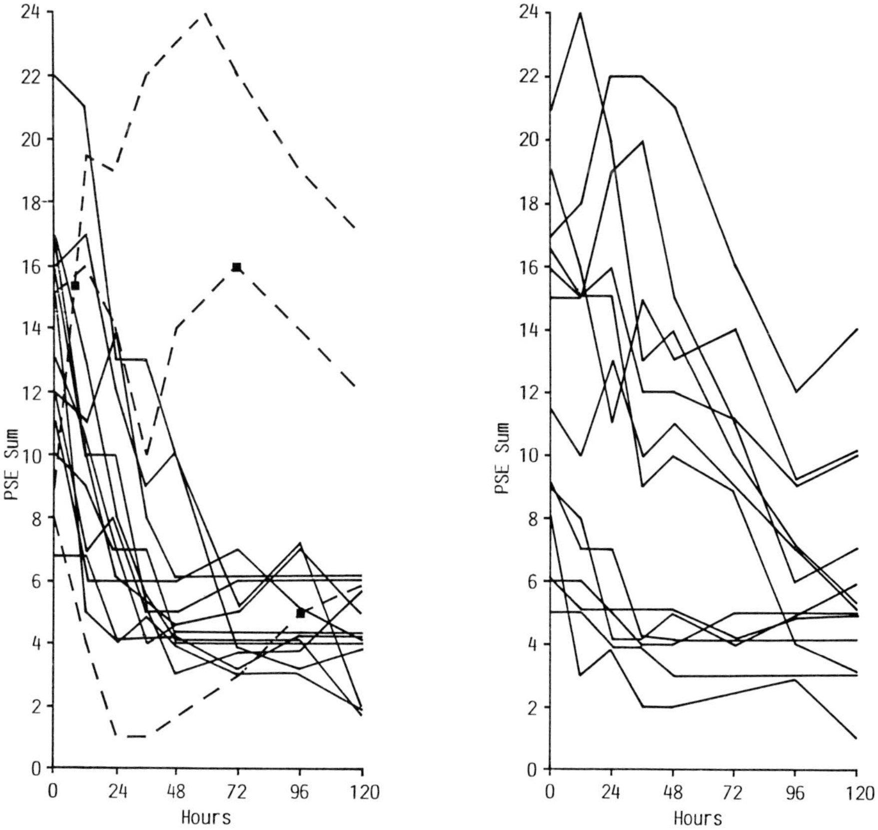

FIGURE 6. Left: Changes occurring in PSE Index in 15 patients with cirrhosis and acute hepatic encephalopathy during five days treatment with lactitol.
- - - Patients withdrawn from treatment but still monitored for entire trial period.
■ Time point of withdrawal from treatment. Right: Changes occurring in PSE sum in 13 patients with cirrhosis and acute hepatic encephalopathy during five days treatment with lactulose.

No other double-blind comparisons of the efficacy of lactitol and lactulose in the treatment of acute hepatic encephalopathy in cirrhotic patients are available with which the results of this trial can be compared. However, Heredia and co-workers (15) have undertaken an open comparison of these two sugars in the treatment of this condition. These workers randomized 40 cirrhotic patients with acute hepatic encephalopathy to treatment with either 48 g of lactitol daily (n=20) or 120 ml of lactulose daily (n=20) for five days. These doses were adjusted to achieve two bowel motions per day. Both groups of patients had comparable demographic variables and similar degrees of neuropsychiatric impairment on entry to the trial. During the time course of the trial, 17 patients (85%) receiving lactitol and 16 patients (80%) receiving lactulose 'improved.' The condition of the remaining seven patients did not change. One patient in each group died because of liver failure. No significant differences were observed in the efficacy of the two treatments as assessed by changes in clinical status, NCT times, blood ammonia concentrations and EEG mean cycle frequencies between the beginning and the end of the study. However, insufficient information was available to enable the rate of improvement to be determined. These authors therefore concluded that lactitol is as effective as lactulose in the treatment of acute hepatic encephalopathy in cirrhotic patients.

Finally, Uribe and colleagues (16) undertook a double-blind comparison of the efficacy of 20% lactitol and lactose enemata with tap water enemata in the treatment of 45 episodes of acute hepatic encephalopathy experienced by 37 patients with cirrhosis. The tap water enemata were discontinued after the first 20 episodes of encephalopathy had been treated because the therapeutic response was so poor. Thereafter the trial was re-randomized to allow comparison of the efficacy of the lactitol and lactose enemata alone. At the end of the study, 22 patients had been treated with lactitol enemata for a mean (±ISD) of 3.7±1.2 days and 18 patients had been treated with lactose enemata for a mean of 3.5 1.2 days. Therapeutic success, defined as a sustained improvement of one grade in mental state during <48 hours or as improvement of more than two grades in mental state, was observed in 19 of the 22 patients treated with lactitol enemata (86%) and in 14 of the 18 patients treated with lactulose enemata (78%).

During the study, 3 of the 18 patients who received lactose enemata (16.6%) experienced adverse effects which were severe enough in two subjects to warrant discontinuation of treatment. Only one of the 22 patients (4.5%) treated with lactitol enemata experienced adverse effects which were not sufficient, however, to require discontinuation of treatment. These authors concluded that lactitol and lactose enemata are equally as effective in the treatment of acute hepatic encephalopathy in cirrhotic patients but caution that, in the presence of diabetes, lactitol enemata should be used in preference as lactose enemata are likely to produce hyperglycemia.

SAFETY MONITORING

Relatively large numbers of patients with hepatic encephalopathy have now been treated with lactitol for periods of three or more years. In a study recently completed at the Royal Free Hospital, London (Morgan MY and Hawley KE, personal communication), 20 patients with chronic hepatic encephalopathy were followed at six-week intervals for up to one year to assess the efficacy and long-term safety of treatment with lactitol. Only patients with proven chronic hepatic encephalopathy who had been maintained on long-term lactulose were eligible for inclusion (Table 6). Four patients were noncompliant with treatment from an early stage; these patients had previously failed to comply with other treatment regimes. The remaining 16 patients were followed for periods of between 4 to 12 months.

During the study, the PSE Index improved or remained the same in the

TABLE 6. Characteristics of the Patients with Chronic Hepatic Encephalopathy Entered into the Long-term Open Study of Lactitol

Number of patients	: 20 (11 men and 9 women)
Mean age (±SEM) (yr)	: 51.5 3.2 (range 19 - 74)
Mean weight (kg)	: 66.6 3.3 (45.9 - 100)
Mean height (cm)	: 166.7 2.3 (147 - 180)

History of hepatic disease		
	Alcoholic cirrhosis	9
	Cryptogenic cirrhosis	4
	Primary biliary cirrhosis	3
	Viral hepatitis	1
	Chronic active hepatitis	2
	Presinusoidal portal hypertension	1
Precipitating factors if known		
	GI tract bleeding	8
	Constipation	1
	Chronic persistent PSE	1
	Shunt surgery	2
	Protein indiscretion	3
	Discontinuation of lactulose	1
	Sepsis	1
No identifiable precipitant		3

majority of patients (Table 7). Thus, during 101 examinations, an improvement in the PSE Index was observed in 58 instances, no change was observed in 22 instances, while deterioration was observed in 21 instances. When deterioration was noted, there was always a valid clinical explanation. Overall, the mean PSE Index gradually improved, although to some extent, this reflects the removal from the trial, by death, of the more severely ill patients.

There was wide variation in the dose of lactitol required to produce two semisoft stools per day, although the average dose was 35 g (range 4 to 108 g). The dose required for a marked laxative effect ranged from 0.65 to 0.86 g per kg per day. The majority of patients adapted to treatment with lactitol very quickly and were able to regulate their stool frequency effectively. The only side effects observed were diarrhea and flatulence. Diarrhea was observed in seven patients at some stage of the study; it was always dose-related for individual patients. Six patients complained of excessive flatulence which was dose-related in four. There was no direct relationship between the amount of lactitol required and the appearance of side effects. High individual lactitol doses were not necessarily accompanied by adverse effects.

During the course of the study, four patients experienced a total of seven episodes of infection requiring treatment with antibiotics. These infections were well tolerated and no adjustments were required in lactitol dosage. Five patients experienced a total of 11 episodes of gastrointestinal bleeding. One patient died following a torrential hemorrhage; the remaining four patients showed deterioration in their PSE Index during each bleeding episode but improved promptly with blood transfusion, continuation of lactitol treatment and the addition of cleansing enemata and short-term dietary protein restriction.

TABLE 7. Number of Patients with Chronic Hepatic Encephalopathy Showing Improvement, No Change or Deterioration in Their PSE Index when Monitored Six-weekly during Treatment with Maintenance Lactitol

	Weeks of trial							
	6	12	18	24	30	36	42	48
Improvement (n)	9	8	8	6	6	8	6	7
No change (n)	3	4	4	4	1	0	3	3
Deterioration (n)	4	4	3	2	4	3	1	0
Total	16	16	15	12	11	11	10	10

During the study, one patient died of liver cell failure following a gastrointestinal bleed and another died following the development of a primary liver cell cancer. Two further patients underwent liver transplantation and died in the perioperative period.

Thus, lactitol proved efficacious in the long-term control of chronic portal-systemic encephalopathy. It was well accepted and well tolerated. The only observed side effects were diarrhea and flatulence and these were usually dose-related.

'MODUS OPERANDI'

Lactulose is used extensively to treat hepatic encephalopathy, although its exact mechanism of action is unknown. It may, however, exert its beneficial effect by: a) lowering colonic pH, thereby suppressing the absorption of nonionized ammonia (17, 18); b) suppressing bacterial and intestinal ammonia generation (19, 20); c) stimulating the incorporation of ammonia into bacterial protein (21); d) decreasing intestinal transit time because of its cathartic properties (22) and hence reducing the time available for both the production and absorption of toxins; and/ or e) increasing fecal nitrogen excretion (23). Lactitol and lactulose undoubtedly share many physico-chemical properties and it might be expected that they would exert their beneficial effects in similar ways. However, the two sugars are distinct and separate compounds so that their modes of action might well differ.

In the double-blind comparison of lactitol and lactulose in the treatment of acute hepatic encephalopathy in cirrhotic patients (12), neuropsychiatric symptoms and signs resolved significantly more rapidly in the patients treated with lactitol. This suggests that the two sugars might act in different ways, although these differences may be quantitative rather than qualitative. Luginbühl has shown recently (24), using a fecal incubation system, that there are distinct differences in the ways in which bacteria metabolize these two sugars. He observed differences both in the speed with which bacteria metabolized the two sugars and in the degree of subsequent gas formation (Table 8). In addition, studies in healthy volunteers, from whom samples of cecal contents were obtained using a capsule technique, have shown that cecal counts of aerobic bacteria and enterococci are lower during ingestion of lactitol, whereas counts of anaerobic bacteria are lower during ingestion of lactulose. Both sugars effectively reduce the cecal ammonia content (Lang O, Wuhl F and Lebek G. Internal Zyma Report 1986. Study LACT-10-8416). These findings suggest that differences may exist in the way in which these two sugars are metabolized by colonic bacteria and this may explain the apparent difference in their speed of action as noted in one clinical study (12).

TABLE 8. Differences in the Bacterial Metabolism of Lactitol and Lactulose (Luginbühl M, 1986)

	Acidification		Gas formation	
	Lactitol	Lactulose	Lactitol	Lactulose
Anaerobic bacteria				
Bacteroides thetaiotaomicron	+	+	-	-
Bacteroides fragilis	+	+	-	-
Clostridium glycolicum	-	+	-	-
Clostridium perfringens	+	++	++	++
Lactobacillus acidophilus	++	+	-	-
Lactobacillus fermentum	-	(+)	-	-
Streptococcus mutans	+	++	-	-
Bifidobacterium bifidum	+	++	-	-
Aerobic bacteria				
Escherichia coli	-	++	-	(+)
Enterobacter	+	++	(+)	+
Enterococci	+	++	-	-
Staphylococcus aureus	(+)	+	-	-
Klebsiella	+	+	(+)	+
Citrobacter	-	+	-	(+)

- not detectable; (+) slight; + moderate; ++ substantial

CONCLUSIONS

Lactitol may be used with effect to treat both acute and chronic hepatic encephalopathy in cirrhotic patients. It is safe and its use is not associated with untoward side effects. Its effectiveness compares well with that of lactulose, but in general, it is better accepted by patients. In a price-sensitive market, it might well become the treatment of choice for this condition.

REFERENCES

1. van Velthuijsen JA. Food additives derived from lactose; lactitol and lactitol palmitate. J Agric Food Chem 1979; 27:680-686.

2. Patil DH, Grimble GK, Silk DBA. Lactitol, a new hydrogenated lactose derivative: intestinal absorption and laxative threshold in normal human subjects. Br J Nutr 1987; 57:195-199.

3. Grimble GK, Patil DH, Silk DBA. Colonic fermentation and caloric value of lactitol in healthy human subjects (Abstract). Gastroenterology 1986; 90:1730.

4. Patil DH, Westaby D, Mahida YR, et al. Comparative modes of action of lactitol and lactulose in the treatment of hepatic encephalopathy. Gut 1987; 28:255-259.

5. Bircher J, Buhrer K, Franz K, van Velthuijsen JA. Erstmaligue Anwendung von Lactitol in der Behandlung der porto-systemischen Enzephalopathie. Schweiz Med Wochenschr 1982; 112:1306-1307.

6. Lanthier PL, Morgan MY. Lactitol in the treatment of chronic hepatic encephalopathy: an open comparison with lactulose. Gut 1985; 26:415-420.

7. Morgan MY, Hawley KE, Stambuk D. Lactitol versus lactulose in the treatment of chronic hepatic encephalopathy. A double-blind, randomized, cross-over study. J Hepatol 1987; 4:236-244.

8. Conn HO, Leevy CM, Vlahcevic ZR, et al. A comparison of lactulose and neomycin in the treatment of portal-systemic encephalopathy: a double blind controlled trial. Gastroenterology 1977; 72:573-583.

9. Heredia D, Terés J, Orteu N, et al. Lactitol vs. lactulose in the treatment of chronic recurrent portal systemic encephalopathy (PSE) (Abstract). J Hepatol 1987; 5, Suppl 1:S143.

10. Balducci G, Riggio O, Ariosto F, et al. Lactitol in the prevention of hepatic encephalopathy (HE) in cirrhotics with porto-systemic anastomosis. A randomized controlled study (Abstract). J Hepatol 1987; 4, Suppl 1:S3.

11. Uribe M, Dibildox M, Malpica S, et al. Treatment of hepatic encephalopathy with a new sugar-alcohol. A double blind controlled trial (Abstract). Gastroenterology 1984; 86:1344.

12. Morgan MY, Hawley KE. A randomized double-blind trial of lactitol and lactulose in acute hepatic encephalopathy in cirrhotic patients. Hepatology 1987; 7:1278-1284.

13. Pugh RNH, Murray-Lyon IM, Dawson JL, et al. Transection of the oesophagus for bleeding oesophageal varices. Br J Surg 1973; 60:646-649.

14. Child CG III, Trucotte JG. Surgery and portal hypertension. In: Child CG III, ed. The liver and portal hypertension. Philadelphia: WB Saunders, 1964: 90.

15. Heredia D, Caballería J, Arroyo V, et al. Lactitol versus lactulose in the treatment of acute portal systemic encephalopathy (PSE). A controlled trial.

J Hepatol 1987; 4:293-298.

16. Uribe M, Campollo O, Vargas F, et al. Acidifying enemas (lactitol and lactose) vs. nonacidifying enemas (tap water) to treat acute portal-systemic encephalopathy: a double-blind, randomized clinical trial. Hepatology 1987; 7:639-643.

17. Castell DO, Moore EW. Ammonia absorption from the human colon. The role of non-ionic diffusion. Gastroenterology 1971; 60:33-42.

18. Bircher J, Haemmerli UP, Trabert E, et al. The mechanism of action of lactulose in portal-systemic encephalopathy. Non-ionic diffusion of ammonia in the canine colon. Rev Eur Etud Clin Biol 1971; 16:352-357.

19. Vince A, Dawson AM, Park N, et al. Ammonia production by intestinal bacteria. Gut 1973; 14:171-177.

20. Van Leeuwen PAM. Lactulose in acute portal-systemic encephalopathy. In: Ammonia generation in the gut and the influence of lactulose and neomycin: Review of the literature and experimental studies in the rat. PhD Thesis, University of Maastricht, The Netherlands, 1985: 39-40.

21. Vince AJ, Burridge SM. Ammonia production by intestinal bacteria: the effects of lactose, lactulose and glucose. J Med Microbiol 1980; 13:177-191.

22. Agostini L, Down PF, Murison J, et al. Faecal ammonia and pH during lactulose administration in man: comparison with other cathartics. Gut 1972; 13:859-866.

23. Weber FL Jr. The effect of lactulose on urea metabolism and nitrogen excretion in cirrhotic patients. Gastroenterology 1979; 77:518-523.

24. Luginbühl M. Effects of lactitol and lactulose on cultures of obligate and facultative anaerobic intestinal bacteria. Study to explain the effectiveness of lactitol and lactulose in the treatment of portal-systemic encephalopathy. Inaugural dissertation for the Doctorate of Medicine, University of Berne. 1986.

18

LONG-TERM TREATMENT WITH CRYSTALLINE LACTULOSE

F. Rossi-Fanelli, M.D., C. Cangiano, M.D., F. Ceci, M.D., M. Familiari, M.D., M. Muscaritoli, M.D., O. Riggio, M.D., A. Cascino, M.D.

More than twenty years of therapeutic success have amply shown the value of lactulose in the treatment and prevention of hepatic encephalopathy (HE) (1-4). Although different therapeutic approaches may be considered in the treatment of acute episodes of HE in patients with chronic liver disease (5-7), lactulose remains the drug of choice in the long-term treatment of chronic HE (1-5, 8).

Lactulose, however, is only available as a syrup that contains small amounts of other sugars, mainly lactose and galactose (9), which contribute to its excessively sweet taste and, perhaps, to the appearance of symptoms often complained of by patients, including nausea, heartburn, epigastric pain, distension and diarrhea (1-4, 8, 10). Occasionally, the patient's discomfort may require suspension of treatment.

On theoretical grounds, a preparation containing only lactulose might be free of the undesirable side effects observed with impure preparations. Recently, chemically pure lactulose (crystalline lactulose) has been made available on the market (Zambon Pharmaceuticals, Milan, Italy). It is dispensed as a powder which can be diluted in water or juice. Its sweetness varies depending on its concentration, but it is always less sweet than lactulose syrup.

We performed a crossover study in 14 consecutive cirrhotic patients, in whom the long-term tolerance to lactulose syrup and to pure crystalline lactulose were compared (11). Fourteen biopsy-proven cirrhotic patients completed two months of treatment. Five patients were treated for acute episodes of grade II encephalopathy. Details of these patients are presented in Table 1. Three patients were included who were treated to prevent recurrences of severe HE (grade III to IV) that had occurred previously. Seven were patients with portal-systemic shunts who were treated to prevent the initial occurrence of PSE. All patients were maintained on a protein-restricted diet (0.5 g per kg body weight) during the study. Eight had

TABLE 1. Clinical Features

Sex	9 male, 5 female
Age	39-68 years
Type cirrhosis	10 cryptogenic, 4 alcoholic
Acute PSE (grade II)	5
Prior PSE* (grade III-IV)	4
No prior PSE*	5
Surgical portal-systemic shunts	7
Spontaneous portal-systemic shunting	7

*Grade 0 at time of study

been receiving lactulose chronically before the study was started. The daily dose of lactulose given in three equal doses was adjusted in each patient to insure at least two soft bowel movements per day (18 to 27 g per day; mean 22.5 g). Seven patients received lactulose syrup during the first month and crystalline lactulose during the second month. The order was reversed in the remaining seven patients.

The order of administration was not randomly determined. To evaluate the tolerance to the treatment, patients reported weekly on the presence of the following symptoms: dyspepsia, epigastric pain, distension, dysphagia and diarrhea. Liver blood tests and plasma ammonia concentrations were monitored throughout the study. Careful clinical examination and Number Connection Tests (NCT) (12) were performed weekly throughout the study, which was conducted outside the hospital. Patients' families were instructed to report the appearance of symptoms indicative of HE, i.e., slurred speech, bizarre behavior, etc.

With the exception of diarrhea, which was reported by two of the 14 patients (14%) during the crystalline lactulose period, no other symptoms were noted. Conversely, during the lactulose syrup treatment period, three patients (21%) complained of epigastric pain, six (43%) of heartburn, three (21%) of dysphagia, four (29%) of abdominal distention and three (21%) of diarrhea. The differences in the prevalence of symptoms between the two treatment periods are significant.

The results of this trial confirm what had been expected. With the exception of diarrhea, which occurred in only two patients and which was severe enough to discontinue treatment in one patient, no other symptoms were reported by the remaining patients while receiving pure lactulose. All five patients who had shown signs of encephalopathy (grade II) on admission regained normal mental state (grade 0) and improved their psychometric performance (NCT) within 48 hours of initiation of crystalline lactulose treatment. Neither mental state nor Number Connection Tests showed further changes throughout the duration of therapy (Table 2).

A comparison between the tolerance to lactulose syrup and crystalline lactulose was made in the eight patients who had been receiving lactulose syrup

TABLE 2. NCT Scores during Treatment with Crystalline Lactulose

Hepatic encephalopathy at onset	No. patients	Basal	After month's treatment
		Mean ±SD in seconds	
Grade 0	9	66±27	60±30
Grade II	5	108±53	96±54

before starting the study (Table 3). The daily dose of lactulose ranged from 30 to 60 ml per day (mean 41.8 ml), corresponding to 18 to 36 g of pure lactulose (mean 25.1 g). The incidence of symptoms with the exception of diarrhea was significantly lower during crystalline lactulose treatment than with lactulose syrup. Diarrhea, defined as more than four bowel movements per day, was reported by one patient receiving crystalline lactulose and by two patients taking the syrup. The dosage of both preparations was then tapered to restore two bowel movements per day. Blood chemistry and ammonia levels did not change significantly during the trial.

The data from this study suggest that the cause of intolerance to lactulose syrup may be the presence of contaminating sugars. Neither crystalline lactulose nor lactulose derived from the syrup is absorbed or metabolized in the small intestine (13). Both are rapidly hydrolyzed in the colon by bacterial beta-galactosidases to form small molecular weight organic acids, such as lactic, acetic or formic acid and small amounts of carbon dioxide (14). Reducing colonic pH with its consequent reduction in ammonia absorption is probably the most important way by which lactulose exerts its pharmacological effects. Although the stool pH was not measured in the present study, a significant increase in fecal acidity has been reported with the administration of lactulose syrup (2-4, 8) and of crystalline lactulose in children (15).

The popularity of this compound is amply justified by its efficacy and safety. The minor drawbacks with long-term lactulose syrup treatment, such as the appearance of gastrointestinal symptoms, may easily be minimized or overcome by utilizing crystalline lactulose instead.

TABLE 3. Comparison of Lactulose Syrup and Crystalline Lactulose in Inducing Side Effects

Side effect	No. patients	Number of side effects (%)	
		Lactulosesyrup	Pure lactulose
Epigastric pain	8	2 (25%)	0 (0%)
Dyspepsia	8	4 (50%)	0 (0%)
Dysphagia	8	2 (25%)	0 (0%)
Distention	8	3 (38%)	0 (0%)
Diarrhea	8	2 (25%)	1 (12%)

REFERENCES

1. Bircher J, Muller J, Guggenheim P, et al. Treatment of chronic portal-systemic encephalopathy with lactulose. Lancet 1966; 1:890-893.
2. Conn HO, Leevy CM, Vlahcevic ZR, et al. A comparison of lactulose and neomycin in the treatment of portal-systemic encephalopathy: a double-blind controlled trial. Gastroenterology 1977; 72:573-583.
3. Atterbury CE, Maddrey WC, Conn HO, et al. Neomycin-sorbitol and lactulose in the treatment of acute portal-systemic encephalopathy: a controlled, double-blind clinical trial. Am J Dig Dis 1978; 23:398-406.
4. Orlandi F, Freddara U, Candelaresi MT, et al. Comparison between neomycin and lactulose in 173 patients with hepatic encephalopathy. A randomized clinical study. Dig Dis Sci 1981; 26:498-506.
5. Rossi-Fanelli F, Riggio O, Cangiano C, et al. Branched-chain amino acids vs. lactulose in the treatment of hepatic encephalopathy. Dig Dis Sci 1982; 27:929-935.
6. Fast B, Wolfe S, Stormont J, et al. Antibiotic therapy in the management of hepatic coma. Arch Intern Med 1958; 101:467-475.
7. Kunin C, Chalmers T, Leevy C, et al. Absorption of orally-administered neomycin and kanamycin with special reference to patients with severe hepatic and renal disease. N Engl J Med 1960; 262:380-385.
8. Conn HO, Lieberthal MM. The Hepatic Coma Syndromes and Lactulose. Baltimore: Williams and Wilkins, 1979.
9. Avery GS, Davies EF, Brogden RN. Lactulose: a review of its therapeutic and pharmacological properties with particular reference to ammonia metabolism and its mode of action in portal systemic encephalopathy. Drugs 1972; 4:7-48.
10. Kaupke C, Sprague T, Gitnick G. Hypernatraemia after the administration of lactulose. Ann Intern Med 1977; 86:745-746.
11. Rossi-Fanelli F, Attili A, Cascino A, et al. Valutazione dell'efficacia e della tollerabilita' del lattulosio in forma purificata nella profilassi e nel trattamento dell'encefalopatia porto-sistemica. Gaz Med It 1980; 139:267-270.
12. Conn, HO. Trailmaking and number-connection tests in the assessment of mental state in portal systemic encephalopathy. Am J Dig Dis 1977; 22:541-550.
13. Dahlqvist A, Gryboski J. Inability of the human small-intestinal lactase to hydrolyze lactulose. Biochim Biophys Acta 1965; 110:635-636.
14. Brown R, Gibson J, Sladen G, et al. Effects of lactulose and other laxatives on ileal and colonic pH as measured by a radiotelemetry device. Gut 1974; 15:999-1004.
15. Besana R, Cicchetti N. Lattulosio cristallino e dispepsi putrefattive: studio clinico preliminare con controlli batteriologici delle feci. Aggiornamento Pediatrico 1981; 32:1-12.

19

EFFECT OF LACTITOL AND LACTULOSE ON HUMAN INTESTINAL FLORA IN PORTAL-SYSTEMIC ENCEPHALOPATHY

G. LEBEK, M.D., AND M. LUGINBÜHL, M.D.

Lactulose, a nonfermentable disaccharide of galactose and fructose, has been used successfully to treat portal-systemic encephalopathy (PSE) for 20 years. It is sweet, syrupy and sometimes distasteful, and may induce nausea, which reduces compliance, especially in long-term administration. Therefore, an alternative, lactitol, a disaccharide of galactose and sorbitol, was devised. It turned out to be equally effective, but didn't have these disadvantages. First used in 1982 by Bircher et al. in chronic PSE (1), it seems to be as effective as lactulose in acute PSE, too (2).

In order to know more about the mechanism of action of these two disaccharides, we attempted to answer the following questions in parallel studies *in vitro* and *in vivo*:

1. Which species of intestinal bacteria ferment lactulose and which ferment lactitol?
2. How does lactulose or lactitol effect pH, NH_3 concentration and the number of microorganisms in stool suspensions of healthy subjects?
3. How do these same parameters behave in cecal and in stool samples of healthy subjects taking lactulose or lactitol?

FERMENTABILITY OF LACTULOSE AND LACTITOL BY THE MAJOR INTESTINAL MICROORGANISMS

Strains of the most common species of intestinal bacteria were incubated in a liquid culture medium containing 0.03 M lactitol, lactulose or glucose. A sugar-free medium was used as a control. Gas formation and pH were measured at regular intervals. After the inoculation of the test media with 10^8 microorganisms, facultative anaerobic species were incubated at 37°C for four days with daily measurements. Obligate anaerobes were incubated for two and six days, respectively, at the same temperature in a BBL Gaspak system with measurements carried out at the end of each incubation. When fermentation occurred, the pH of the medium dropped, often accompanied by an increase in gas formation. The results are summarized in Table 1.

E. coli, citrobacter and Hafnia fermented only lactulose and induced lower pH values with lactulose than with lactitol. The species with the greatest acid production were *Lactobacillus acidophilus*, *Bifidobacterium bifidum* and anaerobic Lactobacillus species. They reduced pH from levels of 6 and 5, respectively, by 1.0 and 1.8. Among facultative anaerobes, Klebsiella, S*treptococcus epidermidis* and enterococci reduced pH from 7.0 to 5.0 (3).

CHANGES IN pH, NH_3 CONCENTRATION AND THE NUMBERS OF MICROORGANISMS IN STOOL SUSPENSIONS AFTER THE ADDITION OF LACTITOL, LACTULOSE OR GLUCOSE

Using the method of Vince et al. (4), samples of eight stools from one healthy subject were diluted 1:3 with 0.9% NaCl solution. Aliquots of the resulting suspension were mixed with lactulose, lactitol or glucose to achieve final concentrations of each disaccharide of 0.03, 0.06, and 0.09 M, and for glucose of 0.06 M. A carbohydrate-free suspension was used as a control. We studied four stools from different bowel movements for each sugar concentration. The incubation was carried out under pure nitrogen with continuous shaking for 48 hours at 37°C. Ammonia and pH were measured at the beginning and after 3, 6, 24 and 48 hours and the numbers of obligate and facultative anaerobic microorganisms determined after 24 and 48 hours. We analyzed the pH of the fluids from sterile Wrong *in vivo* dialysis bags filled with Rheomacrodex (5). At the times indicated, the bags were removed and the NH_3 concentration was determined in the dialysate by the method of Berthelot (6). Blood ammonia concentrations and pH values were averaged and standard deviations calculated. In order to determine the number of microorganisms, 0.1 ml of stool suspension was removed under sterile conditions at the times indicated and series of dilutions with Crowther transport medium were made. These suspensions were incubated on blood agar (aerobes) and Schaedler-Kanamycin Agar (obligate anaerobes) for 24 hours, the number of organisms determined and median values calculated. We observed a marked decline in pH and an inhibition of NH_3 production with all sugars (Figures 1-4). Acid formation occurred more slowly from lactitol than from lactulose, and low concentrations of lactitol inhibited NH_3 production to a lesser degree than the other sugars. All sugars, however, reduced ammonia production significantly. The numbers of both aerobic and anaerobic organisms were decreased (Table 2). The number of aerobes was reduced to a greater degree than that of anaerobes.

TABLE 1. Fermentability of Lactulose, Lactitol and Glucose by Intestinal Microorganisms [1]

A. Obligate Anaerobic Microorganisms

Species	Lactitol			Lactulose			Glucose			Sugar-free control
	No.[2] positive	Mean pH on day 2	Gas	No.[2] positive	Mean pH on day 2	Gas	No.[3] positive	Mean pH on day 2	Gas	Mean pH on day 2
Bacteroides thetaiotaomicron	7/8	5.6±0.5	0	8	5.3±0.3	0	8	5.3±0.7	0	6.6
Bacteroides fragilis	5/8	5.6±0.4	0	8	5.1±0.4	0	8	5.1±0.4	0	6.4±0.4
Bacteroides distasonis	8/8	6.1±0.6	0	8	5.5±0.3	0	8	5.4±0.6	0	6.6±0.3
Bifidobacterium bifidum	1/1	5.5	0	1	4.5	0	1	4.0	0	6.5
Clostridium perfringens	6/8	5.7±0.6	+++	8	4.8±0.5	+++	8	5.1±0.4	+++	6.8±0.4
Lactobacillus acidophilus	7/9	4.7±0.6	0	9	5.5±1.0	0	9	5.0±0.9	0	6.4±0.5
Lactobacillus species	2/2	5.3±1.7	0	2	5.3±1.7	0	2	5.0±1.4	0	6.8±0.4
Streptococcus mutans	5/7	5.3±0.4	0	7	4.3±0.3	0	7	4.0	0	6.6±0.5
Clostridium glycolcium	0/1	—	0	1	5.5	0	1	5.0	+++	6.5
Propionibacterium species	1/2	6.5	0	1	6.5	0	1	5.5±0.7	0	7.0
Lactobacillus fermentum	0/1	—	0	1	6.0	0	1	6.0	0	6.5

[1] All experiments done at least in triplicates; [2] number of positive strains per number of examined strains; [3] all examined strains were positive.

TABLE 1, continued.

B. Facultative Anaerobic and Obligate Anaerobic Microorganisms

Species	Lactitol			Lactulose			Glucose			Sugar-free control
	No.[2] positive	Mean pH on day 2	Gas	No.[2] positive	Mean pH on day 2	Gas	No.[2] positive	Mean pH on day 2	Gas	Mean pH on day 2
Enterobacter	2/7	7.0	+	3/7	5.5	++	7/7	6.8±0.4	+++	7.8±0.4
Klebsiella	14/15	5.6±0.4	+	15/15	5.5±0.2	++	15/15	5.4±0.4	++	6.3±0.3
E. coli	0/2	—	0	2/2	6.0±1.4	+	2/2	4.7±0.4	++	7.5
Proteus mirabilis	0/1	—	0	0/1	—	0	1/1	4.5	+	7.5
Proteus morgani	0/2	—	0	0/2	—	0	2/2	4.5	++	7.7±0.4
Proteus vulgaris	0/2	—	0	0/2	—	0	2/2	5.0	+	7.5
Serratia	0/2	—	0	0/2	—	0	2/2	6.2±0.4	++	7.7±0.4
Citrobacter	0/2	—	0	2/2	6.5±1.4	+	2/2	5.0±0.7	+	7.7±0.4
Hafnia	0/2	—	0	2/2	6.2±0.4	0	2/2	4.5	0	7.0
Pseudomonas aeruginosa	0/2	—	0	0/2	—	0	0/2	—	0	8.5
Candida albicans	0/2	—	0	0/2	—	0	2/2	6.2±0.4	0	7.7±0.4
Enterococci	8/9	5.7±0.4	0	9/9	5.0	0	9/9	4.1±0.2	0	7.0±0.2
Staphylococcus epidermidis	5/10	5.5±0.4	0	5/10	5.0	0	10/10	4.8±0.3	0	7.8±0.4
Staphylococcus aureus	4/8	6.3±0.3	0	8/8	5.4±0.5	0	8/8	4.9±0.5	0	6.5±0.4

Disaccharide fermentation by Fusobacteria and *Clostridium difficile* negative; Gas formation: 0 = not detectable; + = slight; ++ = moderate; +++ = substantial; [2]number of positive strains per number of examined strains.

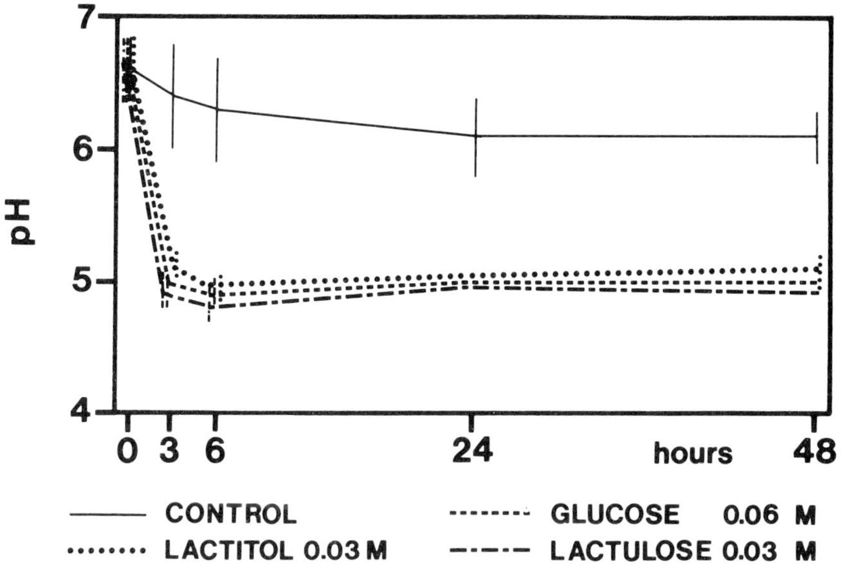

FIGURE 1. A marked decline in pH is noted in each of eight stool suspensions after the addition of lactulose 0.03 M, lactitol 0.03 M, or glucose 0.06 M as compared to control.

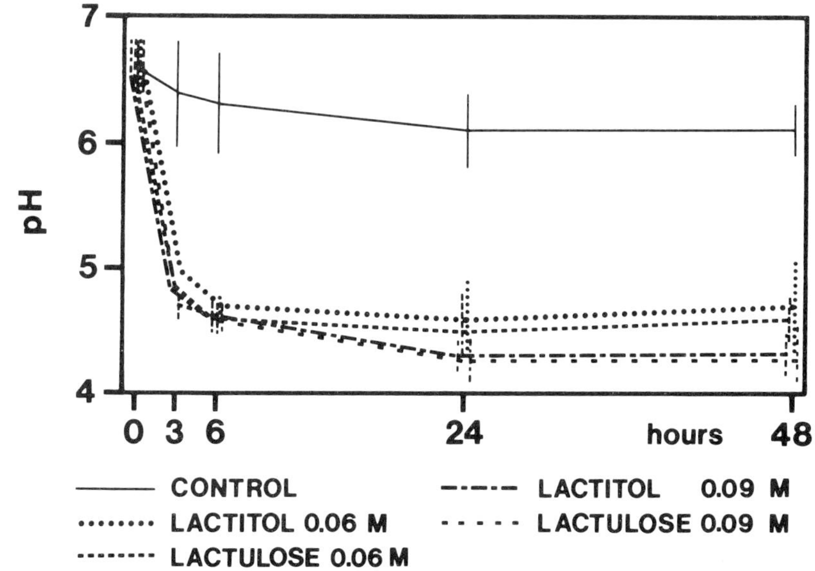

FIGURE 2. A decline in pH similar to that shown in Figure 1 is noted in each of eight stool suspensions after the addition of lactulose 0.06 M, lactitol 0.06 M, or glucose 0.09 M as compared to control.

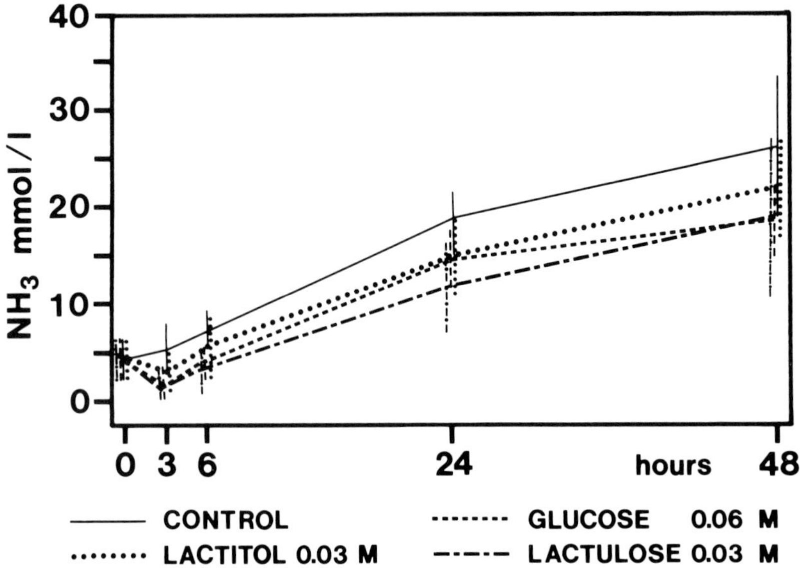

FIGURE 3. A decline in ammonia concentration is noted in each of eight stool suspensions after the addition of lactulose 0.03 M, lactitol 0.03 M, or glucose 0.06 M as compared to control.

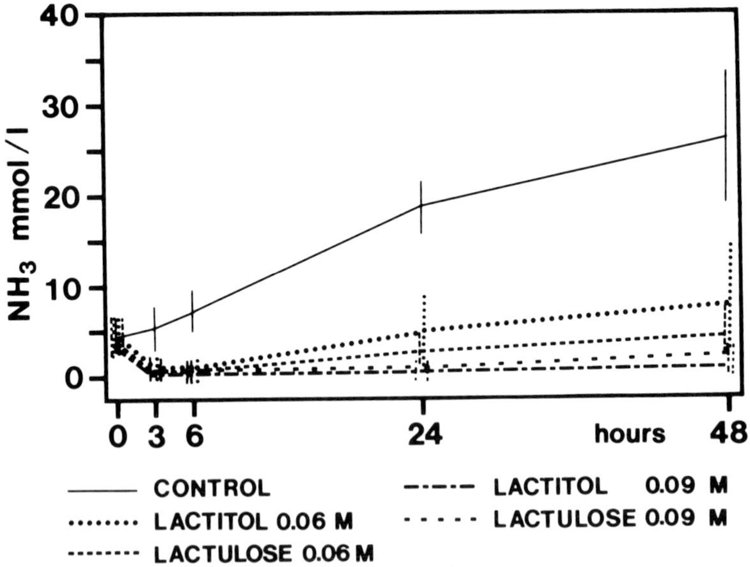

FIGURE 4. A decline in ammonia concentration is noted in each of eight stool suspensions after the addition of lactulose 0.06 M, lactitol 0.06 M, or glucose 0.09 M as compared to control.

TABLE 2. Numbers of Aerobic and Anaerobic Microorganisms in a 25% Stool Suspension after the Addition of Glucose, Lactulose and Lactitol. Median numbers of microorganisms per ml of stool suspension (8 samples).

		Aerobes			Anaerobes		
		0 h	24 h	48 h	0 h	24 h	48 h
Control		$1x10^9$	$4x10^8$	$4x10^8$	$4x10^{10}$	$2x10^{10}$	$4x10^9$
Glucose	0.06 M	$1x10^9$	$1x10^9$	$2x10^8$	$4x10^{10}$	$4x10^9$	$6x10^8$
Lactulose	0.03 M	$1x10^9$	$1x10^9$	$4x10^8$	$4x10^{10}$	$4x10^9$	$7x10^8$
	0.06 M	$1x10^9$	$2x10^7$	$4x10^6$	$4x10^{10}$	$1x10^8$	$1x10^8$
	0.09 M	$1x10^9$	$3x10^5$	$7x10^5$	$4x10^{10}$	$1x10^8$	$1x10^7$
Lactitol	0.03 M	$1x10^9$	$1x10^9$	$3x10^8$	$4x10^{10}$	$2x10^9$	$6x10^8$
	0.06 M	$1x10^9$	$6x10^6$	$1x10^7$	$4x10^{10}$	$1x10^9$	$3x10^8$
	0.09 M	$1x10^9$	$1x10^6$	$1x10^5$	$4x10^{10}$	$3x10^8$	$6x10^7$

CHANGES IN pH, NH_3 CONCENTRATION AND NUMBERS OF MICROORGANISMS IN CECAL CONTENTS AND STOOL SAMPLES OF TWO HEALTHY SUBJECTS TAKING LACTITOL OR LACTULOSE.

Two healthy male volunteers took part in a parallel experiment. After a three-week, drug-free period on their normal diet, lactitol was added for three weeks followed by lactulose for three weeks. The dose of the disaccharide was chosen to produce two soft stools daily. It amounted to 60 g of lactitol and 80 g of lactulose for subject A and 60 g of either disaccharide for subject B. Since the change from one disaccharide to the other took place without a washout period, no analyses were made during the first five days of each period to permit the intestinal flora to adapt. In order to obtain samples of cecal contents, we used Pyxigraphy, a method developed by Perrenoud et al. (7, 8): sterile capsules (30 x 9 mm) were swallowed and transported by peristalsis to the desired position in the bowel. By introducing the subject into an oscillating magnetic field, aspiration of 0.1 to 0.2 ml of intestinal contents into the capsules was accomplished. After aspiration the capsules were closed, then they were excreted. Pyxigraphy is a noninvasive, relatively nonstressful method of obtaining intestinal contents. However, it has certain disadvantages.

First, localization of the capsule is inaccurate since it depends on the image intensifier and barium contrast. Second, the interval between aspiration of the samples to processing varies with the bowel transit time. Since we could not justify localizing each capsule by X-ray, we determined at the beginning of the study the approximate transit time from swallowing the capsule to its appearance in the ascending colon by image intensifier. In subject A it was 12 hours; in subject B, 18 hours. In the following experiments the localization was determined both by the noise produced by the aspiration process and by the appearance and pH of the aspirate. If the sound of aspiration wasn't heard in the right lower abdomen, the aspirate wasn't of the typical yellowish color (8) and if the pH differed greatly from those of other samples taken during the same period, that capsule was excluded from further processing. Therefore, we analyzed different numbers of samples in the different periods. Ten carbohydrate-free control specimens were analyzed for subject A and five for subject B. Ten lactulose specimens for subject A and eight for subject B were studied. Ten lactitol specimens for subject A and eight for subject B were analyzed. After excretion, the surface of the capsule was disinfected with 70% ethanol and the contents immediately processed. The capsules were washed out with a known volume of 0.9% NaCl, and the pH was measured with Merck indicator paper strips. After centrifugation, the NH_3 concentration of the supernatant was determined. One part of the suspension was used to prepare a series of dilutions with Crowther transport solution to count the numbers of aerobes, anaerobes, Bacteroides, enterococci and enterobacteriaceae. Stool samples were diluted 1:4 with 0.9% NaCl solution. Further processing was performed in the same manner as for the cecal samples. Mean values and standard deviations were calculated for pH and NH_3 concentrations and median values for the bacterial counts.

The results are summarized in Table 3. We found marked reductions in the mean pH values of cecal contents and stool samples of both subjects during administration of glucose, lactulose and lactitol. The reductions of NH_3 concentration correlated well with the decrements in pH. In subject A, NH_3 decreased to 18% of basal values with lactulose and to 23% with lactitol. In subject B they decreased to 34% and 26%, respectively. In stool samples the ammonia decreased to 48% of the initial value in subject A after administration of lactulose and to 52% after lactitol. In subject B, reductions of 70% and 80% of the initial values were found, respectively.

Since subject B was often constipated on a normal diet, the transit time of the capsules to the colon was prolonged, which seemed to correlate with the number of microorganisms in the contents of the capsules. Major differences in cecal flora were noted between the two subjects. Only anaerobic organisms could be recovered from the contents of the capsules from subject B while he was on the carbohydrate-free control diet. When disaccharides were given, the intestinal activity of subject B became normal and anaerobic microorganisms could be recovered in normal numbers.

In the cecal contents, lower numbers of microorganisms were almost always found in subject B than in A (Table 3). We noted a relative increase of anaerobic bacteria in the cecal contents as was found in the *in vitro* stool suspensions. In subject A, anaerobes rose by one order of magnitude with lactulose and two orders with lactitol, whereas the aerobes remained constant on lactulose and fell by two orders of magnitude on lactitol. In subject B the anaerobes remained constant with both disaccharides. We have no data about aerobes in subject B. During administration of disaccharides, however, the numbers of anaerobic bacteria exceeded those of aerobes by one or two logs.

In the stool samples the numbers of anaerobes rose by a factor of ten in both subjects after administration of either disaccharide. The aerobes, however, fell by one log with lactulose and by two logs with lactitol in subject A. They remained

TABLE 3. pH, NH_3 Concentration and Numbers of Microorganisms in Cecal Contents and Stool Samples from Two Healthy Subjects Taking Lactulose or Lactitol and Normal Diet

	Subject A			Subject B		
Cecal contents	Normal diet	Lactulose	Lactitol	Normal diet	Lactulose	Lactitol
pH	5.5±0.5	4.5±0.5	4.4±0.4	5.1±0.5	4.6±0.4	4.6±0.6
NH_3 conc.(mmol/L)	46±22	8±2	11±6	15±10	5±2	4±3
Aerobes (total)	$2.5x10^6$	$1.4x10^6$	$2.5x10^4$	$<9x10^4$	$3.6x10^6$	$1.2x10^4$
Anaerobes (total)	$7.8x10^7$	$4.4x10^8$	$2.3x10^9$	$8.0x10^6$	$5.0x10^7$	$4.2x10^6$
Bacteroides	$2.0x10^6$	$1.7x10^8$	$1.9x10^8$	$<9x10^4$	$4.1x10^6$	$1.1x10^5$
Enterobacteria	$1.2x10^7$	$1.2x10^8$	$1.6x10^8$	$<7x10^4$	$1.1x10^6$	$1.7x10^4$
Enterococci	$1.7x10^6$	$1.8x10^6$	$4.6x10^3$	$<6x10^4$	$4.3x10^6$	$6.2x10^4$
Stool						
pH	7.4±0.3	6.4±0.4	6.8±0.3	7.5±0.3	6.9±0.3	7.3±0.3
NH_3 conc.(mmol/L)	40±11	19±9	21±7	28±11	20±7	25±8
Aerobes (total)	$8.8x10^7$	$1.5x10^6$	$9.6x10^5$	$1.3x10^8$	$3.8x10^8$	$4.2x10^8$
Anaerobes (total)	$2.6x10^9$	$3.2x10^{10}$	$3.2x10^{10}$	$7.9x10^{10}$	$4.6x10^{11}$	$4.4x10^{11}$
Capsule transit time (days in gastro-intestinal tract)	1.7±0.6	2.1±1.5	2.6±0.8	6.0±2.4	6.9±2.0	6.3±3.3

Enterobacter and Enterococci on selective media using anaerobic procedures.
Numbers of determinations: subject A, 10; subject B, 5 (normal diet), 8 (disaccharide diet).
Mean values and standard deviations of pH and NH_3 concentration.
Median values of numbers of microorganisms per ml of stool.

constant in subject B. In both subjects a marked increase of Bacteroides was noted in the cecal contents in the presence of both disaccharides. Enterobacteria, too, rose in subject A with lactulose and lactitol, whereas it increased only with lactulose in subject B. Enterococci did not change on lactulose in subject A, but rose markedly in subject B. On lactitol, however, they fell in subject A and remained constant in subject B.

CONCLUSIONS

The following conclusions can be reached from these results:

1. Lactitol and lactulose are both fermented by the major species of intestinal flora.
2. The numbers of aerobic and anaerobic bacteria are decreased by increasing concentrations of both disaccharides (9).
3. A progressive decrease in pH and ammonia concentration paralleled the decrease in the number of organisms (10). Bacteriodes, the most frequent species and the most active NH_3 producer as well, metabolizes both disaccharides.
4. Lactitol and lactulose reduce pH, NH_3 concentration and bacterial counts in *in vitro* stool suspensions.
5. Similar results were found in our *in vivo* study. Increased flatulence during the first few days of lactulose administration was observed in our subjects. It may be related to vigorous gas formation by Clostridia, Klebsiella and Enterobacter noted in our *in vitro* experiments. Thus, lactitol and lactulose appear to act by the same mechanism and seem to have equal effects *in vitro* and *in vivo*.

REFERENCES

1. Bircher J, Bührer M, Franz K, et al. Erstmalig Anwendung von Lactitol in der Behandlung der porto-systemischen Enzephalopathie. Schweiz Med Wochenschr 1982; 112:1306-1307.
2. Heredia D, Caballeria J, Orteu N, et al. Lactitol versus lactulose in the treatment of acute portal-systemic encephalopathy. A controlled trial (Abstract). J Hepatol 1985; Suppl 1:65.
3. Luginbühl M, Kitler ME, Lang O, et al. Lactitol and lactulose in portal-systemic encephalopathy therapy: a comparison in vivo and in vitro of their effect on the human intestinal flora (In preparation).
4. Vince A, Killingley M, Wrong OM. Effect of lactulose on ammonia production in a fecal incubation system. Gastroenterology 1978; 74:544-549.
5. Wrong O, Metcalfe-Gibson A, Morrison RBI, et al. Dialysis of feces as a

method of stool analysis. Clin Sci 1965; 28:357-375.

6. Richterich R. Klinische Chemi, Theorie und Praxis. Basel, Switzerland: Karger, 1968.

7. Perrenoud JP. La Pyxigrafie, procédé d'exploitation du contenu du tube digestif au moyen de capsules de prélevement. Gastroenterologia 1957; 87:349-355.

8. Perrenoud JP, Ruedi B, Rossel J, et al. Pyxigrafie. Med Chir Dig 1983; 12:173-179.

9. Drasar BS. Some factors associated with geographical variations on the intestinal microflora. In: Skinner FA, Carr JG, eds. The Normal Microbial Flora of Man. London: London Academic Press, 1974: 187-196.

10. Vince A, Burridge SM. Ammonia production by intestinal bacteria: the effects of lactose, lactulose and glucose. J Med Microbiol 1980; 13:177-191.

20

MANAGEMENT OF PORTAL-SYSTEMIC ENCEPHALOPATHY WITH LACTOSE

Misael Uribe, M.D.

Lactulose, a semisynthetic lactose derivative has been widely and successfully used for the treatment of patients with portal-systemic encephalopathy (1-3). The rationale for the use of lactulose was to induce disaccharide malabsorption (4) due to the absence of its respective disaccharidase, lactulase. Lactulose, after arriving in the colon, is digested by bacterial disaccharidases and metabolized to fatty acids, acetoacetic acid, lactic acid, and hydrogen gas. It is believed that the change in colonic pH decreases both the absorption and the production of nitrogen derivatives, mainly ammonia (5, 6).

It is a paradox that a lactose derivative was first used to treat portal-systemic encephalopathy, particularly since lactose malabsorption occurs in the vast majority of the world's populations (7). Therefore, both lactose in lactase-deficient populations and lactulose in all populations are able to induce acidic diarrhea, which favors cleansing of the large bowel. In this work, we will present evidence of controlled trials on the similar benefits of lactose, lactulose and the recently developed, new disaccharide, lactitol, for the treatment of chronic and acute portal-systemic encephalopathy (PSE).

THE COLONIC ECOSYSTEM

The idea to change the colonic ecosystem, pH and colonic flora to treat PSE was first suggested by Macbeth et al. (8) in 1965. This group attempted to manipulate the intestinal flora by the administration to two cirrhotic patients of high doses of oral *Lactobacillus acidophilus*. These authors concluded that the human colonic flora can be manipulated, but not easily. However, their experiments demonstrated that the increase of acidophilic flora was associated with decreased intestinal urease activity, and with a reduction in blood ammonia levels.

A year later, in a limited number of cirrhotic patients with PSE, Fenton et al. (9) tested the tolerance of protein from several sources. This group administered a variety of proteins (vegetable, meat, eggs and dairy products), and concluded that, gram for gram, dairy proteins were better tolerated than meat and egg-derived proteins. In the three individuals in whom the dairy protein was administered, psychometric improvement of PSE was noted compared with the other diets. These authors thought that the apparent psychometric improvement was due to less putrefactive degradation and to less ammonia production during the digestion of dairy protein.

More recently Welsh and coworkers (10) for the first time used powdered lactose to treat PSE in an open trial. In that study they administered 100 g per day of lactose to American Indians with lactase deficiency and PSE. These investigators assessed mental state, EEG, and stool pH before and after each week of treatment with or without lactose. In this breakthrough clinical experiment, the patient recovered from deep PSE, and the EEG tracings improved, while his stools became more numerous and more acid. With lactose, the stool pH decreased from 6.0 and 6.4 to 4.0 and 5.9, respectively. Clinical improvement was associated with stool acidification.

Although preliminary, these exciting findings prompted us to perform a number of controlled trials with lactose in our Mexican patients with PSE, the majority of whom are lactase-deficient. To our knowledge these are the only controlled trials so far carried out with lactose.

PHARMACOLOGY OF LACTOSE

Lactose is a disaccharide composed of the monosaccharides glucose and galactose. It is the primary carbohydrate in mammalian milk. Lactose constitutes less than 5% (wt/volume) of bovine milk. In human milk, lactose may achieve even higher concentrations. After hydrolysis by its natural disaccharidase, lactase, lactose yields equimolar amounts of glucose and galactose, which are rapidly absorbed by the intestine. Hydrolysis does not occur in the small intestine in the absence of lactase. Lack of lactase favors the presence of undigested lactose in the colon where it is fermented by colonic bacteria (Figure 1).

The presence of undigested lactose in the colon exerts a hyperosmotic effect. The hyperconcentration of sugar draws water into the intestinal lumen. In the colon lactose undergoes bacterial degradation to acidic metabolites (Figure 1). Thus, as a result of hyperosmosis and fermentation, the clinical picture of acidic diarrhea, flatulence, distention, and abdominal pain is produced. This is the typical clinical pattern of carbohydrate malabsorption (11).

Lactose is the most abundant (>90%) carbohydrate and the most important

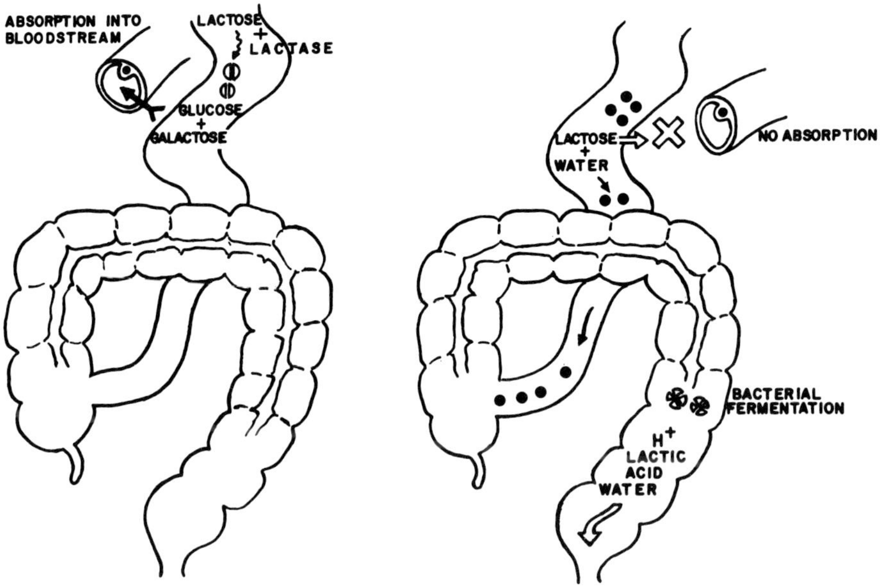

FIGURE 1. Lactose digestion in normal patients with adequate lactase (left) and with lactase deficiency (right).

caloric source in human milk. Lactose differs from other disaccharides like maltose and sucrose. In lactose, the monosaccharides are linked by a beta-glycosidic bond, while maltose and sucrose have alpha-glycosidic linkages.

Whole milk contains a large amount of both sodium and protein (Table 1), which limit its use in patients with advanced liver disease, particularly those with fluid retention and/or PSE, in whom salt and protein must be restricted.

TABLE 1. Human and Bovine Milk Composition

	Human milk		Condensed milk	
	Range	Mean	Range	Mean
Lactose (g per dl)	49-95	71	45-50	42
Protein (g per dl)	7-20	16	30-46	32
Sodium (mEq per L)	64-430	172	390-1300	760

ABSORPTION AND COLONIC DIGESTION BY FECAL FLORA

To be absorbed, lactose must be split into its two monosaccharides, glucose and galactose. Lactase is the specific disaccharidase that performs this task. Lactase is synthesized by the cells that line the surface of the small intestine. Absent or reduced amounts of this enzyme lead to lactose malabsorption.

The molecular weight of lactase is 280,000. Its optimal pH for milk fermentation is 5.5 - 6.0, which is that of the duodenum. Although the enzyme is found in all parts of the small intestine, its concentration and activity are more important before the angle of Trietz (13). Some drugs, like colchicine and neomycin, are able to decrease lactase activity.

Bacteria normally present in the colon play a major role in the digestion of sugar. These bacteria use lactose as a source of energy, thus promoting their growth. It is believed that bacterial growth assimilates the ammonia produced by degradation and putrefaction of ingested proteins as a source of nitrogen (6).

The main bacterial strains involved in lactose fermentation are those that are adaptable to an acidic environment, i.e.: *Lactobacillus acidophilus*, *Lactobacillus bifidus*, *Clostridium perfringens*, *E. coli* and some types of staphylococci (14). The fermentation of disaccharides occurs very rapidly. Instillation of lactulose near the ileal valve causes an increase of H_2 in the breath in less than 5 minutes (15). Perhaps, this is the explanation for the very rapid cathartic response that occurs in some patients with PSE.

In humans, intestinal lactase activity is high in all newborns and during infancy. In mammalians including man, lactase activity declines as the individual ages. The loss of enzyme activity in adulthood is called primary adult lactase deficiency. This deficiency occurs in the vast majority of the populations of the world (7) (Figure 2). However, in central and northern Europeans, and in their descendants worldwide, lactase activity remains high during adulthood, and they do not develop lactose malabsorption.

Many experts believe that lactose malabsorption is inherited, since ethnic groups that live in different parts of the world have similar prevalence of lactose malabsorption. For instance, Jews living in the United States have a similar prevalence of lactase deficiency as those living in Israel or eastern Europe. Also, the prevalence of lactase deficiency in American blacks and Mexican Americans is similar in African blacks or Mexicans living in Mexico.

Before attempting to treat PSE with oral lactose, the presence of lactase deficiency must be established. However, in acute PSE (see below), the administration of lactose enemas does not require such evaluations since by the rectal route lactose is directly deposited in the colon and the effect of bacterial fermentation promptly produces acidification and diarrhea.

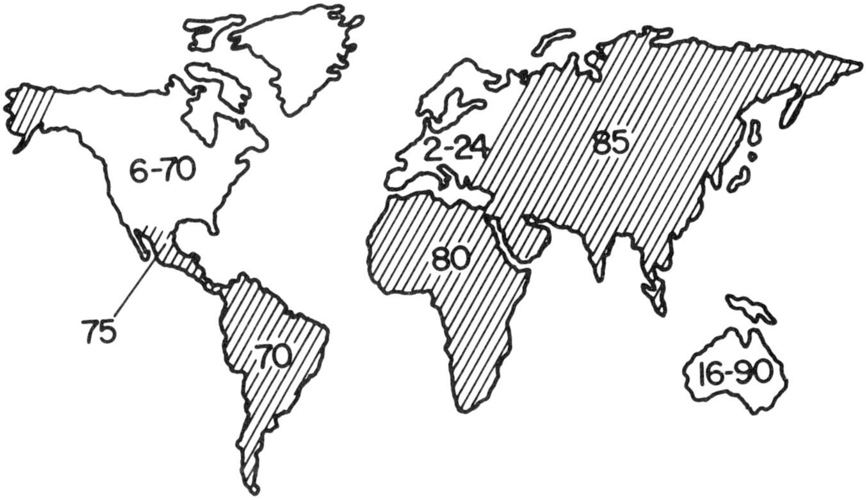

FIGURE 2. Worldwide distribution of lactase deficiency (adulthood).

LACTOSE TOLERANCE TEST (LTT)

The lactose tolerance test (LTT) is the most common, simplest and least expensive test for documenting lactose malabsorption. The test, however, is nonspecific. LTT consists of the administration of lactose powder (50 g) dissolved in 100 ml of water. Blood samples are drawn at 15 and 30 minutes after the ingestion of the disaccharide. After digestion, lactose yields significant amounts of glucose and galactose. Analysis of blood glucose in normal subjects demonstrates an elevation of more than 25 mg per dl. When this occurs, the individual is considered lactase-sufficient. With glucose elevations of 20 to 25 mg per dl, the test is considered inconclusive and should be repeated. Blood glucose elevations below 20 mg per dl are indicative of lactase deficiency (16).

Other more sophisticated tests to assess lactase deficiency are the breath hydrogen test and the enzymatic analysis of intestinal lactase activity in a peroral biopsy of the intestine. In our experience these tests are rarely needed to prove lactase deficiency. The oral LTT is an office procedure. Glucose determinations using a reflectometer give an immediate result and, in the majority of the cases in which the test is positive, it is accompanied by clinical signs of lactose maldigestion (abdominal pain, diarrhea, flatulence, etc.)

USE OF ORAL LACTOSE IN CHRONIC PSE

The efficacy and safety of oral lactose was evaluated in a controlled trial in patients with lactose malabsorption and chronic PSE (17). The trial included ten patients with PSE who had previously responded to standard therapy with neomycin and milk of magnesia. The study compared two 2-week periods of conventional treatment and two periods of lactose therapy. Because of the different nature of the treatments, the study was not blinded for the patients, but the investigator who evaluated the PSE was not informed of the nature of the treatment the patients were receiving. Therefore, the study design was a double, cross-over, single-blind trial.

During control periods I and II with standard treatment, the patients received neomycin (3 g per day) plus approximately 70 ml of milk of magnesia per day to induce two to four soft bowel movements each day. After each control period patients received lactose treatment for two weeks. In lactose periods I and II the patients were treated with 50 g of lactose dissolved in 100 ml of water bid. Dietary intake was maintained at 40 g per day and the total calories at 1800 kcal per day.

PSE parameters included the evaluation of mental state, EEGs, psychometric tests (Number Connection Tests), asterixis and blood ammonia levels. These

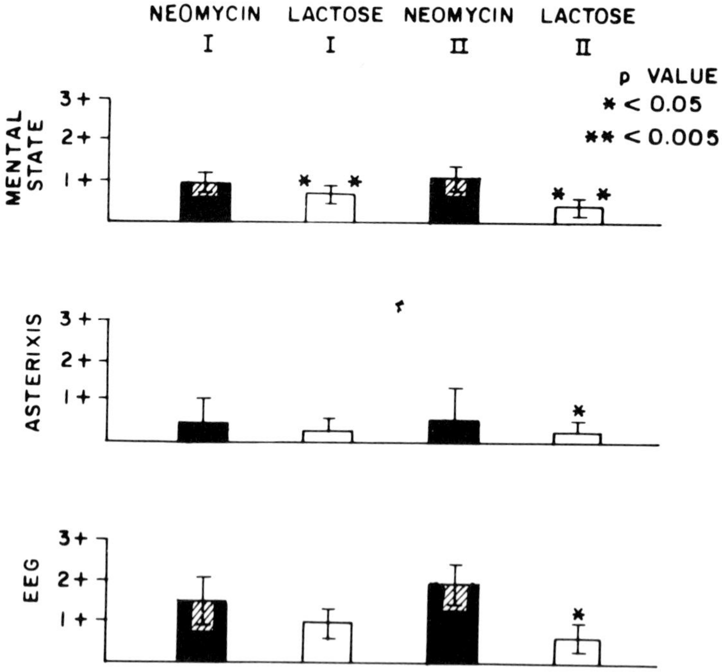

FIGURE 3. The effects of oral lactose (50 g bid) in ten patients with chronic PSE

parameters of PSE were assessed blindly.

The overall results of therapy on PSE are shown in Figures 3 and 4. Mental state was significantly better during both lactose periods than during standard therapy, and in some cases lactose therapy improved other aspects of PSE. 'The only side effects were associated with lactose maldigestion, i.e., mild abdominal pain, flatulence, etc. Several patients were continued on treatment with lactose for up to seven months; no serious side effects were noted.

Since the therapeutic response with lactose resembles the response obtained with lactulose, we have since used lactose in all PSE patients who have an abnormal LTT. Most patients prefer lactose rather than lactulose because the powder is easier to carry; lactose syrup is much less sweet than lactulose syrup and is less expensive. In terms of cost-benefit in our country, lactose, gram for gram, is only 5% of the cost of lactulose and 20% as expensive as neomycin.

Unfortunately, in many places the use of lactose is limited by the erroneous impression that lactose malabsorbers are uncommon and that complicated tests are needed to assess lactose maldigestion. Even countries like the United States, with a fast-growing minority population, have large numbers of patients in whom lactose can be used. Lactase deficiency in American minorities occurs in 75% of blacks, 70% of Jews, 95% of Asians, 60% of American Indians and more than 60% of Mexican Americans. Cost versus benefit should be considered in those populations.

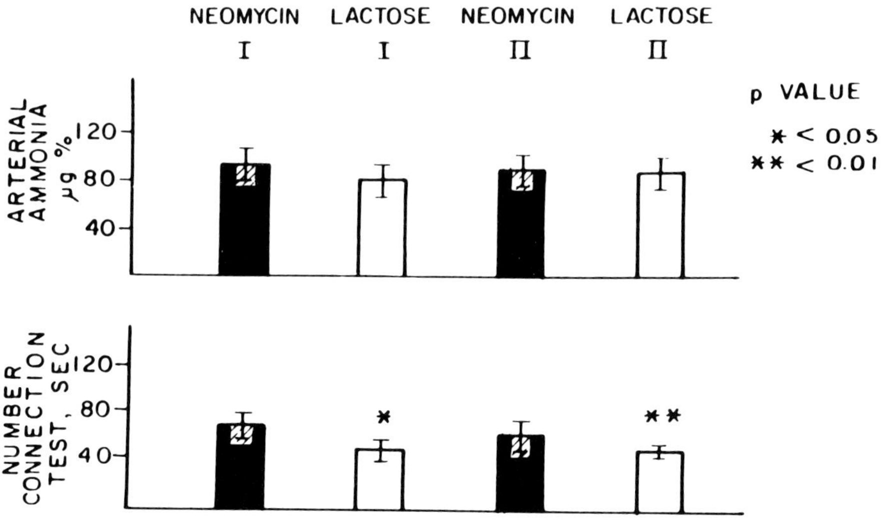

FIGURE 4. The effects of oral lactose on asterixis, ammonia and Number Connection Test times (same legend as in Figure 3). Clear improvement in NCT was observed after both lactose periods.

LACTOSE VERSUS LACTITOL

Lactitol is a new derivative of lactose that can be prepared in crystalline form. It is less sweet than lactulose, but is sweeter than lactose. A number of recent controlled trials (18, 19) suggest that the taste of lactitol makes this disaccharide the treatment of choice for PSE.

Since lactitol is available as a powder it can be blindly compared with lactose. Both sugars theoretically may exert a similar therapeutic effect, but compliance and adherence to both treatments must be established.

We, therefore, decided to evaluate in a double-blind, double cross-over fashion, the efficacy and safety of these two sugars versus the standard therapy of neomycin and milk of magnesia (20). The trial was performed in 18 patients with chronic PSE and lactase deficiency. The study consisted of four periods: two for washout and two for lactitol or lactose treatment. Each period lasted two weeks; thus the total length of the trial was eight weeks.

During washout periods, patients were stabilized with neomycin (3 g per day) plus milk of magnesia (70 ml per day), an amount sufficient to induce two to four bowel movements per day. Ten patients were randomly assigned to receive lactose and eight patients to receive lactitol first. The components of the PSE syndrome were assessed before and biweekly during therapy. Stool pH was assessed after each period of treatment. The dose of disaccharides was adjusted individually to achieve two to four bowel movements each day. Patients required an average of 39 ± 14 g per day of lactitol and 65 ± 12 g per day of lactose to achieve 2.7 ± 1 and 2.9 ± 1.3 bowel movements, respectively.

The results demonstrated that both sugars were equally effective in controlling PSE. During the first and second periods of administration, mental state, Number Connection Test times and blood ammonia concentrations were very similar regardless of the nature of the treatment administered (Figure 5). The overall response as indicated by the PSE Index was also similar after lactose and lactitol and both were comparable with neomycin treatment (Figure 6). In both cases, the administration of lactitol and lactose induced significant stool acidification (Figure 7).

Nine of the 18 patients preferred lactitol, five preferred lactose; the rest declared no preference. Lactitol exerted a more predictable and tolerable effect. However, since lactitol is not yet available in our country, cost-benefit considerations cannot be discussed.

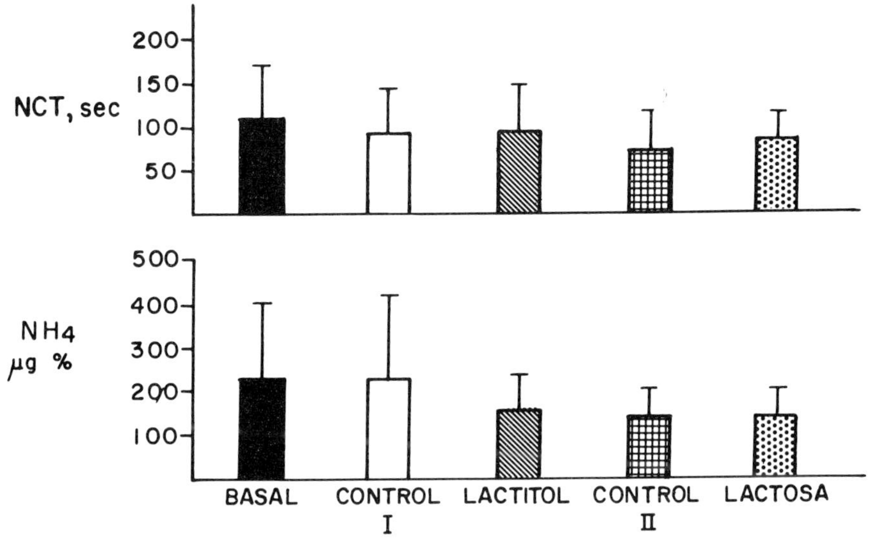

FIGURE 5. Results from a group of 18 patients who received oral lactose and lactitol (see text). NCTs and blood ammonia levels were similar after the lactose (lactosa) and lactitol periods.

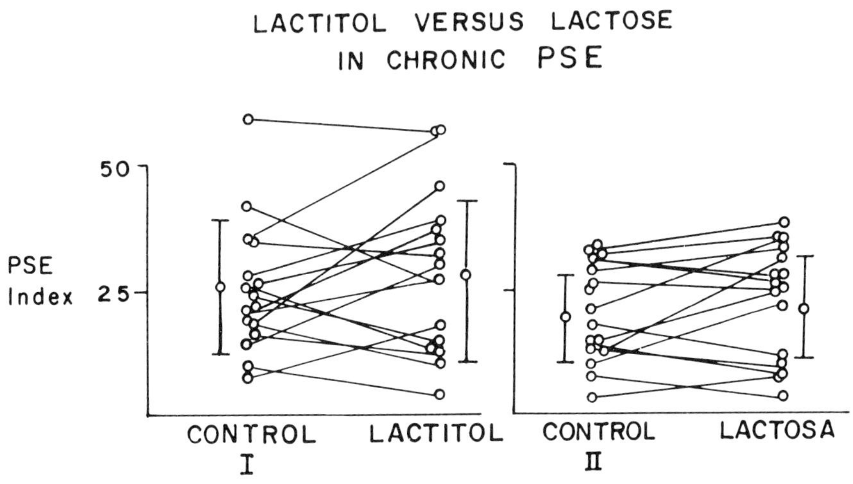

FIGURE 6. The PSE Index was very similar after oral lactitol and oral lactose (lactosa) in 18 patients with chronic PSE.

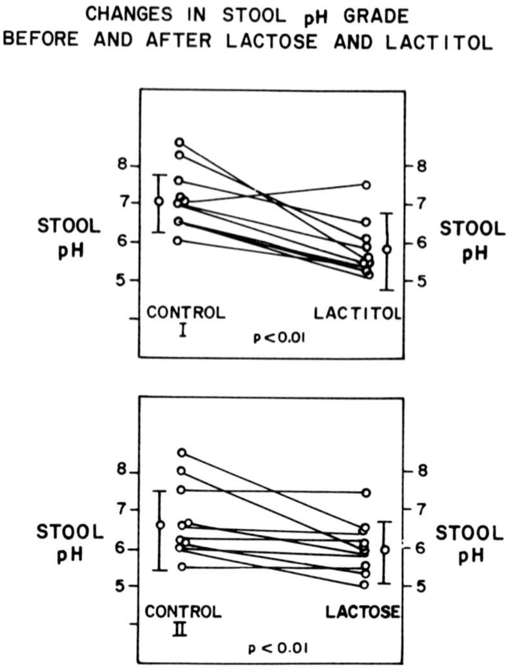

FIGURE 7. Both lactitol and lactose produced a similar degree of stool acidification in patients with chronic PSE.

LACTOSE PLUS NEOMYCIN

The combination of neomycin and disaccharides has been proposed for the treatment of PSE. This recommendation is supported by the finding that when neomycin alone is administered, incomplete sterilization of the large bowel is obtained. Thus, many bacteria remain that are able to ferment disaccharides even though the patient is receiving neomycin. Thus, theoretically, the beneficial effects of both medications may be additive. Other reasons to support this concept are that many cirrhotic patients have received neomycin repeatedly, and some have developed resistance to neomycin and other antibiotics. Antibiotic-resistant bacterial strains are able to ferment disaccharides.

Neomycin, however, may in many cases inhibit the bacteria that degrade disaccharides and thus prevent intestinal acidification. To clarify this important point a number of *in vitro* and *in vivo* studies have been performed.

In vitro, stool culture studies (simulating the colonic conditions) were performed to investigate the effect of lactose, lactulose and lactitol on stool pH, ammonia generation *in vitro* and on the total counts of aerobes and anaerobes. Significant acidification of stools and a reduction in ammonia generation *in vitro* occurred after the addition of the three disaccharides. The addition of neomycin to stool cultures with disaccharides reduced the effect of acidification (21).

In a recent study, Patil et al. (22) compared the metabolism of lactitol and lactulose with and without the addition of neomycin, using an *in vitro* fecal incubation system. Both sugars were readily metabolized by fecal bacteria, producing volatile fatty acids. The metabolism was inhibited by neomycin. *In vivo*, colonic pH was monitored by telemetry in a group of six healthy individuals after the administration of oral lactulose and lactitol in amounts sufficient to induce two to three soft stools per day (30 to 180 g per day). Both sugars significantly lowered the right colon pH (basal 6.5±0.4 versus lactitol 5.6±0.5; lactulose 5.18±0.8, $p<0.05$). The pH of the rest of the colon was unaffected. *In vivo*, the simultaneous administration of neomycin (2 to 4 g per day) reversed the effect, and the colonic pH remained at 6.4±0.9 (NS).

In vivo, we have recently examined the effect of the addition of neomycin on 40 patients receiving lactose (n=16), lactulose (n=8) or lactitol (n=16) (23). The patients had mild, chronic PSE that had been controlled with disaccharides and protein restriction. After a basal 10-day period of disaccharide therapy the patients received neomycin tablets (3 g per day) or an identical placebo for two weeks. The components of PSE, the PSE Index (4) and stool pH were assessed biweekly during the trial. The results showed that in mild PSE the addition of neomycin does not significantly improve PSE (Figure 8) or the PSE Index. In our study the patients showed stool acidification regardless of the simultaneous administration of neomycin. In a previous study Conn et al. (24) reported that a group of patients showed wide individual variations in stool pH after the administration of the combination of lactulose and neomycin. They concluded that neomycin inhibited stool acidification in one-third of the cases, produced no significant changes in one-third, and in the remaining one-third, stool pH remained acidic.

Based on these *in vivo* and *in vitro* studies, we believe that neomycin may inhibit the bacterial metabolism of disaccharides and in some cases negates the

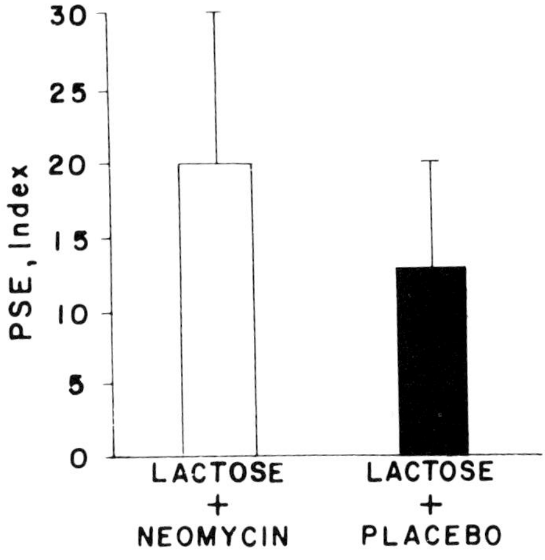

FIGURE 8. Results on the PSE Index in a group of 16 patients with chronic PSE receiving 3 grams of lactose plus 3 g neomycin per day or identical placebo during two-week periods of therapy. The differences are not significant statistically. (The bars express mean ± SD).

effect of disaccharides on the pH of the right colon. Differences in response to the addition of neomycin can be explained by wide variations of fecal flora composition and antibiotic resistance. From the clinical side, in mild PSE the addition of neomycin is unable to significantly improve PSE in patients already receiving disaccharides. On the other hand, adding neomycin to disaccharides increases the cost of treatment and, more important, exposes the patients to the well-known, untoward, antibiotic side effects (ototoxicity and nephrotoxicity). The combination of disaccharides plus neomycin has not been explored in controlled fashion in severe chronic PSE or in acute PSE and, therefore, no objective recommendations can be made.

LACTOSE PLUS ANTACIDS

In preliminary, uncontrolled trials it was noted that antacids sometimes prevent lactulose-induced acidification of the stool, the basis of its therapeutic effect. It is not clear, however, whether this effect is due to neutralization of acid in the intestinal lumen, or to the prevention of the degradation of the disaccharide.

We have recently performed a number of controlled trials (25) in lactase-deficient volunteers and have demonstrated that two antacids (Gelusil® and Amphogel®) diminish the intensity of the symptomatic response and the reduction in stool pH. Therefore, we suggest that, if needed, other medications such as H_2 antagonists may be preferred when PSE is being treated with lactulose in patients with peptic ulcer disease.

LACTOSE ENEMAS IN ACUTE PSE

The rectum has been used as an alternate route for a number of purposes. It appears to be advantageous for the administration of medications to uncooperative children or to adults who are unable to take oral medications. In addition, in the case of patients with PSE, the effects of disaccharides may be enhanced by direct deposition into the colon.

To exert their therapeutic effects, disaccharides need to reach the lower intestine where bacterial fermentation and colonic acidification occur. The time to reach the colon under normal conditions varies from 1 hour to 8 hours or more. This interval is radically reduced if the disaccharide is given by enema. Further indication for rectal use is the comatose condition of patients with acute PSE. A nasogastric tube is mandatory in such patients. The risk of severe nausea from the sweetness of the syrup, vomiting and bronchial aspiration should also be kept in mind. Using the rectal route permits the deposition of as much as 200 g lactose in the colon immediately. This massive amount of disaccharide via the oral route is unlikely to be tolerated by patients.

Based on these concepts we have established in our intensive care unit the use of lactose enemas as the treatment of choice for acute PSE. Cost versus benefit favors lactose enemas against any other therapy of acute PSE.

LACTOSE ENEMAS VERSUS NEOMYCIN IN ACUTE PSE

Several years ago (26) we decided to investigate the efficacy and safety of lactose enemas versus oral neomycin in acute PSE. To maintain the double-blind status of the study, it was necessary to use a double-drug design. Eight patients with acute PSE received 1-liter enemas of 20% lactose and simultaneously two placebo tablets tid, which were identical to 0.5 g neomycin tablets. Ten patients received 1-liter starch enemas tid, plus two 0.5 g neomycin tablets tid. Both groups were comparable in demographic characteristics and liver function.

After the treatment, both groups showed significant improvement in their asterixis, blood ammonia levels and EEGs. In addition, patients treated with lactose enemas showed a significant improvement in the time required to perform the Number Connection Test.

After therapy, stool pH decreased from 6.0±0.8 to 5.6±0.7 with the starch enema-neomycin group (Figure 9), but this change was not statistically significant. In contrast, fecal pH significantly decreased in the lactose-treated group (6.0±0.8 to 4.8±1.0; $p<0.05$). Overall clinical and biochemical improvement was observed in 87% and 70% of lactose and neomycin groups, respectively. These differences are not statistically significant.

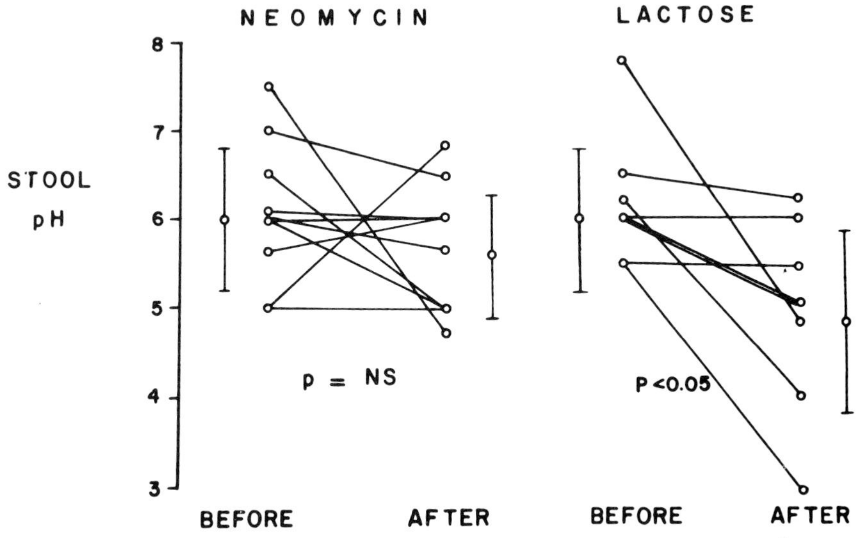

FIGURE 9. Stool pH after neomycin (3 g per day) plus starch enemas or lactose enemas.

LACTOSE ENEMAS VERSUS TAP WATER AND LACTITOL ENEMAS

Most investigators believe that acidification and diarrhea induced by disaccharide maldigestion is the mechanism of therapeutic action in PSE. However, there are at least two main factors involved in the effects of disaccharides. One is the degree of colonic acidification; the other is the emptying of the intestinal contents. The cleansing of the colon, which is obtained with the application of purgatives or with enemas, raises the possibility that the cleansing factor *per se* may be responsible for the improvement observed in these patients. In fact, the effect of cleansing the colon has not been subjected to controlled trials in patients with PSE.

Therefore, we decided to investigate the efficacy and safety of acidifying and non-acidifying enemas in patients with acute PSE (27). Enemas were tested in 45 episodes of acute PSE. Patients included in the study had encephalopathy of at least grade II+ severity, prolongation of the time required to perform the Number Connection Test and hyperammonemia. Originally the design predicted that 23 patients per group would be needed to achieve statistically significant differences. However, sequential analysis performed after the first 20 patients demonstrated that tap water enemas were associated with a high frequency of treatment failure (Table 2). Thus, this group was discontinued, and the study was continued with the lactose and lactitol groups. As consequence of this re-randomization, only five patients

TABLE 2. Treatment Response During the Trial

First 20 patients	Tap water group (n=5)	Lactose group (n=5)	Lactitol group (n=10)
Response*	1	3	10
Failure	4	2	0
Deaths	3	1	0

Lactose versus Lactitol (after Re-randomization)	Lactose group (n=18)	Lactitol group (n=22)
Response**	14	19
Failure	4	3
Deaths	1	0

* Lactose vs lactitol p=0.095; lactose vs water p=0.26; lactitol vs water p=0.0037.
** Lactose vs lactitol p=0.38.

received tap water enemas (1 liter tid), 18 received lactose enemas (1 liter 20% tid) and 22 received lactitol (1 liter 20% tid).

A favorable response to therapy was obtained in 18 (86%) of the patients receiving lactitol enemas versus 14 (78%) of those receiving lactose enemas (Table 2). Similar significant improvements in the PSE parameters were observed after both disaccharides, but not after the tap water enemas (Figures 10 and 11). Both sugars reduced stool pH whereas top water enemas exerted no such effect. In general, the response to treatment paralleled the degree of stool acidification.

Based on these results we suggest that acidifying enemas are superior to nonacidifying tap water enemas in the treatment of patients with acute PSE and that lactose and lactitol are equally effective.

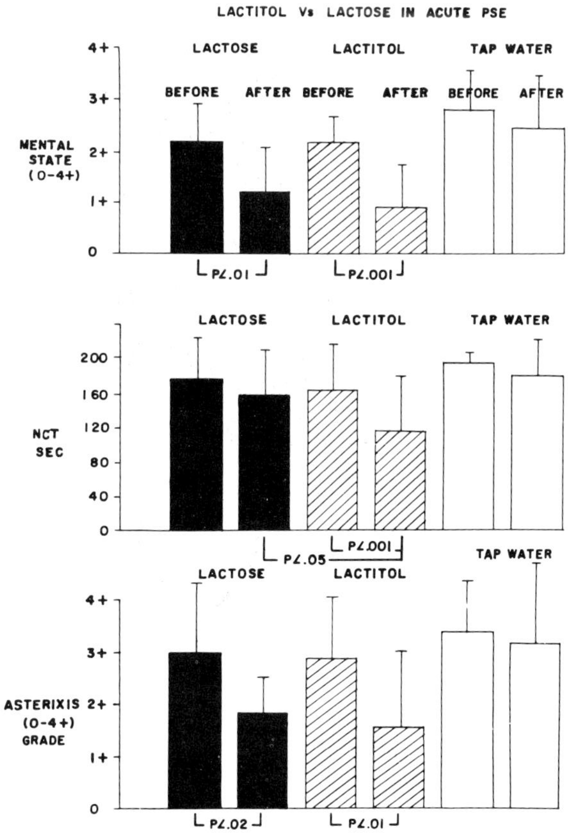

FIGURE 10. Changes in mental state, Number Connection Tests and asterixis after lactose, lactitol and tap water enemas in 18, 22 and 5 patients respectively, with acute PSE. The bars represent mean ±SD.

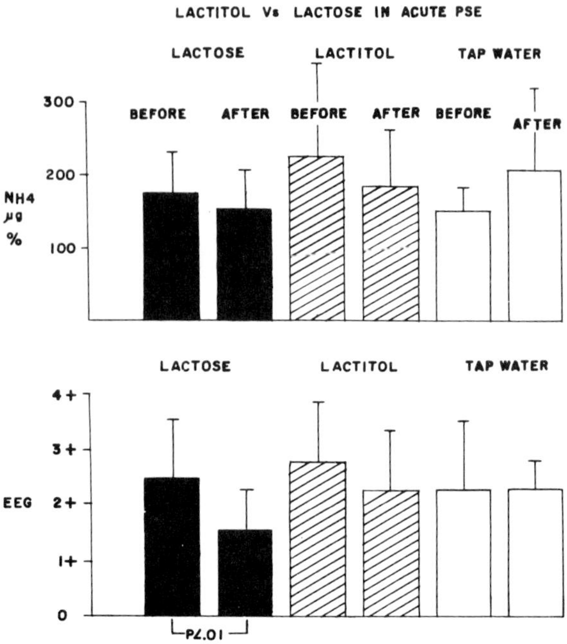

FIGURE 11. Changes in blood ammonia levels and EEG tracings after lactose, lactitol and tap water enemas (same legend as in Figure 10).

REFERENCES

1. Conn HO, Leevy CM, Vlahcevic RZ, et al. Comparison of lactulose and neomycin in the treatment of chronic portal-systemic encephalopathy. A double blind controlled trial. Gastroenterology 1977; 72:573-583.
2. Bircher J, Muller J, Guggenheim P, et al. Treatment of chronic portal systemic encephalopathy with lactulose. Lancet 1966; 1:890-893.
3. Atterbury CE, Maddrey WC, Conn HO, et al. Neomycin, sorbitol and lactulose in the treatment of acute portal systemic encephalopathy. A double blind clinical trial. Am J Dig Dis 1978; 23:398-406.
4. Conn HO. Lactulose: a drug in search of a modus operandi. Gastroenterology 1978; 74:624-626.
5. Lewis H, Rohas S, Uribe M. Similar effect of lactose and lactulose on in vitro fecal ammonia generation and bacterial flora (Abstract). Gastroenterology 1980; 78:1206.
6. Vince AJ, Burridge SM. Ammonia production by intestinal bacteria: The effects of lactose, lactulose and glucose. J Med Microbiol 1980; 13:177-192.
7. Lisker R, Lopez Habib G, Daltabuit M. Lactase deficiency in a rural area of Mexico. Am J Clin Nutr 1974; 27:756-759.

8. Macbeth WAAG, Kass EH, McDermott WB. Treatment of hepatic encephalopathy by alteration of intestinal flora with Lactobacillus acidophilus. Lancet 1965; 1:399-403.

9. Fenton JCB, Knight EJ, Humpherson PL. Milk and cheese diet in portal systemic encephalopathy. Lancet 1966; 1:164-166.

10. Welsh JD, Cassidy D, Prigatano, et al. Chronic hepatic encephalopathy treated with oral lactose in a patient with lactose malabsorption. N Engl J Med 1974; 291:240-241.

11. Dehesa M. Sindromes de malabsorption. In: Uribe M, ed. Tratado de Medicina Interna, Chapter 157. Mexico: Editorial Medica Panamericana, 1987: 1089-1106.

12. Gabuzda GJ. Relation of potassium depletion to renal ammonium metabolism and hepatic coma. Medicine 1966; 45:481-490.

13. Kretchmer N. Memorial lecture: Lactose and lactase, a historical perspective. Gastroenterology 1971; 61:805-813.

14. Doell RG, Kretchmer N. Studies of small intestine during development. Distribution of activity of ß-galactosidase. Biochim Biophys Acta 1962; 6:353-362.

15. Bond JH, Levitt MD. Use of pulmonary hydrogen measurement to quantify carbohydrate absorption. J Clin Invest 1972; 51:1219-1225.

16. Lisker R, Lopez Habib G, Mora MA. Correlation in the diagnosis of intestinal lactase deficiency between the radiological method and the lactose tolerance test. Rev Invest Clin (Mex) 1975; 27:1-5.

17. Uribe M, Marquez MA, Garcia Ramos G, et al. Treatment of chronic portal systemic encephalopathy with lactose in lactase-deficient patients. Dig Dis Sci 1980; 25:924-929.

18. Lanthier PL, Morgan MY. Lactitol in the treatment of chronic hepatic encephalopathy: an open comparison with lactulose. Gut 1985; 26:415-420.

19. Heredia D, Caballeria J, Arroyo V, et al. Lactitol versus lactulose in the treatment of acute portal systemic encephalopathy (PSE). J Hepatol 1987; 4:293-298.

20. Uribe M, Toledo H, Garcia Ramos G, et al. Lactitol, a second disaccharide for the treatment of chronic portal systemic encephalopathy: a double blind controlled trial. Dig Dis Sci 1987; (in press).

21. Uribe M, Gill S, Galvan E. Neomycin plus disaccharides in portal systemic encephalopathy: Beneficial or deleterious? (Abstract). Gastroenterology 1984; 86:1344.

22. Patil DH, Westaby D, Mahida YR, et al. Comparative modes of action of lactitol and lactulose in the treatment of hepatic encephalopathy. Gut 1987; 28:255-259.

23. Uribe M, Gil S, Garcia Ramos G, et al. Disaccharides plus neomycin to treat chronic portal systemic encephalopathy: a double blind controlled trial. Submitted for publication.

24. Conn HO, Lieberthal MM. Lactulose and neomycin-combined therapy. In: The Hepatic Coma Syndromes and Lactulose, Chapter 15. Baltimore: Williams and Wilkins, 1979: 340-345.

25. Uribe M, Conn HO. Effects of antacids on intestinal response and stool acidification induced by lactulose and lactose in lactose intolerant subjects (Abstract). Gastroenterology 1982; 82:1248.

26. Uribe M, Moreno Berthier J, Lewis H. Lactose enemas plus placebo tablets vs neomycin tablets plus starch enemas in acute portal systemic encephalopathy. A double blind randomized controlled study. Gastroenterology 1981; 81:101-106.

27. Uribe M, Campollo O, Vargas F, et al. Acidifying enemas (lactitol and lactose) vs nonacidifying enemas (tap water) to treat acute portal systemic encephalopathy: a double blind randomized clinical trial. Hepatology 1987; 7:639-643.

SUNDRY ASPECTS OF LACTULOSE

21

CATHARTIC PROPERTIES OF LACTULOSE

JOHN HAMILTON, M.D., AND PAUL BASS, M.D.

Laxatives have been used throughout history in the form of herbal and folk remedies. Claims have been made for their efficacy in the treatment of numerous diseases unrelated to the gastrointestinal tract. These claims extend even to the present day in the belief that dietary fiber, because of its laxative action, will be useful in the prevention of diseases as diverse as diabetes and varicose veins (1). The search for the mechanisms of laxative action has evolved throughout history from superstition to empiricism and, in recent years, to scientific evaluation (2). This chapter characterizes the pathophysiology of constipation and provides objective assessment of its correction.

Before discussing any drug used for the treatment of constipation, it is important first to obtain an objective definition for constipation so that the effectiveness of the drug can be assessed against these criteria. *Constipation* is from the Latin *con-stipo*: to press together. Therefore, constipation might be viewed as an excess processing of the stool. From another point of view, the Dorland medical dictionary defines constipation as "A condition in which bowel movements are infrequent or incomplete." Completeness of evacuation is certainly a difficult parameter to evaluate clinically, but there are data on stool frequency in normal subjects (3). In a study of 1,055 industrial workers (655 women and 400 men) and 400 patients of a private practitioner (266 women and 134 men) in Great Britain, a bowel movement frequency of three per week to three per day was defined as normal. This encompassed 98% of all the so-called "normal" subjects. A similar study by Rentorff has supported this range of frequency as normal (4). However, many patients consider themselves to be constipated even when they have more than three bowel movements per week. Some even perceive themselves to be "constipated" while having a stool every day. Therefore, factors other than frequency alone should be considered as attributes of constipation. In addition to frequency, patients may also complain of excessively hard or small stools as manifestations of their constipation. There are some data on normal stool weight. In the study by Rentorff on normal people, the average weight of 8,267 stools was 123 g (4). In our own study of normal volunteers, we found the average individual stool weight to be 112±15 g (5). In contrast, constipated subjects in our studies have a lower *mean* daily fecal weight, but the weight of their *individual* stools is not significantly different from that of a normal population. This suggests that total weight of the stool produced may need to approach a certain critical weight, i.e., approximately 100 g, before a bowel movement will be passed. The decrease in fecal frequency in constipated individuals may thus be a reflection of a decrease in average of daily production of colonic excrement.

If frequency is normal and individual stool weight does not accurately differentiate between patients, what other factors may be perceived by patients as constipation? Perhaps constipation may also be a manifestation of the character of the stool. In our recent study we found that constipated subjects did indeed rate their stools to be firmer than normal subjects, but the differences were not striking. No formal, objective measurements of stool firmness have been made to allow a more definitive evaluation of stool character, and therefore, this parameter is difficult to apply to studies of constipation. In previous studies we have seen that the percent moisture of stools of constipated volunteers is less than 70% and significantly less than those of normal volunteers (6, 7). Therefore, while stool firmness would be a difficult parameter to measure and quantify, stool moisture may be a reflection of this and a much easier parameter to assess.

Lastly, the actual passage of the bowel movement, even if it is regularly timed or of normal consistency, may be difficult and interpreted by the patient as constipation. Recent studies have indicated that a certain group of chronically constipated young women have a problem evacuating their rectums (8). This has been attributed to a lack of perineal descent causing a so-called "outlet obstruction." These subjects had difficulty evacuating balloons of increasing size from their rectums. In these subjects this type of anomaly may be important when considering an ineffective response to bulk laxatives in that a stool of larger size theoretically may not be as easy to pass as a smaller stool. No laxative drug would be expected to correct this functional defect.

In summary, when discussing the laxative effect of any agent, it is important to be aware of these varied considerations in individual patients' perceptions of constipation. It may be that a patient with excessively firm daily bowel movements may respond differently to a particular laxative than a patient complaining of infrequent but otherwise normal bowel movements. In practice, frequency, stool weight and water content are reasonable objective measurements for investigational purposes, but these three parameters may not be altered measurably by laxatives in all real or perceived conditions of constipation.

MECHANISMS OF ACTION OF LACTULOSE

Before discussing the results of lactulose for constipation, an understanding of possible mechanisms of action would be helpful. A single primary mechanism for laxation for lactulose cannot be determined because of multiple possible effects. Conn has also speculated on a similar multifactorial action for the effects of lactulose in hepatic encephalopathy (9). The multiple effects of lactulose include metabolism by the colonic bacteria to yield short-chain fatty acids (SCFA), reduction of colonic pH, and production of gases (hydrogen and carbon dioxide). Additionally, there can be an increased intraluminal osmolarity from either lactulose or the products of its metabolism by bacteria, and finally, a shortened transit time may occur in both the small intestine and colon. It is well documented that lactulose is not enzymatically metabolized in nor absorbed from the small intestine. As a result, at best it may exert only a mild osmotic effect in the small intestine as it moves toward the colon. Thus, its primary site of laxation is the colon. In this organ, the drug is rapidly broken down by bacteria to its component short-chain fatty acids. The speed with which this metabolism occurs supports the idea that the laxative activity of lactulose is most likely due to the resultant short-chain fatty acids and/or intestinal acidification which alters normal colonic function.

Bacterial Degradation. a) Gas production: Carbohydrates entering the lower small bowel and colon undergo anaerobic metabolism by the colonic bacteria. These carbohydrates range from the disaccharides, e.g., lactose, to the complex polysaccharides, e.g., bran and psyllium. Lactulose, a disaccharide that is not metabolized by human small intestinal mucosal enzymes, is readily broken down by the colonic bacteria. The ability of colonic bacteria to metabolize lactulose was dramatically demonstrated by Levitt et al. (10). In an *in vitro* experiment, they mixed various carbohydrate products with human fecal homogenates. Lactulose was equivalent to starch and glucose in its ability to be broken down to yield hydrogen gas (Figure 1). Levitt has used the lack of small intestinal absorption of lactulose and subsequent production of hydrogen gas by colonic bacteria as a marker of oral to ileal transit times (10). Intestinal gas travels quickly through various portions of the gastrointestinal tract (11). Gas production by bacteria may contribute to defecation by causing colonic distention (12). Presently, it is not possible to quantify the relationship between gas production, colon distention, and the urge to defecate.

b) Short-chain fatty acid production: The laxative action of lactulose could also be explained by fermentation that yields a mixture of SCFAs, i.e., acetate, propionate, lactate, and butyrate. Hoppert and Clark and, subsequently, Stephens and Cummings have presented evidence that certain types of indigestible matter that reach the colon foster the growth of bacteria (12, 13). As postulated by Stephens and Cummings, the SCFAs (as produced from lactulose) become substrate for the resident bacteria. This availability of enriched substrate stimulates a logarithmic

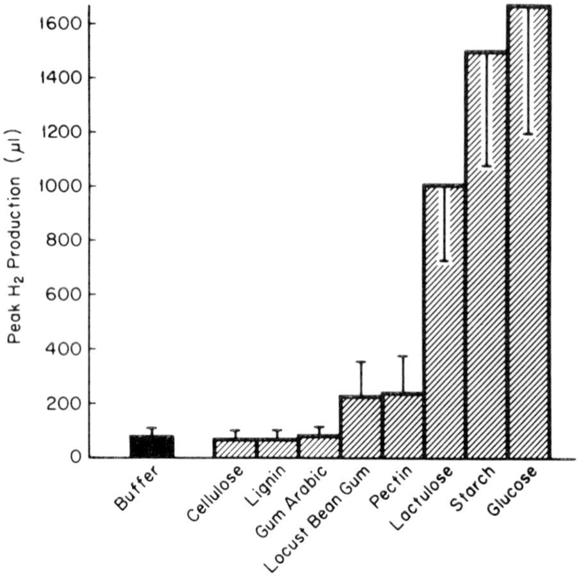

FIGURE 1. *In vitro* hydrogen gas accumulation over a 4-hour period of fermentation of various carbohydrates, fibers or control (buffer). Note that lactulose is readily metabolized by stool (1 g per ml of stool homogenate).

rate of growth of the colonic bacteria. Since stool composition is more than 50% bacteria, the increase in the bacterial population is reflected in an increase in stool bulk.

Luminal osmolality. It is well established in perfusion studies that the human colon readily absorbs SCFAs (14, 15). However, the simultaneous presence of several different SCFAs in the colon may require a more complex interaction that is not present in perfusion studies with single fatty acids. Neither the rates of production nor the ratios of the respective SCFAs have been documented for the fermentation of lactulose. It is quite possible that the presence of the fatty acid mixture may inhibit the selective absorption of different individual fatty acids. Thus, as shown by Ruppin, et al., while single fatty acids may readily cross the colonic membrane, "mixtures" may not (14). Experimentally, acetates are effective in inhibiting propionates from the absorption of perfused rat jejunum (16). If SCFAs accumulate in the colon the luminal osmolarity would increase. This would cause an early laxation effect, i.e., within 8 hours, while the bacterial proliferation effects may occur later, i.e., 48-hour laxation.

Colonic acidification. The SCFAs produced by bacterial fermentation of the lactulose may lower the pH of the colonic contents. As indicated above, SCFA perfusion studies tend to decrease luminal pH; however, objective evidence that lactulose can lower colonic pH has been presented by Bown et al. (17). Using a pH-sensitive radio telemetering device, they showed that 30 to 40 grams of lactulose daily decreases the pH of the right colon from control levels of 6.0 to 4.9. In animal studies, Bennett and Eley have shown that lowering luminal pH can drastically shorten colonic transit time (18). A highly significant relationship between acidorrhea and fecal matter volume has been documented (19). Thus, a decrease in colonic pH produced by acidic by-products of lactulose metabolism may be a causative factor in inducing defecation and diarrhea. Additionally, the low colonic pH may decrease fermentation leading to accumulation of undigested sugars or complex carbohydrates which also may obligate water retention and enhance defecation. Although the pH in the distal colon eventually increases even with lactulose to 6.5 or greater, the pH effects of lactulose could still contribute to laxation by the above mechanisms in the proximal colon.

Thus, the presence of SCFAs from bacterial degradation of lactulose in the colon may play a pivotal role in inducing laxation. They may: a) cause gas production; b) increase bacterial growth; c) increase intraluminal osmolarity; and/or d) decrease stool pH.

Decreased Transit Time. Transit times for the entire GI tract are shortened by the ingestion of dietary fiber (2). Lactulose has been used for measuring oral-cecal transit time. However, does it, itself, possess sufficient gastrointestinal activity to alter stomach emptying and small intestinal transit? This has not been evaluated. Clearly, it alters colonic function, but the effects on actual transit time in the colon have not been documented.

In summary, there are a number of potential mechanisms by which lactulose could exert its effect of laxation. It is difficult to separate these varied effects to know which is the most important.

CLINICAL TRIALS

There are a number of studies that have shown the efficacy of lactulose for constipation. However, most of the studies are neither blinded nor controlled.

In an early double-blind comparison trial by Wesselius-De Casparis, 103 elderly patients were entered into a comparison of lactulose vs. glucose (20). An initial dose of 15 ml (10 g) of lactulose was used. Using subjective criteria of "truly constipated patients," successful therapy was defined by the patient not requiring other laxatives. By this criterion, lactulose was found to be effective in 80% whereas glucose was effective in only 33% of the subjects.

In another double-blind, placebo-controlled trial of lactulose 30 ml (20 g) vs. glucose, Sanders evaluated 47 elderly (mean age greater than 80) constipated patients in a nursing home (21). Lactulose restored fecal frequency into the normal range of more than three bowel movements per week in 53% vs only 17% in the glucose control group. There was also a striking decrease in the number of fecal impactions with only 6 occurring in the lactulose group and 66 in the glucose control group during a 12-week period of observation.

In a subsequent comparison of lactulose 15 ml (10 g) twice a day to a laxative which the individual patients had previously used (usually senna, or other anthraquinones, or bisacodyl) (22), lactulose led to the passage of a "normal" stool in 58% of patients as compared to 42% of patients on their previous laxative.

Lactulose 20 ml (10 g) has been compared to anthraquinones in 37 patients in a nursing home (23). The laxative appeared to be equally effective and better tolerated than placebo. This study compared the 80% transit time of small radiopaque markers. This was defined as the time in days that it took 80% of the markers to disappear on x-ray examination of the abdomen. In most patients, 80% transit time remained longer than six days, but a few patients treated with the laxatives were improved. In another small trial, lactulose was effective in doses of 20 ml (10 g) three times a day in a group of patients with constipation induced by vincristine (24).

In the above studies no systematic evaluations of fecal weight or consistency were performed. In the only study that has been published with full evaluation of fecal parameters, Bass and Dennis compared the effects of lactulose syrup to 5% sucrose syrup in a group of normal subjects and also in a group of chronically constipated, young volunteers (7). In this study of 42 healthy, normal volunteers (22 men and 20 women aged 18 to 54 years), doses of 30 and 60 ml (20 and 40 g, respectively) of lactulose were compared. Both doses of lactulose led to increased fecal weight, fecal volume, fecal frequency and a decreased consistency score (Table 1). They also reported a separate study of constipated subjects which included 24 subjects (2 male and 22 female) who met the criteria of three or fewer bowel movements per week (7). As occurs in double-blind studies, there was a significant placebo response. However, the lactulose in a dose of 60 ml (40 g) per day led to an even greater fecal frequency (4.5 vs 2.8 bowel movements per week). There was also a significant increase in fecal weight, percent moisture and consistency (Table 2). There were only very minor changes in output of fecal

TABLE 1. Mean Responses to Treatment in Normal Subjects. Bass et al. (7).

Stool response	15g Dose (n=22) Treatment			30g Dose (n=20) Treatment		
	Lactulose	Placebo	p-Value[b]	Lactulose	Placebo	p-Value[b]
Frequency (per day)	1.0	0.8	<0.03	1.2	0.8	<0.01
Volume (ml/day)	79.0	50.5	<0.02	109.0	63.0	<0.01
Wet weight (g/day)	92.5	62.1	<0.02	124.5	78.0	<0.02
Consistency score	3.2	4.0	<0.01	2.2	3.8	<0.01

Lactulose-placebo difference from crossover analysis.
Stool consistency score: 1 - liquid . . . . 7 - very hard.

TABLE 2. Mean Responses to Treatment in Constipated Subjects (Bass et al. [7])

	Treatment group (30 g medication)				
	Lactulose (n=10)		Placebo (n=14)		
	Pretreatment	Treatment	Pretreatment	Treatment	p-Value[a]
Frequency (per week)	1.6	4.5*	1.4	2.8*	<0.05
Volume (ml/day)	13.8	54.4*	15.8	39.6*	<0.06
Wet weight (g/day)	17.7	65.7*	20.5	46.9*	<0.05
Dry weight (g/day)	5.3	15.0*	6.6	13.3*	>0.10
Percent moisture	64.2	73.2*	67.6	69.8*	<0.02
Consistency score[b]	4.9	3.8*	4.7	4.3	<0.01

* Significantly different from respective pretreatment value ($p<0.05$).

[a] p-Value for the differences of the lactulose treatment period vs placebo treatment period.

[b] Stool consistency score: 1 - liquid . . . 7 - very hard.

sodium, potassium and chloride. This study clearly shows that lactulose produces significant laxation.

In children, two studies have shown lactulose to be effective and well tolerated (25, 26). Nine of eleven patients in the report by Bush found the laxative to be palatable. The two other patients were felt to have problems interacting with their parents which probably played a role in their disfavor of the laxative (25). In a larger study by Perkins, 21 children under 15 years of age were treated in a three-week, cross-over, single-blinded protocol (26). Lactulose was given in a dose of 10 to 15 ml (5 to 7.5 g) per day, while senna syrup was given in a dose of 10 to 20 ml per day. There were no differences in the number of stools passed on either medication, but there was a striking difference in side effects. During one week of observation on no medication, 4 of 21 patients reported colic or distention. On lactulose, only one patient complained of colic. In the senna group, 11 of 21 complained of colic, 3 had diarrhea, and 1 distention. These differences are highly significant.

These studies indicate that lactulose is an effective agent in increasing stool frequency, volume and water content. Low values for these are important criteria of constipation. Lactulose is also effective in decreasing patient complaints and complications of constipation. It should be pointed out that there are portions of the population that do not seem to have bacteria in their colon that will metabolize lactulose (27). The effect of this deficiency on the laxation properties of lactulose is not known, but, presumably, lactulose would be less effective or ineffective under such circumstances.

SIDE EFFECTS

Because lactulose is a non-absorbed disaccharide that is metabolized in the colon by intestinal bacteria, the most common side effects of lactulose may be considered to be excessive efficacy, i.e., diarrhea and gas production with colic. In several of the above studies, colic was usually more common in the placebo or active controls than it was with lactulose treatment. Lactulose-induced diarrhea is controllable by reducing the amount of drug. Some patients find lactulose syrup to be unpalatably sweet.

OTHER DISACCHARIDES

It should be kept in mind that many poorly absorbed sugars such as mannitol and sorbitol are also transported to the colon intact and produce effects similar to those of lactulose. However, detailed clinical studies have not been conducted on mannitol or sorbitol. Lactitol is a newly available disaccharide with a ß-galactosido-sorbitol structure that, like lactulose, is neither absorbed nor cleaved in the upper intestinal tract. Lactitol may be administered as a tablet and may be better tolerated by some individuals who do not like the sweetness of lactulose syrup. Lactulose is sweeter than sucrose while lactitol is only 35% as sweet as sucrose. Its mechanism of action appears to be similar to lactulose (29). In a preliminary study on 21 healthy volunteers, lactitol caused laxation at a dose of 40 g per day (30). Five patients with encephalopathy conveniently titrated themselves daily with 48 to 84 g of lactitol to achieve two semi-soft stools per day (31). An extension of that study showed that lactitol and lactulose both induced catharsis, but lactulose was more potent on a per gram basis (32). Lactitol is not yet approved in the United States as a laxative nor as treatment for portal-systemic encephalopathy.

Finally, in lactase-deficient individuals lactose induces pathophysiologic effects similar to lactulose. Lactose has been shown to release hydrogen in expired air and to lower stool pH (33, 34). Since patients with lactase deficiency may not have a total deficiency of lactase, it may take more lactose on a weight or molar basis to produce an effect similar to lactulose. Kolars et al. have shown the breath hydrogen effect of 20 g of lactose or one glass of milk (18 g lactose) to be similar to the effect of 10 g of lactulose (35). Lactose has been shown to induce laxation in lactase-deficient individuals with a mean effective dose of approximately 15 to 20 g (36). It should be kept in mind that lactose is a much less expensive laxative agent in lactase-deficient patients than is lactulose. Indeed, in Mexico where lactase deficiency is the rule and lactulose is not available commercially, lactose has been shown to be at least as effective as lactulose in PSE when administered orally (37) or by enema (38).

CONCLUSION

Constipation is at least perceived to be a major problem by millions of Americans as is shown by the large number of proprietary formulations on the market and an estimated annual expenditure for laxatives of over $400 million. Patients must be carefully counselled that a goal of routine frequency (the American Dream of a bowel movement per day after breakfast) is not required and that "normality" can be as few as three bowel movements per week. Accepting this definition, a large number of patients still complain about "constipation." The initial approach to such patients should be to increase dietary fiber. One hopes that fiber can be tolerated with minimal side effects and can be recommended as a lifelong therapy. No laxative has been scrutinized for long periods of time, which is a pertinent shortcoming since constipation is usually a chronic problem. Theoretically, in a chronic treatment program lactulose may increase the bacterial mass in stool as do diets containing digestible fiber. The short-chain fatty acids produced from lactulose should be absorbed; no knowledge of long-term adverse effects of lactulose metabolism is known. Other nonabsorbed disaccharides may act similarly, but only preliminary studies have yet been performed. They show that other such disaccharides do have therapeutic potential.

REFERENCES

1. Burkitt DP, Trowell HC. Refined carbohydrate foods and disease: some implications of dietary fiber. London: Academic Press, 1975: 356-360.

2. Gullikson GW, Bass P. Mechanisms of action of laxative drugs. In: Csaky TZ, ed. Handbook of experimental pharmacology, Vol 70/II. Berlin Heidelberg: Springer-Verlag, 1984: 419-459.

3. Connel AM, Hilton C, Irvine G, et al. Variation in bowel habit in two population samples. Br Med J 1965; 2:1095-1099.

4. Rentorff RC, Kashgarian M. Stool patterns of healthy adult males. Dis Colon Rectum 1967; 10:222-228.

5. Hamilton JW, Wagner J, Burdick BB, et al. A clinical evaluation of methylcellulose as a bulk laxative. Dig Dis Sci, in press.

6. Marlett JA, Li BUK, Patrow CJ, et al. Comparative laxation of psyllium with and without senna in an ambulatory constipated population. Am J Gastroenterol 1987; 82:333-337.

7. Bass P, Dennis S. Laxative effects of lactulose in normal and constipated subjects. J Clin Gastroenterol 1981; 3(Suppl 1):23-28.

8. Schouler P, Keighley MRB. Changes in colorectal function in severe

idiopathic chronic constipation. Gastroenterology 1986; 90:414-420.

9. Conn HO. Lactulose: a drug in search of a modus operandi. Gastroenterology 1978; 74:624-626.

10. Levitt MD, Hirsh P, Fetzer CA, et al. H_2 excretion after ingestion of complex carbohydrates. Gastroenterology 1987; 92:383-389.

11. Bennett DR, Bass P. The action of inhalation anesthetics on the gastrointestinal tract. In: Chenoweth MB, ed. Modern inhalation anesthetics. New York: Springer, Berlin, Heidelberg, 1972: 318.

12. Hoppert CA, Clark AJ. Digestibility and effect on laxation of crude fiber and cellulose in certain common foods. J Am Diet Assoc 1945; 21:157-160.

13. Stephen AM, Cummings JH. Mechanisms of action of dietary fibre in the human colon. Nature 1980; 284:283-284.

14. Ruppin H, Bar Meir S, Soergel KH, et al. Absorption of short-chain fatty acids by the colon. Gastroenterology 1980; 78:1500-1507.

15. Wrong OM, Edmonds CJ, Chadwick VS. Short-chain organic acids. In: The Large Intestine: Its Role in Mammalian Nutrition and Homeostasis. New York: Halsted Press, John Wiley & Sons, 1981: 113-121.

16. Watson AJM, Kelly MJ, Wilks M. Mechanism of acetate absorption in normal rat jejunum (Abstract). Gut 1985; 26:A1109.

17. Bown RL, Gibson JA, Sladen GE, et al. Effects of lactulose and other laxatives on ileal and colonic pH as measured by a radiotelemetry device. Gut 1974; 15:999-1004.

18. Bennett DR, Eley KG. Intestinal pH and propulsion: an explanation of diarrhoea in lactase deficiency and laxation by lactulose. J Pharm Pharmacol 1976; 28:192-195.

19. Fernandez LB, Gonzalez E, Marzi A, et al. Fecal acidorrhea. N Engl J Med 1971; 284:295-298.

20. Wesselius-De Casparis A, Braadbaart S, Bergh-Bohlken GE, et al. Treatment of chronic constipation with lactulose syrup: results of a double-blind study. Gut 1968; 9:84-86.

21. Sanders JF. Lactulose syrup assessed in a double-blind study of elderly constipated patients. J Am Geriatr Soc 1978; 26:236-239.

22. Connolly P, Hughes IW, Ryan G. Comparison of 'Duphalac' and 'Irritant' laxatives during and after treatment of chronic constipation: a preliminary study. Curr Med Res Opin 1975; 2:620-625.

23. Bocklehurst JC, Kirckland JL, Martin J, et al. Constipation in long-stay elderly patients: its treatment and prevention by lactulose, poloxalkol-dihydroxyanthroquinolone and phosphate enemas. Gerontology 1983; 29:181-184.

24. Harris AC, Jackson SM. Lactulose in vincristine-induced constipation. Med J Aust 1977; 22:573-574.

25. Bush RT. Lactulose: an ideal laxative for children. NZ Med J 1970; 71:364-365.

26. Perkin JM. Constipation in childhood: a controlled comparison between

lactulose and standardized senna. Curr Med Res Opin 1977; 4:540-543.

27. Bond JH, Levitt MD. Investigation of small bowel transit time in man utilizing pulmonary hydrogen (H_2) measurements. J Lab Clin Med 1975; 85:546-555.

28. van Velthuijsen JA. Food additives derived from lactose: lactitol and lactitol palmitate. J Agric Food Chem 1979; 27:680-686.

29. Patil DH, Westaby D, Mahida YR, et al. Comparative modes of action of lactitol and lactulose in the treatment of hepatic encephalopathy. Gut 1987; 28:255-259.

30. Patil DH, Grimble GK, Silk DBA. Intestinal absorption and laxative threshold of lactitol - a new hydrogenated derivative of lactose (Abstract). Gut 1985; 26:A1114.

31. Lanthier PL, Morgan MY. Lactitol in the treatment of chronic hepatic encephalopathy: An open comparison with lactulose. Gut 1985; 26:415-420.

32. Morgan MY, Hawley KE, Stambuk D. Lactitol versus lactulose in the treatment of chronic hepatic encephalopathy. J Hepatol 1987; 4:236-244.

33. Christopher NL, Bayless TM. Role of the small bowel and colon in lactose-induced diarrhea. Gastroenterology 1971; 60:845-852.

34. Bond JH, Levitt MD, Use of pulmonary hydrogen (H_2) measurements to quantitate carbohydrate absorption. J Clin Invest 1972; 51:1219-1225.

35. Kolars JC, Levitt MD, Aouji M, et al. Yogurt—an autodigesting source of lactose. N Engl J Med 1984; 310:1-3.

36. Gudmand-Høyer, Simony K. Individual sensitivity to lactose in lactose malabsorption. Dig Dis Sci 1977; 22:177-181.

37. Uribe M, Masquez MA, Garcia-Ramos G, et al. Treatment of chronic portal systemic encephalopathy with lactose in lactase deficient patients. Dig Dis Sci 1980; 25:924-928.

38. Uribe M, Campollo O, Vargas F, et al. Acidifying enemas (lactitol and lactose) vs. nonacidifying enemas (tap water) to treat acute portal-systemic encephalopathy: a double-blind, randomized clinical trial. Hepatology 1987; 7:639-643.

22

LACTULOSE IN PEDIATRICS

Dieter Ullrich, M.D., and Johannes Bircher, M.D.

The synthetic disaccharide lactulose (ß-galactosido-fructose) is produced from lactose during the processing and heating of milk. Therefore, lactulose is a component of commercial infant milk feedings (up to 6% of total disaccharides) (1-3). As described first by Petuely in infants, the ingestion of lactulose stimulates preferential colonization of the intestine with *Lactobacillus bifidus*. Hence, lactulose and human breast milk are considered to be potent bifidus-factors (4-7).

The human organism is unable to absorb lactulose from the upper intestinal tract or to metabolize it. Thus, in the colon it is utilized by bacteria with the following consequences: a) acidification of the colonic contents; b) production of short-chain fatty acids; c) preferential colonization by *Lactobacillus bifidus*; and d) osmotic diarrhea. Based on these properties, lactulose may be used in pediatrics for diagnostic purposes in gastrointestinal diseases, and for the treatment of constipation and of hyperammonemia (5-14).

LACTULOSE IN THE INVESTIGATION OF INTESTINAL ABSORPTION

Since lactulose is not hydrolyzed by intestinal disaccharidases (15, 16) and since there is no transport system for disaccharides, oral doses pass through the small bowel largely unabsorbed and have ample opportunity to move across the mucosal barrier wherever permeability of the intestinal wall is increased. It is generally accepted that permeability of the human intestine decreases progressively from the duodenum to the colon. Studies of intestinal permeability in normal adults have revealed that passive transport of neutral hydrophilic compounds is inversely related to their molecular weight. Due to its molecular weight of 342 and its radius of 0.52 nm, only minute amounts of lactulose pass across the mucosa, presumably either via tight junctions or via gaps left by extruded cells (17-24). Once in the blood, lactulose is not metabolized, but is excreted unchanged in the urine. On the basis of these qualities, lactulose has been proposed as a marker for the assessment of small bowel permeability associated with immaturity or disease.

The smaller molecule mannitol (molecular weight: 164; radius: 0.4 nm) has been chosen as a reference compound, because a small amount is thought to pass freely across the mucosa via aqueous pores (radius: 0.4 nm). Therefore, mannitol is regarded as an absorption index of the intestinal surface area in different conditions. Like lactulose, mannitol is excreted in urine intact (16, 24, 25).

As expected, intestinal permeability, as expressed by the urinary lactulose/mannitol ratio, was found to be increased in some preterm newborns (less than 37 weeks gestation) presumably due to immaturity of the intestine. However, the normalization of mucosal permeability within four days after the onset of oral feeding indicates rapid maturation of the digestive tract. In contrast, normal permeability was observed in full-term newborns (26-28) (Table 1).

In disorders of the gastrointestinal tract such as tropical sprue, Crohn's disease, celiac disease and toxic damage of the small bowel mucosa due to drugs (e.g., methotrexate) lactulose/mannitol ratios reveal enhanced permeability. The various studies indicate that these test procedures are highly sensitive although nonspecific. Due to overlapping ranges of test results, tests of absorption are not able to discriminate reliably between normal and pathologic conditions. They are, however, valuable tools for noninvasive, serial follow-up examinations of intestinal diseases, e.g., for the evaluation of the results of various treatments (Table 2) (29-37).

TABLE 1. Lactulose/Mannitol Ratios based on Urinary Spot Samples during Steady State Conditions in Newborns (28) Expressed as Median (Range)

Gestational age (weeks)	No.	Days after starting oral feeding	Ratio Lactulose/mannitol
27 - 33	13	1	2.10 (0.75 - 5.10)
		4	0.80 (0.50 - 1.60)
		7	0.80 (0.15 - 1.60)
34-37	13	1	0.80 (0.40 - 3.30)
		4	0.50 (0.40 - 1.20)
		7	0.55 (0.30 - 1.20)
>37	7	1	0.56 (0.28 - 0.94)
		4	0.59 (0.28 - 1.59)

TABLE 2. Mean Percentage Lactulose Output in 5-hour Urine Samples and Corresponding Lactulose/Mannitol Ratios in Different Gastrointestinal Diseases

Disease	No.	Age (years)	Renal output of lactulose (%/5h)	Lac/Man[1] ratio	Reference
Controls	16	17-52	0.30	0.026[2]	29
Controls	16	20-65	0.11	0.009	32
Controls	25	19-65	0.13	0.010	30
Controls	31	2-13	0.25	0.018	31, 33
Controls				0.070	34
Controls	10	2-9		0.050[2]	35
Tropical Sprue	5	19-44	0.52	0.200[2]	29
Tropical diarrhea	9	23-77	0.31	0.031[2]	29
Celiac disease	22	22-74	0.92	0.170	30
Celiac disease	5	2-14	0.25	0.100	31
Colonic Crohn's disease	7	17-75	0.29	0.033	32
Ileal Crohn's disease	13	17-75	0.43	0.045	32
Crohn's disease	8	9-16	1.10	0.100	31
Chronic ulcerative colitis	6	24-65	0.13	0.009	32
Acute lymphoblastic leukemia before treat-	16	2-13	0.25	0.018	33
ment induct. period[3]			0.35	0.065	33
Acute gastroenteritis	14	2-15[4]		0.430[2]	34
Chronic diarrhea	14	4-19[4]		0.120[2]	34
Food allergy	10	2-9		0.056[3]	35

[1] Lactulose/mannitol (mean values)

[2] Ratios were calculated with rhamnose instead of mannitol. The results are presumably the same.

[3] Cytostatic therapy consisted of mercaptopurine, methotrexate, vincristin and prednisone.

[4] Age is given in months.

Another diagnostic use of lactulose is the "lactulose-hydrogen breath test," which is a well-established procedure to investigate either small intestinal transit time or small intestinal bacterial overgrowth in the adult. The method is based on the observation that bacterial metabolism of carbohydrates results in the formation of molecular hydrogen (H_2) which is partially absorbed and eliminated in exhaled air (38-44).

Studies with the lactulose hydrogen breath test have shown that infants have longer transit times (105±14 min, n=12) than adults (80±20 min, n=12) (45). In view of the importance of hydrolysis of lactose by intestinal lactase, prolonged contact of intestinal contents with small bowel mucosa appears physiologically purposeful. Another important observation made with the lactulose hydrogen breath test is that the transit time is prolonged in patients with cystic fibrosis (median: 245 min, range: 160 to 390 min) when compared to age-matched controls (median: 80 min, range: 50 to 150 min) (46). In view of the normal small bowel transit time in adults with pancreatic insufficiency, it is unlikely that the slow transit in patients with cystic fibrosis is a consequence of the lack of pancreatic enzymes. Rather, it may reflect increased viscosity of the small bowel contents due to excessive secretion of highly viscous mucus (47). Postnatal episodes of obstructive ileus, so-called meconium ileus equivalents, are well described in the pediatric literature and represent a major complication of cystic fibrosis (48-50).

LACTULOSE IN THE TREATMENT OF PEDIATRIC CONSTIPATION

Although not universally agreed upon in the pediatric literature, constipation is generally diagnosed when less than one bowel movement occurs every three days and when moderate to large amounts of solid feces are palpable upon rectal examination. The list of possible explanations is long, yet the most frequent causes are anal achalasia (about 75%) and Hirschsprung's disease (about 15%) (50, 51-56). Since the pathogenesis of anal achalasia is as yet ill-defined, treatment usually is symptomatic, including psychologic counselling, high residue diet, increased fluid intake, enemas and anal dilatations (57-59).

When responses to such therapy are inadequate, many pediatricians empirically try lactulose. Doses are usually titrated according to individual needs and vary between 0.5 and 1.5 ml per kg per day of the 60% w/v commercial lactulose preparations corresponding to about 0.3 to 1.0 g per kg per day of lactulose. This treatment has been widely used and appears to be well accepted by patients and physicians. Inadequate dose titrations and noncompliance seem to be the most important causes for failure (16, 60-62).

Perkin studied the laxative effects of lactulose in chronically constipated children younger than 15 years (63). The patients were randomized and treated either with lactulose or with senna alkaloids in a crossover trial for one week each.

In regard to both its cathartic actions as well as to its lower frequency of side effects, lactulose was found to be superior to the senna preparation.

Unfortunately, no further controlled trials have been performed. Consequently, even for indications such as constipation the need for controlled studies is apparent (64, 65). Nevertheless, compared to the generally recommended alternatives such as repeated enemas, which may be physiologically and psychologically inappropriate, and mineral oil, which may deplete fat-soluble vitamins, chronic treatment with lactulose appears to have the most favorable benefit/risk ratio (16).

Pediatricians have also used lactulose largely in an uncontrolled manner for the symptomatic treatment of conditions other than anal achalasia, such as postoperative Hirschsprung's disease and constipation due to neurological disorders.

TREATMENT OF HYPERAMMONEMIC SYNDROMES IN PEDIATRICS

The most important sources of ammonia are protein catabolism (1 g protein is equivalent to 0.15 to 0.2 g ammonia), renal deamination of glutamine and intestinal bacterial and nonbacterial degradation of urea and amino acids. Most of the ammonia is cleared by the liver with a high extraction ratio and is utilized mainly for the synthesis of urea. Hyperammonemia is thought to contribute to hepatic encephalopathy and occurs whenever hepatic elimination of ammonia is decreased, and particularly when its formation is increased simultaneously. Clinical observations and histomorphological findings indicate that the immature, infantile brain seems to be highly susceptible to ammonia toxicity. However, due to its great capacity for regeneration it tends to recover once hyperammonemia is corrected. Nevertheless, mental defects have occurred and were thought to be related to severity and duration of hyperammonemia (9, 66-79).

Causes for hyperammonemia in pediatrics (Table 3) include not only diseases which are known to be associated with elevated blood ammonia levels in adults, but also a large number of conditions which are specific for infancy and childhood (9, 71-74, 80, 81). The following points require emphasis:

1. Portal-systemic encephalopathy (PSE) due to portal hypertension and liver failure is a rare event in childhood (82-86). In more than 80% of all cases with infantile PSE, the underlying disease was either biliary atresia (about 32%), idiopathic cirrhosis (about 32% or alpha-1-antitrypsin deficiency (17%) (86).

2. Inherited disorders of urea-cycle enzymes generally manifest themselves in the newborn period or infancy. Hyperammonemia and associated clinical symptoms develop during episodes of increased protein ingestion or catabolism. Symptoms are nonspecific and include vomiting, respiratory distress, hyperventilation, hyperexcitability, seizures, somnolence and coma. Prognosis is guarded, because severe hyperammonemia may lead to mental retardation or death (9, 50, 71,

78, 80, 81, 87-94).

3. Hyperammonemia is also observed in patients with inborn errors of amino acid or lipid metabolism. The basic biochemical defects often are unknown. Clinical signs, complications and prognosis resemble those of urea-cycle enzyme defects (9, 50, 72-74, 80, 81, 88, 89, 95-97).

4. Hyperammonemia due to Reye's syndrome is thought to represent an acquired, transient defect of urea-cycle enzymes (i.e., ornithine transcarbamylase and/or carbamylphosphate synthetase). The course and prognosis of Reye's syndrome is closely correlated with the degree of hyperammonemia noted soon after the onset of encephalopathy (9, 98-105).

5. The biochemical basis of "transient hyperammonemia of the newborn" is unknown. In the acute stage it has to be differentiated from the inherited hyperammonemic syndromes. After recovery from hyperammonemic coma, the children appear to be healthy except for possible cerebral residuals (88, 95, 97, 106-108).

The aims of symptomatic treatments of hyperammonemia in children are the same as those in adults, and consist of efforts to reduce ammonia formation and to increase ammonia elimination. Conventional measures in hyperammonemic syndromes include (71-74, 88, 93, 95-97, 109, 110): a) infusion of glucose to normalize protein catabolism (up to 30 g glucose per kg body weight per day as hypertonic solutions; this amount is equivalent to 120 kcal per kg body weight per day); b) reduction of dietary protein intake sometimes to as low as zero; c) neomycin by mouth 100 mg per kg body weight per day in six doses (to reduce bacterial ammonia production).

In children with inborn errors of urea synthesis the additional application of the following substances as priming infusions has been recommended to facilitate alternative routes of nitrogen metabolism: a) sodium benzoate (0.25 g per kg body weight); b) sodium phenylacetate (0.25 g per kg body weight) (both substrates should be administered in argininosuccinase deficiency); c) arginine hydrochloride (0.21 g per kg body weight), (0.84 g per kg body weight is recommended in patients with argininosuccinic acid synthetase and argininosuccinase deficiencies).

The above infusions are given as shown in Table 4. In cases in which these therapeutic efforts do not lower plasma ammonia levels sufficiently, peritoneal dialysis or hemodialysis is advisable. These last-mentioned measures may transiently lower plasma ammonia levels as summarized in Table 5 (88, 89, 93, 95-97, 111, 112).

Long-term treatment of moderate hyperammonemia is based primarily on the reduction of dietary proteins (in infants 1.5 g per kg body weight per day and less). Additional measures include oral doses of neomycin and the treatments summarized in Tables 4 and 5. In organic acidemias the dietary regimen has to be tailored in each individual according to his specific biochemical defect. In some conditions (i.e., propionic acidemia, multiple carboxylase deficiencies, meth-

TABLE 3. Hyperammonemic Syndromes in Newborns and Infants

I Acquired hyperammonemias
- A. Acute hepatic failure
- B. Portal hypertension with chronic liver failure
- C. Reye's syndrome
- D. Transient hyperammonemia of the newborn

II Hereditary hyperammonemias
- A. Inherited urea-cycle enzyme deficiencies
  - 1) Ornithine transcarbamylase deficiency
  - 2) Argininosuccinase deficiency
  - 3) Argininosuccinate synthetase deficiency
  - 4) Carbamylphosphate synthetase deficiency
  - 5) Arginase deficiency
  - 6) Citrullinemia
  - 7) N-acetylglutamate synthetase deficiency
- B. Transport defects of urea-cycle metabolites
  - 1) Lysinuric protein intolerance
  - 2) Hyperornithinemia-homocitrullinuria-hyperammonemia syndrome
- C. Inherited hyperammonemic non-urea-cycle enzyme deficiencies
  - 1) Methylmalonic acidemia
  - 2) Hyperlysinemia
  - 3) Ornithinemia
  - 4) Multiple carboxylase deficiency
  - 5) Glutaric acidemias type II
  - 6) ß-ketothiolase deficiency
  - 7) Isovaleric acidemia
  - 8) Defective isoleucin metabolism
  - 9) Methylcrotonglycinuria
  - 10) 3-hydroxy-3-methyl glutaric aciduria

ylmalonic acidemia) megadoses of vitamins are thought to be helpful. All these therapeutic endeavors, however, are associated with important side effects, such as dystrophy and delayed psychomotor development due to protein restriction and oto- and neurotoxicity due to chronic administration of neomycin (9, 16, 50, 82-86, 88-93, 95, 113-115).

In view of the drawbacks of the described conventional therapy, it is difficult to understand why the use of lactulose for the control of hyperammonemia in infancy and childhood is not better documented. In those conditions, only the occasional use of lactulose has been described and only in an uncontrolled manner (87, 92, unpublished observations cited from 80). Chronic application of lactulose

TABLE 4. Conventionally Recommended Long-term Treatments of Hyperammonemia due to Urea-cycle Enzyme Deficiencies (88-93)

Calories	100 - 120 kcal/kg/d
Protein	0.6 - 1.5 g/kg/d
Essential amino acids	0.7 g/kg/d
Folate p.o.	0.1 mg/d
Pyridoxine p.o.	5 mg/d
Sodium benzoate[1] p.o.; i.v.	0.25 - 0.5 g/kg/d
Sodium phenylacetate[1] p.o.; i.v.	0.25 - 0.5 g/kg/d
Arginine[2] p.o.; i.v.	0.21 g/kg/d
Citrulline[3] p.o.	0.18 g/kg/d
Lactulose p.o.	not documented

[1] Omitted in organoacidopathies and argininosuccinase deficiencies

[2] 0.84 g/kg/d in argininosuccinic acid synthetase and argininosuccinase deficiencies.

[3] Should be given instead of arginine in carbamyl phosphate synthetase and ornithine transcarbamylase deficiencies.

may decrease colonic bacterial ammonia production and increase ammonia utilization. In addition, acidification of colonic contents leads to ammonia trapping. These pharmacological properties of lactulose should reduce blood ammonia levels also in the infantile hyperammonemias. According to our limited experience, therapy with lactulose might improve hyperammonemia without requiring protein restriction (Figure 1) (9, 80, 87). Due to the favorable risk/benefit ratio of lactulose, it might represent an important improvement in the treatment of pediatric hyperammonemias. In view of the rarity of these syndromes, a critical evaluation of this hypothesis by classical methods appears difficult. The principles of controlled trials in single patients might therefore be the best method to document unequivocally the risk/benefit ratio of lactulose (117, 118).

SUMMARY

Significant amounts of lactulose (up to 5 g per liter) are included in infant formulas. Biochemical and physiological properties and the excellent risk/benefit ratio render lactulose useful for the following diagnostic and therapeutic purposes in pediatric disorders:

In immaturity of the intestine and in some pathological conditions,

TABLE 5. Effects of Exchange Transfusion, Peritoneal Dialysis, Hemodialysis and Benzoate in the Treatment of Pediatric Hyperammonemic States

Treatment	Age	Initial ammonia values (µmol/L)	% decrease	Reference
Exchange transfusion	Neonates	1068±160	34±21	89
	Neonates	681±115	16±11	89[2]
	Neonate	1830±210	14±7	96
Peritoneal dialysis	Neonates	1068±159	49±9	89[2]
	Neonates	1235±299	85±6	89
	Neonate	735	59	112
	Children	599±123	33±18	89
Hemodialysis	Neonate	1375±35	77±6	111
	Neonate	1434±569	61±21	96
Sodium benzoate	Neonates[1]	700±529	52±21	89
	Children	188±55	52±29	89
Lactulose		not documented		

[1] In 2 neonates, therapy was successful; in 1 neonate, it failed.

[2] Summarized from various reported cases.

mucosal permeability for lactulose may be enhanced. In these cases increased amounts of lactulose excreted in urine may serve as an indicator of this abnormality. Noninvasive lactulose absorption tests may give valuable information about maturity and integrity of the intestinal mucosa, although they are not able to differentiate among various diseases.

Common causes for constipation in pediatrics are anal achalasia and Hirschsprung's disease. Although not based on controlled studies, lactulose has been introduced empirically as medical treatment of constipation irrespective of its pathogenesis. Doses should be titrated individually depending on the desired cathartic effects.

Although the efficacy of lactulose in lowering plasma ammonia levels has been well documented in adults, its use in pediatrics for this purpose is not well established. In infantile hyperammonemic conditions due to liver failure or inherited hyperammonemic syndromes, lactulose may be an important addition to our therapeutic armamentarium. Lactulose may lower plasma ammonia levels without the necessity of severe restriction of dietary protein in children with chronic hepatic disorders.

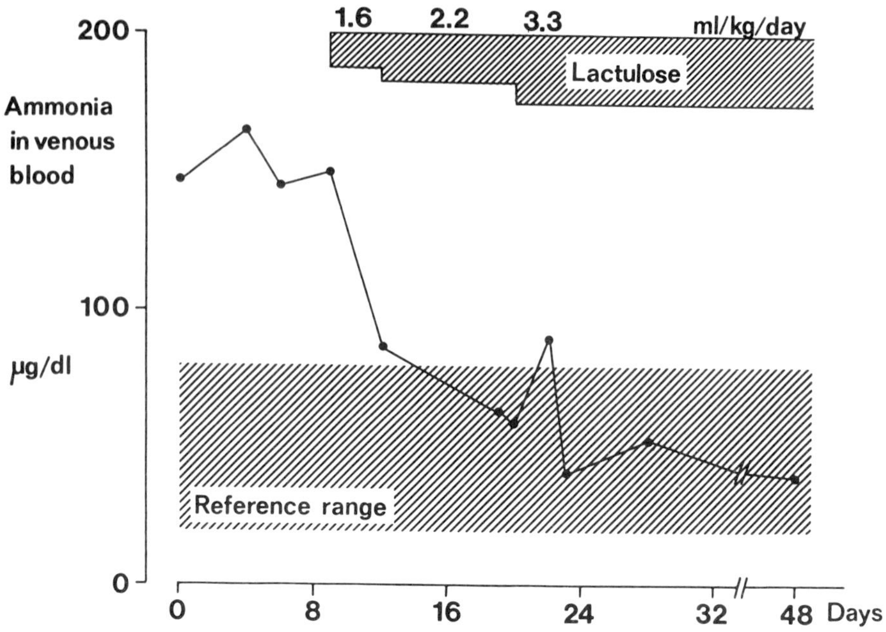

FIGURE 1. Treatment of hyperammonemia with lactulose in a 6-month-old infant with biliary cirrhosis after an unsuccessful operation of a biliary atresia. The shaded area corresponds to the normal range of venous ammonia concentration (determined according to [116]). Nutrition was not changed during treatment with lactulose. The parents noted improvement in vitality. Growth, however, has remained unchanged.

REFERENCES

1. Ersser RS, Mitchell JD. Automated anion-exchange chromatographic method for the quantitation of lactulose in physiological fluids and processed milks. J Chromatogr 1984; 307:393-398.

2. Hendrickse RG, Wooldridge MAW, Russell A. Lactulose in baby milks causing diarrhea simulating lactose intolerance. Br Med J 1977; 7:1194-1195.

3. Beach RC, Menzies IS. Lactulose and other non-absorbable sugars in infant milk feeds (Letter). Lancet 1983; 1:425-426.

4. Braun OH. Effects of consumption of human milk and other formulas on intestinal bacterial flora. In: Lebenthal E, ed. Textbook of Gastroenterology and Nutrition in Infancy, Vol 1. New York: Raven Press, 1981: 247-253.

5. Petuely F. Bifidusflora bei Flaschenkindern durch bifidogene Substanzen

(Bifidusfaktor). Z Kinderheilk 1957; 79:174-179.

6. Petuely F. Der Heutige Stand unseres Wissens über das Bifidusproblem in bakteriologischer, chemischer und klinischer Hinsicht. Arch Kinderheilk 1962; 165:209-218.

7. Petuely F. Der Bifidusfaktor. Dtsch Med Wochenschr 1957; 82:1957-1960.

8. Weber FL. The effect of lactulose on urea metabolism and nitrogen excretion in cirrhotic patients. Gastroenterology 1979; 7:518-523.

9. Conn HO, Lieberthal MM. The Hepatic Coma Syndromes and Lactulose. Baltimore: Williams and Wilkins Company, 1979: 122-168, 306-339.

10. Vince A, Killingley M, Wrong OM. Effect of lactulose on ammonia production in a fecal incubation system. Gastroenterology 1978; 74:544-549.

11. Pomare EW, Branch WJ, Cummings JH. Carbohydrate fermentation in the human colon and its relation to acetate concentrations in venous blood. J Clin Invest 1985; 75:1448-1454.

12. Agostini L, Down PF, Murison J, et al. Faecal ammonia and pH during lactulose administration in man: comparison with other cathartics. Gut 1972; 13:859-866.

13. Castell DO, Moore EW. Ammonia absorption from the human colon. The role of nonionic diffusion. Gastroenterology 1971; 60:33-42.

14. Bircher J, Haemmerli UP, Trabert E, et al. The mechanism of action of lactulose in portal-systemic encephalopathy. Non-ionic diffusion of ammonia in the canine colon. Rev Europ Etudes Clin Biol 1971; 16:352-357.

15. Dahlquist A, Gryboski JD. Inability of the human small intestinal lactase to hydrolyse lactulose. Biochim Biophys Acta 1965; 110:635-636.

16. Reynolds EF, ed. Martindale—The Extra Pharmacopeia, 28th ed. London: The Pharmaceutical Press, 1982: 1365.

17. Loehry CA, Axon ATR, Hilton PH, et al. Permeability of the small intestine to substances of different molecular weight. Gut 1970; 11:466-470.

18. Loehry CA, Kingham J, Baker J. Small intestinal permeability in animals and man. Gut 1973; 14:683-688.

19. Cornell R, Walker WA, Isselbacher KJ. Small intestinal absorption of horseradish peroxidase. Lab Invest 1971; 25:42-48.

20. Fordtran JS, Rector FC, Ewton MF, et al. Permeability characteristics of the human small intestine. J Clin Invest 1965; 44:1935-1944.

21. Chadwick VS, Phillips SF, Hofmann AF. Measurements of intestinal permeability using low molecular weight polyethylene glycols (PEG 400) - Chemical analysis and biological properties of PEG 400. Gastroenterology 1977; 73:241-246.

22. Chadwick VS, Phillips SF, Hofmann AF. Measurements of intestinal permeability using low molecular weight polyethylene glycols (PEG 400) - Chemical analysis and biological properties of PEG 400. Gastroenterology 1977; 73:247-251.

23. Wheeler PG, Menzies IS, Creamer BM. Effect of hyperosmolar stimuli and coeliac disease on the permeability of the human gastrointestinal tract. Clin Sci Mol Med 1978; 54:495-501.

24. Windholz M, ed. The Merck Index, 10th ed. Rahway/USA: Merck and Co Inc, 1983: 770, 818.

25. Nasrallah M, Iber FL. Mannitol absorption and metabolism in man. Am J Med Sci 1969; 258:80-88.

26. Weaver LT, Laker MF, Nelson R. Enhanced intestinal permeability in preterm babies with bloody stools. Arch Dis Child 1984; 59:280-281.

27. Beach RC, Menzies IS, Clayden GS, et al. Gastrointestinal permeability changes in the preterm neonate. Arch Dis Child 1982; 57:141-145.

28. Weaver LT, Laker MF, Nelson R. Intestinal permeability in the newborn. Arch Dis Child 1984; 59:236-241.

29. Cook GC, Menzies IS. Intestinal absorption and unmediated permeation of sugars in post-infective tropical malabsorption (tropical sprue). Digestion 1986; 33:109-116.

30. Ukabam SO, Cooper BT. Small intestinal permeability to mannitol, lactulose, and polyethylene glycol 400 in celiac disease. Dig Dis Sci 1984; 29:809-816.

31. Pearson AD, Eastham EJ, Laker MF, et al. Intestinal permeability in children with Crohn's disease and coeliac disease. Br Med J 1982; 85:20-21.

32. Ukabam SO, Clamp JR, Cooper BT. Abnormal small intestinal permeability to sugars in patients with Crohn's disease of the terminal ileum and colon. Digestion 1983; 27:70-74.

33. Pearson AD, Craft AW, Pledger JV, et al. Small bowel function in acute lymphoblastic leukaemia. Arch Dis Child 1984; 59:460-465.

34. Ford RP, Menzies IS, Phillips AD, et al. Intestinal sugar permeability: relationship to diarrhoeal disease and small bowel morphology. J Pediatr Gastroenterol Nutr 1985; 4:568-574.

35. DuMont GC, Beach RC, Menzies IS. Gastrointestinal permeability in food-allergic eczematous children. Clin Allergy 1984; 14:55-59.

36. Weaver LT, Chapman PD, Madeley CR, et al. Intestinal permeability changes and excretion of micro-organisms in stools of infants with diarrhoea and vomiting. Arch Dis Child 1985; 60:326-332.

37. Ukabam SO, Cooper BT. Small intestinal permeability as an indicator of jejunal mucosal recovery in patients with celiac sprue on a gluten-free diet. J Clin Gastroenterol 1985; 7:232-236.

38. Metz G, Drasar BS, Gassull MA, et al. Breath hydrogen test for small intestinal bacterial colonisation. Lancet, 1976; 1:668-669.

39. Rhodes JM, Middleton P, Jewell DP. The lactulose H_2 breath test as a diagnostic test for small intestinal bacterial overgrowth. Scand J Gastroenterol 1979; 14:333-336.

40. Davidson GP, Robb TA, Kirubakaran CP. Bacterial contamination of the

small intestine as an important cause of chronic diarrhea and abdominal pain: diagnosis by breath hydrogen test. Pediatrics 1984; 74:229-235.

41. Robb TA, Goodwin DA, Davidson GP. Faecal hydrogen production in vitro as an indicator for in vivo hydrogen producing capability in the breath hydrogen test. Acta Paediatr Scand 1985; 74:942-944.

42. Corbert CL, Thomas S, Read NW, et al. Electrochemical detector for breath H_2 determination: measurement of small bowel transit time in normal subjects and patients with the irritable bowel syndrome. Gut 1981; 22:836-840.

43. Caride VJ, Prokop EK, Troncale FJ, et al. Scintigraphic determination of small intestinal transit time: comparison with the hydrogen breath technique. Gastroenterology 1984; 86:714-720.

44. King CE, Toskes PP. Comparison of the 1-gram (^{14}C) xylose, 10-gram lactulose-H_2, and 80-gram glucose-H_2 breath tests in patients with small intestine bacterial overgrowth. Gastroenterology 1986; 91:1447-1451.

45. Breuer N, Ptok A, Götze H, et al. Methodische Aspekte zur Anwendung des Wasserstoff (H_2)-Atemtestes. Z Gastroenterologie 1986; 24:80-84.

46. Bali A, Stableforth DE, Asquith P. Prolonged small intestinal transit time in cystic fibrosis. Br Med J 1983; 287:1011-1013.

47. Schiff, L. The small intestine. In: Sodeman WA, Sodeman WA Jr., eds. Pathologic Physiology, 4th ed. Philadelphia and London: Saunders Company, 1969: 594-636.

48. Matseshe JW, Go VLW, DiMagno EP. Meconium ileus equivalent complicating cystic fibrosis in postneonatal children and young adults. Report of 12 cases. Gastroenterology 1977; 72:732-736.

49. Rubinstein S, Moss R, Lewiston N. Constipation and meconium ileus equivalent in patients with cystic fibrosis. Pediatrics 1986; 78:473-479.

50. Behrman RE, Vaughan III VC, eds. Nelson—Textbook of Pediatrics, 12th ed. Philadelphia: W B Saunders Company, 1983: 417-443, 889, 1086-1099.

51. Loening-Baucke V, Younoszai MK. Abnormal anal sphincter response in chronically constipated children. J Pediatr 1982; 100:213-218.

52. Corazziari E, Cucchiara S, Staiano A, et al. Gastrointestinal transit time, frequency of defecation, and anorectal manometry in healthy and constipated children. J Pediatr 1985; 106:379-382.

53. Bentley JFR. Faecal soiling and anal achalasia. Arch Dis Child 1978; 53:185-186.

54. Abrahamian FP, Lloyd-Still JD. Chronic constipation in childhood: a longitudinal study of 186 patients. J Pediatr Gastroenterol Nutr 1984; 3:460-467.

55. Bentley JFR. Progress report: constipation in infants and children. Gut 1971; 12:85-90.

56. Arhan P, Devroede G, Jehannin B, et al. Idiopathic disorders of fecal continence in children. Pediatrics 1983; 71:774-779.

57. Levine MD, Bakow H. Children with encopresis; a study of treatment outcome. Pediatrics 1976; 58:845-852.

58. Clayden GS, Lawson JON. Investigation and management of longstanding chronic constipation in childhood. Arch Dis Child 1976; 51:918-923.

59. Loening-Baucke V, Younoszai MK. Effect of treatment on rectal and sigmoid motility in chronically constipated children. Pediatrics 1984; 73:199-205.

60. Bush RT. Lactulose: an ideal laxative for children. NZ Med J 1970; 71:364-365.

61. Roy CC, Silverman A, Cozetto FJ. Pediatric Clinical Gastroenterology, 2nd ed. St. Louis: C V Mosby Company, 1975: 320-336.

62. Palmie PE. Zur Behandlung der Obstipation im Kindes- und Jugendalter. Therapiewoche 1980; 30:4045-4049.

63. Perkin JM. Constipation in childhood: a controlled comparison between lactulose and standardized senna. Curr Med Res Opin 1977; 4:540-543.

64. Bass P, Dennis S. The laxative effects of lactulose in normal and constipated subjects. J Clin Gastroenterol 1981; 3(Suppl. 1):23-28.

65. Wesselius-de Casparis A, Broadbaart S, Bergh-Bohlken GE v d, et al. Treatment of chronic constipation with lactulose syrup: results of a double-blind study. Gut 1968; 9:84-86.

66. Voorhies TM, Ehrlich ME, Duffy TE, et al. Acute hyperammonemia in the young primate: physiologic and neuropathologic correlates. Pediatr Res 1983; 17:970-975.

67. Gaull GE. Early nutrition and brain development. In: Arima M, Suzuki Y, Yabuuchi H, eds. The Developing Brain and Its Disorders. Basel: S. Karger, 1985: 279-290.

68. Friede RL. Developmental Neuropathology. Wien: Springer-Verlag, 1975: 488-504.

69. Davison AN, Dobbing J, eds. Applied Neurochemistry. Oxford, London: Blackwell Scientific Publications, 1968: 253-316.

70. Swaiman KS, Menkes JH, DeVivo CD, et al. Metabolic disorders of the central nervous system. In: Swaiman KS, Wright FS, eds. The Practice of Pediatric Neurology, 2nd ed. St. Louis: C V Mosby Company, 1982: 472-600.

71. Walser M. Urea cycle disorders and other hereditary hyperammonemic syndromes. In: Stanbury JB, Wyngaarden JB, Fredrickson DS, et al., eds. The Metabolic Basis of Inherited Disease, 5th ed. New York: McGraw Hill Book Company, 1983: 402-438.

72. Tanaka K, Rosenberg LE. Disorders of branched chain amino acid and organic acid metabolism. In: Stanbury JB, Wyngaarden JB, Fredrickson DS, et al., eds. The Metabolic Basis of Inherited Disease, 5th ed. New York: McGraw Hill Book Company, 1983: 440-473.

73. Rosenberg LE. Disorders of propionate and methylmalonate metabolism. In: Stanbury JB, Wyngaarden JB, Fredrickson DS, et al., eds. The Metabolic Basis of Inherited Disease, 5th ed. New York: McGraw Hill Book Company, 1983: 474-497.

74. Valle D. Simell O. The hyperornithinemias. In: Stanbury JB, Wyngaarden

JB, Fredrickson DS, et al., eds. The Metabolic Basis of Inherited Disease, 5th ed. New York: McGraw Hill Book Company, 1983: 382-401.

75. Lewis PD, Miller AL. Argininosuccinic aciduria. Brain 1970; 93:413-422.

76. Ebels EJ. Neuropathological observations in a patient with carbamyl phosphate-synthetase deficiency and in two sibs. Arch Dis Child 1972; 47:47-51.

77. Brutton CJ, Corsellis JAN, Russell A. Hereditary hyperammonaemia. Brain 1970; 93:423-434.

78. Msall M, Batshaw ML, Suss R, et al. Neurological outcome in children with inborn errors of urea synthesis. N Eng J Med 1984; 310:1500-1505.

79. Msall M, Batshaw ML, Brusilow SW. Neurologic outcome of children with complete urea cycle enzyme deficiencies surviving the first year of life (Abstract). Pediatr Res 1983; 17:365 A.

80. Hsia YE. Progress in gastroenterology—inherited hyperammonemic syndromes. Gastroenterology 1974; 67:347-374.

81. Colombo JP. Hyperammonemia due to inherited deficiencies of urea cycle enzymes. In: Bianchi L, Gerok W, Landmann L, eds. Liver in Metabolic Disease. Boston: MTP Press Limited, 1983: 169-173.

82. Alagille D, Odievre M. Liver and Biliary Tract Disease in Children. New York: J Wiley and Sons Inc, 1978: 262-295.

83. Vorhees AB, Chaitman E, Schneider S. Portal-systemic encephalopathy in the noncirrhotic patient. Arch Surg 1973; 107:659-663.

84. Hassall E, Benson L, Hart M, et al. Hepatic encephalopathy after portocaval shunt in a noncirrhotic child. J Pediatr 1984; 105:439-441.

85. Psacharopoulos HT, Mowat AP, Davies M, et al. Fulminant hepatic failure in childhood. Arch Dis Child 1980; 55:252-258.

86. Bernard O, Alvarez F, Brunelle F, et al., eds. Portal hypertension in children. In: Benhamou JP, Lebrec DC, eds. Clin Gastroenterol 1985; 14:33-73.

87. Campbell AGM, Rosenberg LE, Snodgrass P, et al. Ornithine transcarbamylase deficiency - a cause of lethal neonatal hyperammonemia in males. N Eng J Med 1973; 288:1-6.

88. Brusilow SW, Batshaw ML, Waber L. Neonatal hyperammonemic coma. In Barness LA: Advances in Pediatrics, Vol 29. Chicago: Year Book Medical Publishers Inc, 1982: 69-103.

89. Batshaw ML, Brusilow SW. Treatment of hyperammonemic coma caused by inborn errors of urea synthesis. J Pediatr 1980; 97:893-900.

90. Batshaw ML. Long-term treatment of inborn errors of urea synthesis. In: Kleinberger G, Ferenci P, Riederer P, et al., eds. Advances in Hepatic Encephalopathy and Urea Cycle Diseases. Basel: S. Karger, 1984: 187-195.

91. Snyderman SE, Sansaricq C, Phansalkar SV, et al. The therapy of hyperammonemia due to ornithine transcarbamylase deficiency in a male neonate. Pediatrics 1975; 56:65-73.

92. DiMagno EP, Lowe JE, Snodgrass PJ, et al. Ornithine transcarbamylase deficiency - a cause of bizarre behavior in man. N Engl J Med 1986; 315:744-747.

93. Brusilow SW, Danney M, Waber LJ, et al. Treatment of episodic hyperammonemia in children with inborn errors of urea synthesis. N Engl J Med 1984; 310:1630-1634.

94. Batshaw ML, Msall M, Beaudet AL, et al. Risk of serious illness in heterozygotes for ornithine transcarbamylase deficiency. J Pediatr 1986; 108:236-241.

95. Goodman StI. Inherited metabolic disease in the newborn: approach to diagnosis and treatment. In: Barness LA, ed. Advances in Pediatrics, Vol 33. Chicago, London: Year Book Medical Publishers Inc, 1986: 197-223.

96. Wiegand C, Thompson T, Bock GH, et al. The management of life-threatening hyperammonemia: a comparison of several therapeutic modalities. J Pediatr 1980; 96:142-144.

97. Bachmann C, Colombo JP. Hyperammonämie: Ein Vorschlag Für das diagnostische un therapeutisch Vorgehen. Pädiatr und Pädol 1982; 17:141-148.

98. Heubi JE, Daugherty CC, Partin JS, et al. Grade I Reye's syndrome - outcome and predictors of progression to deeper coma grades. N Engl J Med 1984; 311:1539-1542.

99. Mowat AP. Reye's syndrome: 20 years on. Br Med J 1983; 286:1999-2000.

100. Jenkins G, Glasgow JFT, Black GW, et al. Reye's syndrome: assessment of intracranial monitoring. Br Med J 1987; 294:337-338.

101. Glasgow JFT. Clinical features and prognosis of Reye's syndrome. Arch Dis Child 1984; 59:230-235.

102. Brown T, Hug G, Lansky L, et al. Transiently reduced activity of carbamyl phosphate synthetase and ornithine transcarbamylase in liver of children with Reye's syndrome. N Engl J Med 1976; 294:861-867.

103. Snodgrass PJ, DeLong GR. Urea-cycle enzyme deficiencies and an increased nitrogen load producing hyperammonemia in Reye's syndrome. N Engl J Med 1976; 294:855-860.

104. Latham PS, LaBrecque DR, McReynolds JW, et al. Liver ultrastructure in mitochondrial urea cycle enzyme deficiencies and comparison with Reye's syndrome. Hepatology 1984; 4:404-407.

105. Heubi JE, Partin JC, Partin JS, et al. Reye's syndrome: current concepts. Hepatology 1987; 7:155-164.

106. Hudak ML, Jones MD, Brusilow SW. Differentiation of transient hyperammonemia of the newborn and urea cycle enzyme defects by clinical presentation. J Pediatr 1985; 107:712-719.

107. Batshaw ML, Brusilow SW. Asymptomatic hyperammonemia in low-birth-weight infants. Pediatr Res 1978; 12:221-224.

108. Batshaw ML, Wachtel R, Cohen L, et al. Developmental outcome of asymptomatic hyperammonemia of the preterm infant (Abstract). Pediatr Res 1983; 17:93A.

109. Batshaw ML, Brusilow SW, Waber L, et al. Treatment of inborn errors of

urea synthesis: activation of alternative pathway of waste nitrogen synthesis and excretion. N Engl J Med 1982; 306:1387-1392.

110. Brusilow SW, Valle DL, Batshaw ML. New pathways of nitrogen excretion in inborn errors of urea synthesis. Lancet 1979; 1:452-454.

111. Donn StM, Swartz RD, Thoene JG. Comparison of exchange transfusion, peritoneal dialysis, and hemodialysis for the treatment of hyperammonemia in an anuric infant. J Pediatr 1979; 95:67-70.

112. Francois D. Peritoneal dialysis and exchange transfusion in a neonate with argininosuccinic aciduria. Arch Dis Child 1976; 51:228-231.

113. Letarte J, Qureshi IA, Quellet R, et al. Chronic benzoate therapy in a boy with partial ornithine transcarbamylase deficiency. J Pediatr 1985; 106:794-797.

114. Batshaw ML, Brusilow SW, Walser M. Long-term management of a case of carbamyl phosphate synthetase deficiency using ketoanalogues and hydroxyanalogues of essential amino acids. Pediatrics 1976; 58:227-235.

115. Simell O, Sipilä I, Rajantie J, et al. Waste nitrogen excretion via amino acid acylation: benzoate and phenylacetate in lysinuric protein intolerance. Pediatr Res 1986; 20:1117-1121.

116. Anken v HC, Schiphorst ME. A kinetic determination of ammonia in plasma. Clin Chim Acta 1974; 56:151-157.

117. McLeod RS, Taylor DW, Cohen Z, et al. Single-patient randomized clinical trial. Lancet 1986; 1:726-728.

118. Guyatt G, Sackett D, Taylor W, et al. Determining optimal therapy — randomized trials in individual patients. N Engl J Med 1986; 314:889-892.

23

EFFECT OF LACTULOSE ON CHOLESTEROL AND BILE ACID METABOLISM

GIANFRANCO SALVIOLI, M.D., AND RUGGERO LUGLI, M.D.

Lactulose is an nonabsorbed disaccharide which retains fluid in the intestinal lumen by osmotic activity. In this way it increases the volume of the intestinal lumen and stimulates intestinal peristalsis. An inverse correlation has been found between the metabolism of lactulose and small intestine transit time (1).

Overall cholesterol balance is influenced by the intake of dietary cholesterol, which is absorbed in the small intestine, and by the loss of cholesterol from the body, which occurs almost entirely via bile in the form of neutral sterol (cholesterol and its metabolites) and bile acids (BA). The output of sterols is inversely related to the efficiency of the absorption, which depends on the small intestine transit time, and the diffusion across the unstirred water layer adjacent to the intestinal mucosal surface (2).

Hypocholesterolemia results from a decrease in dietary intake, an increase in sterol and BA output either by a reduction in intestinal transit time, or by the adsorption of bile acids and cholesterol to fiber components (3, 4).

Diet can induce changes of intestinal flora and, consequently, of the fecal sterol profile (5). Modification of intestinal bile acid degradation induced, for example, by the administration of metronidazole, reduces both the proportion of deoxycholic acid (DCA) and the saturation of cholesterol in bile (6).

Ingested lactulose reaches the colon unchanged where it is rapidly fermented by the colonic bacteria. Short-chain fatty acid concentration increases as does the number of lactic acid-metabolizing bacteria. The consequent reduction of the pH of the right colon (7) influences the activity of bile acid and neutral sterol-degrading enzymes (8). Some studies have reported a reduction of both DCA percentage and cholesterol saturation in bile during lactulose administration (9).

Lactulose acts like dietary fiber which influences some steps in cholesterol and bile acid metabolism. The purpose of the present study was to investigate variations of some aspects of sterol metabolism during short-term administration of lactulose.

MATERIALS AND METHODS

Sixteen men, aged 67 to 75 years, who had no evidence of metabolic or gastrointestinal disease, took part. They gave informed consent to participate in the study. A standard diet (35 kcal per kg per day) containing 500 mg of cholesterol was given for 30 days. On the 15th day, eight subjects received 18 g of lactulose in three daily doses for the next 15 days. The remaining eight subjects, who received no lactulose, represent the control group. All 16 patients were given 500 mg per day of chromium oxide for the last seven days of each 15-day period of stool collection.

Feces were collected during the last two days of each 15-day period and were stored at -20°C until analyzed. Fecal bile acids and neutral sterols were evaluated as previously described (10). Sterol balance was calculated according to Grundy and Ahrens (11), using the formula: sterol balance (mg per day) = daily total fecal sterol (neutral + acidic) daily cholesterol uptake. Cholesterol absorption was measured from the seventh day of the last 15-day period using the plasma isotope ratio method, as previously described (12).

RESULTS

The results are shown in Table 1. Only lactulose-treated subjects showed an increase in the number of bowel movements per day, with little variation in fecal wet weight. No changes in fecal pH were observed in either group. Analysis of the fecal excretion of sterols in the lactulose group showed that bile acid excretion increased, whereas that of neutral sterol did not change. The sterol balance

TABLE 1. Variations of Bowel Movements, Fecal Weight and Fecal pH in Patients Treated with Lactulose and Controls

	Lactulose		Controls	
	Before	After	Before	After
Bowel movements (no. per day)	0.8±0.2	1.6±0.3**	0.7±0.2	0.8±0.3
Fecal weight (g per day)	128±19	177±22*	136±31	141±19
Fecal pH	6.4±0.2	6.0±0.2	6.3±0.3	6.2±0.2

*p<0.02; **p<0.001

increased from 726 to 963 mg per day. No variations were observed in the control group (Figure 1).

In the lactulose group cholesterol absorption was lower than in the control group (mean 40.2% versus 47.6%, $p<0.02$) (Table 2). Table 3 shows the percentage distribution of the individual bile acids. The percentage of DCA decreased significantly in the lactulose group while primary bile acids increased. As a consequence the ratio between primary and secondary bile acids increased in the lactulose-treated subjects. Total bile acid excretion was greater during lactulose administration. The content of bile acids increased from 2.9 to 3.2 mg per g of feces (wet weight). However, DCA content decreased from 1.33 to 1.27 mg per g wet feces.

DISCUSSION

Effects of lactulose on bowel activity and the properties of feces. Lactulose administration increased the number and weight of bowel movements. Because of its osmotic activity, lactulose increases the luminal bulk and stimulates peristalsis. Fecal pH does not change, but this finding does not exclude the possibility that the pH is lower in the first portion of the large intestine,

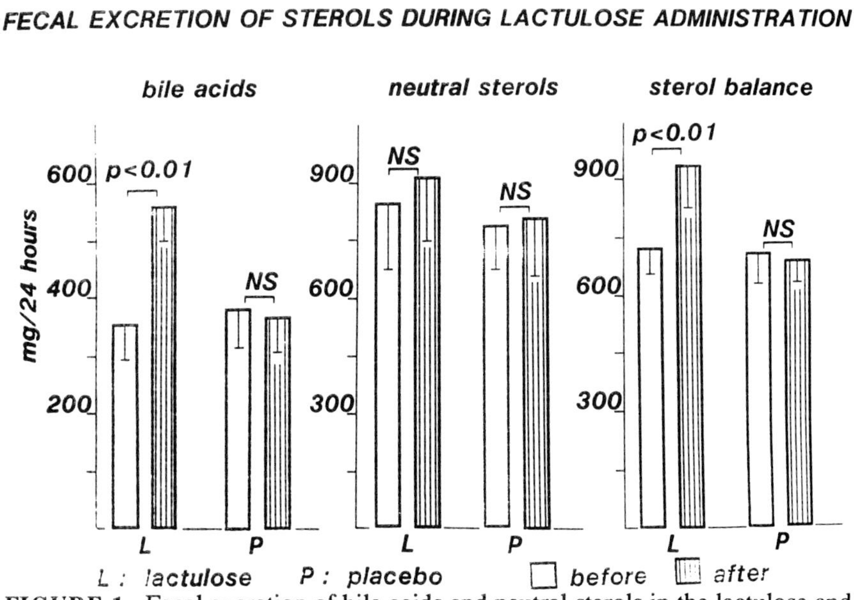

FIGURE 1. Fecal excretion of bile acids and neutral sterols in the lactulose and control groups. Sterol balance values are also reported. Statistical significance is indicated.

TABLE 2. Percentage of Exogenous Cholesterol Absorbed

Patient No.	Placebo (%)	Lactulose (%)
1	46	44
2	47	41
3	51	42
4	50	40
5	48	39
6	48	38
7	47	40
8	46	38
mean	47±2	40±2*

*p<0.02

as shown by Bown et al. (7). At pH levels below 6, the 7-alpha-dehydroxylating activity of intestinal flora on bile acids is reduced (12).

Effects of lactulose on exogenous cholesterol absorption. The subjects taking lactulose showed a lower absorption rate of exogenous cholesterol than did the control group.

Gelling and mucillagenous dietary fibers reduce plasma cholesterol levels and increase neutral and acidic sterol loss (3). Mechanisms that may regulate cholesterol absorption are the time available for the process, which is influenced by the diffusion to the intestinal surface (2, 13, 14), and the adsorption of bile acid and other micellar lipids to components of the intestinal contents (4, 15). Lactulose does not have binding capacity, but accelerates intestinal transit time probably by increasing the luminal bulk by its osmotic activity and by decreasing intraluminal pH. Moreover, the intestinal uptake of cholesterol and fatty acids is a passive diffusion process that is reduced by the physicochemical properties of carbohydrates (2). It is possible that high concentrations of lactulose may interfere with intestinal permeability.

Few data are available about the effect of lactulose feeding on circulating cholesterol levels. Conti et al. (16) treated 62 subjects with serum cholesterol concentrations higher than 280 mg per dl with 10 to 20 g per day of lactulose for 30 days and observed a 21% reduction in cholesterol levels. In animals lactulose feeding exerts a favorable effect on circulating cholesterol (17).

In our study we did not find any significant alterations in serum lipid levels despite variations in sterol balance. The composition of the bile acids, especially the percentage of DCA, seems to influence cholesterol metabolism. Its increase enhances biliary cholesterol secretion and reduces both cholesterol absorption and synthesis. Although a reduction of serum cholesterol has been described during

TABLE 3. Percentage Distribution of Individual Bile Acids in Fecal Bile Acids (mean±SD)

	LCA	DCA	CDCA	UDCA	CA	Others
Control group, n=8						
Before	31±6	48±8	7±2	1±1	1±1	10±2
After	33±6	45±8	8±2	1±1	1±1	11±1
Lactulose group, n=8						
Before	31±6	46±7	9±2	2±1	2±1	10±1
After	28±6	40±8*	15±2*	2±1	6±1*	10±1

LCA, lithocholic acid; DCA, deoxycholic acid; CDCA, chenodeoxycholic acid; UDCA, ursodeoxycholic acid; CA, cholic acid. *p<0.02;

DCA administration (18), no changes were observed in 17 hypercholesterolemic subjects treated with 1 g per day of DCA for two weeks (19). Therefore, the possible reduction in serum cholesterol appears to occur by a mechanism that is different from simply varying the bile acid pattern in bile.

Effect of lactulose on fecal bile acid excretion. Bile acids are excreted as glycine and taurine conjugates or their sulfate esters into the intestine where they are degraded during enterohepatic circulation. The conjugates are rapidly deconjugated to free bile acids. Secondary bile acids (deoxycholic and lithocholic acid, LCA) are formed from primary BA (cholic and chenodeoxycholic acid) by 7-alpha-dehydroxylation. The OH groups of DCA are commonly oxidized at pH 7 to form keto-derivatives, which are poorly absorbed (20). At pH levels higher than 7, the reduction of keto groups is dominant (2, 21).

After the reabsorption of most BA in the proximal colon, their fecal composition and concentration and their transit time, both of which are influenced by diet, may be relevant to colon carcinogenesis (21, 22).

Epidemiologic studies have shown increased bacterial degradation of bile acids with higher LCA and DCA concentration in high risk groups for colon cancer (21). These bile acids can be co-carcinogenic (22) and co-mutagenic (23). Unconjugated bile acids represent the most important fraction (about 80% to 90%). They are partially bound (about 30%) to nonabsorbed, undigested dietary fiber undergoing fermentation and degradation in the proximal colon. Other important factors are the pH of the intestinal contents, the regulation of BA solubility in the aqueous phase, and the calcium concentration which may minimize the toxic effect of BA by forming insoluble BA soaps (24). Even though other studies have found no variations in either total or secondary bile acid levels in patients with colonic cancer (25), there is considerable evidence that bile acid profiles and especially high concentrations of secondary bile acids influence the morphology of the colonic mucosa.

The prevalence of cancer of the cecum and ascending colon is 10% to 20% higher in women than in men (26), and women show a high concentration of bacterially degraded BA in bile (27).

Lactulose administration reduces 7-alpha-dehydroxylase activity which in turn decreases deoxycholic acid formation from cholic acid (9, 28). In our subjects lactulose decreased the percentage of DCA in feces from 36% to 27% after 15 days of therapy. Lactulose feeding seems to reduce the risk of cholesterol gallstone formation in high-risk groups via the reduction in cholesterol saturation in bile and in the percentage of DCA (9).

The lithogenic index of bile remained unchanged after 10 mg per kg per day of DCA administration for four to eight weeks in healthy subjects even though its percentage in bile increased from 26% to 74% (18). Metronidazole administration reduced the relative concentration of deoxycholic acid and of cholesterol saturation of bile (5). Recently Van Berge Henegouwen et al. demonstrated that 60 g per day of lactulose during a 12-week period did not change the biliary cholesterol saturation in eight healthy women with colonic, adenomatous polyps and slightly elevated lithogenic indices (28). During lactulose administration the percentage of biliary deoxycholate was reduced and that of chenic acid increased. Other data support the importance of DCA in the pathogenesis of cholesterol supersaturation of bile. In 548 patients with gallstones in the National Cooperative Gallstone Study a positive correlation was found between the proportion of biliary DCA and the molar percentage of cholesterol in bile (29).

The ratio of secondary to primary bile acids is greater in the bile of women, who have higher prevalence of cholesterol gallstones than do men (27). This difference might be due to a higher pH in the colon and a longer bowel transit time which tends to increase production and reabsorption of deoxycholate (30). Cholesterol cholelithiasis is an age-related disease; aging is associated with a progressive increase of bacterial metabolic activities of bile acids (31) and on cholesterol saturation of bile (32).

Effects of lactulose on sterol balance. Compared to control subjects lactulose-treated subjects showed greater fecal bile excretion and higher sterol balance, even though neutral sterol excretion did not change (Figure 1). High sterol balance indicates an increase of excretion of sterol from the body. As mentioned above, the mechanisms responsible for such metabolic variations might be either the shorter intestinal transit time or the changes of intestinal flora that influence both sterol absorption and the degradation of bile acids. These variations occur after only a short period of lactulose administration, a duration that is probably too short to establish a steady state.

Nevertheless, the capacity of lactulose to increase sterol balance and to reduce the relative concentrations of secondary bile acids in feces seem to be of great interest in long-term treatment with this drug.

CONCLUSION

What is the clinical and therapeutic importance of these findings? Any treatment that is able to decrease the degradation of primary BA seems to prevent the intestinal availability of possible co-carcinogens. The administration of lactulose, which reduces both the bile acid concentrations and the time of contact of BA with the intestinal mucosa, appears to be such treatment.

Moreover, biliary lipid secretion remained abnormal even after the dissolution of gallstones with deoxycholic acid. In animals fed with an essential fatty acid-deficient diet, gallstones are completely prevented by lactulose (33). Lactulose administration may also be used to prevent the recurrence of cholesterol stones that occurs in about one-third to one-half of successfully treated patients.

REFERENCES

1. Bond JH, Levitt, MD. Investigation of small bowel transit time in man—utilizing pulmonary hydrogen (H_2) measurement. J Lab Clin Med 1975; 85:546-555.
2. Thomson ABR. Uptake of lipids into rabbit jejunum and colon following ileal resection. Effect of variation in dietary content of carbohydrate. Dig Dis Sci 1986; 31:193-201.
3. Kay RM, Truswell AS. Effect of citrus pectin on blood lipids and fecal excretion in man. Am J Clin Nutr 1977; 30:171-175.
4. Birkner NJ, Kern F Jr. *In vitro* adsorption of bile salts to food residues, salicylazosulfapyridine and hemicellulose. Gastroenterology 1974; 67:237-244.
5. Mastromarino AJ, Reddy BS, Wynder EL. Fecal profiles of anaerobic microflora of large bowel cancer patients with nonhereditary large bowel polyps. Cancer Res 1976; 38:4458-4462.
6. Low-Beer TS, Nutter S. Colonic bacterial activity, biliary cholesterol saturation and pathogenesis of gallstones. Lancet 1978; 2:1063-1065.
7. Bown RI, Gibson JA, Sladen GE, et al. Effects of lactulose and other laxatives on ileal and colonic pH as measured by radiotelemetry device. Gut 1974; 15:999-1004.
8. Florent C, Flourie B, Leblond A, et al. Influence of chronic lactulose ingestion on the colonic metabolism of lactulose in man (an in vivo study). J Clin Invest 1985; 75:608-613.
9. Thornton JR, Heaton KW. Do colonic bacteria contribute to cholesterol gall-stone formation? Effects of lactulose in man. Br Med J 1981; 282:1018-1020.
10. Salvioli G, Lugli R, Pradelli JM. Cholesterol absorption and sterol balance

in normal subjects receiving dietary fiber or ursodeoxycholic acid. Dig Dis Sci 1985; 30:301-307.

11. Grundy SM, Ahrens EH Jr. Measurement of cholesterol turnover, synthesis, and absorption in man, carried out by isotope kinetics and sterol balance methods. J Lipid Res 1969; 10:91-107.

12. Macdonald IA, Bokkenheuser VD, Winter J, et al. Degradation of steroids in the human gut. J Lipid Res 1983; 24:675-700.

13. Ponz de Leon M, Iori R, Barbolini G, et al. Influence of small-bowel transit time on dietary cholesterol absorption in human beings. N Engl J Med 1982; 307:102-103.

14. Holgate AM, Read NW. Relationship between small bowel transit time and absorption of solid meal. Influence of metaclopramide, magnesium sulfate, and lactulose. Dig Dis Sci 1983; 28:812-819.

15. Vahouny GV. Dietary fibers and intestinal absorption of lipids. In: Vahouny GV, Kritchevsky D, eds. Dietary Fiber in Health and Disease. New York and London: Plenum Press, 1982: 203-227.

16. Conti D, Bardella MT, Bernardi M, et al. Hypocholesterolemic effect of lactulose in man. Minerva Med 1977; 19:1-4.

17. Rotstein OD, Kay R, Wayman M, et al. Hypocholesterolemic effect of dietary fiber and lactulose. Arteriosclerosis 1981; 1:73-74.

18. LaRusso NF, Szczpanic PA, Hofmann AF. Effect of deoxycholic acid ingestion on bile acid metabolism and biliary secretion in normal subjects. Gastroenterology 1977; 72:132-140.

19. Leuven JAG, Havekes L, Kempen HJ. Effect of deoxycholic acid on lipoprotein and apolipoprotein levels in patients with familial hypercholesterolemia. Atherosclerosis 1986; 62:21-25.

20. Björkhem I, Liljeqvist L, Nilsell K, et al. Oxidoreduction of different hydroxyl groups in bile acids during their enterohepatic circulation in man. J Lipid Res 1986; 27:177-182.

21. Hill MJ. Steroid nuclear dehydroxylation and colon cancer. Am J Clin Nutr 1974; 27:1475-1480.

22. Reddy BS, Narisawa R, Weisburger JH, et al. Promoting effect of sodium deoxycholate on colon adenocarcinomas in germ-free rats. JNCI 1976; 56:441-442.

23. Wilpart M, Mainguet P, Maskens A, et al. Mutagenicity of 1,2-dimethylhydrazine towards Salmonella thyphimurium, comutagenic effect of secondary bile acids. Carcinogenesis 1983; 4:45-48.

24. Wargovich MJ, Eng VWS, Newmark HL, et al. Calcium ameliorates the toxic effect of deoxycholic acid on colonic epithelium. Carcinogenesis 1983; 4:1205-1207.

25. Breuer NF, Dommes P, Jaekel S, et al. Fecal bile acid excretion pattern in colonic cancer patients. Dig Dis Sci 1985; 30:852-859.

26. De Joung UW, Day NE, Muir CS, et al. The distribution of cancer within

the large bowel. Int J Cancer 1972; 10:463-477.

27. Fisher MM, Yousef IM. Sex differences in the bile acid composition of human bile: studies in patients with and without gallstones. Can Med Assoc J 1973; 109:190-193.

28. Van Berge Henegouwen GP, Van der Werf SDJ, Ruben A. Th. Effect of lactulose on biliary lipid composition. J Hepatol 1986; 3:328-332.

29. Hofmann AF, Grundy SM, Lachin JM, et al. Pretreatment biliary lipid composition in white patients with radiolucent gallstone in the National Cooperative Gallstone Study. Gastroenterology 1982; 83:738-752.

30. Van der Werf SD, Huijbregts AW, Lamers HL, et al. Age dependent differences in human bile acid metabolism and 7-alpha dehydroxylation. Eur J Clin Invest 1981; 11:425-431.

31. Huang CTL, Levine MM, Woodward WE, et al. Biohydrogenation of cholesterol as an index of bacterial 7-alpha-dehydroxylation activity. Lipids 1981; 16:670-676.

32. Einarsson K, Nilsell K, Leijd B, et al. Influence of age on secretion of cholesterol and synthesis of bile acids by the liver. N Engl J Med 1985; 313:277-282.

33. Rotstein OD, Kay RM, Wayman M, et al. Prevention of cholesterol gallstones by lignin and lactulose in the hamster. Gastroenterology 1981; 81:1098-1103.

24

LACTULOSE AND ANTIOXIDANT VITAMINS IN THE PREVENTION OF THE RECURRENCE OF ADENOMATOUS POLYPS

Maurizio Ponz de Leon, M.D., Paola di Donato, M.D., Luca Roncucci, M.D., Antonio Manenti, M.D., Gianpiero Rigo, M.D., Mario Perini, M.D., Alberto Ferrari, M.D., Aldo Antonioli, M.D., Marco Gandolfo, M.D., Guido Biasco, M.D., and Luigi Barbara, M.D.

Colorectal cancer is one of the most prevalent cancers that affects both men and women in Western countries (1). The factors leading or predisposing to colorectal cancer are still poorly understood. There are, however, several factors which, all together, make this malignancy of particular interest when compared to other neoplastic disorders. First, the importance of a genetic component for cancer of the large bowel has clearly been demonstrated (2). Several syndromes (Lynch I and II, adenomatosis coli, et al.), characterized by an autosomal dominant pattern of inheritance, have been described. Moreover, recent studies show that genetic factors are not limited to these well-defined clinical syndromes, but might occur commonly, and could be responsible for a consistent proportion of sporadic colorectal cancers (3). Second, it is commonly accepted that environmental factors are somehow implicated in the development of these tumors (4), although there are still several concerns about dietary and/or metabolic factors involved in the process of carcinogenesis. Third, evidence has been provided by Morson and coworkers and others that a large proportion of human colorectal cancer develops from benign adenomas (5). It follows that the endoscopic removal of colorectal polyps might reduce the incidence of cancer and this has now become the routine procedure in treating these tumors. Polyps, however, tend to reappear and their recurrence rate has been estimated in various studies to be between 5% and 30% per year (6).

After endoscopic polypectomy the patients are usually left without any specific therapy but are invited to return for endoscopic examination at regular intervals. Although it is still unproven that any therapy will reduce the prevalence (or the recurrence rate) of polyps, there are suggestions from the literature which suggest that many substances should be considered for the prevention of recurrent polyps.

THEORETIC BASIS FOR THE PREVENTION OF THE RECURRENCE OF LARGE BOWEL POLYPS

In theory, the formation of polyps might be prevented by the acidification of the large bowel contents (7). At a pH value lower than 6.5 the degradation of primary bile acids to more toxic, cocarcinogenic, secondary bile acids is greatly reduced (8). In support of this view it is known from the literature that vegetarians who excrete feces more acidic than normal are at reduced risk of developing colorectal cancer (9). Fecal pH lower than 6.5 can be induced by taking lactulose (or other nonabsorbable sugars) as well as by eating a vegetable diet. It is reasonable to believe that lactulose administration may render the bowel resistant to the development of polyps.

In recent years considerable attention has been given to the possible role of micronutrients in tumor prevention (10). Selenium and the antioxidant vitamins A, C and E are among the factors most frequently identified as potential modifiers of the process of carcinogenesis. There are studies showing that selenium supplementation can inhibit chemical carcinogenesis in the skin and liver (11). Similarly, epidemiologic studies have shown that the intake of selenium is inversely related to the overall cancer mortality. Similar results were observed for each of the most common cancers, i.e., lung, large bowel and breast. Selenium is necessary for the activity of glutathione peroxidase; thus, it might inhibit the development of tumors by protecting cells against aberrant oxidations (11).

Vitamin A and retinoids in general, including the precursor beta-carotene, seem able to protect mice and other animals against colorectal tumors induced by chemical compounds (12). Moreover, epidemiologic studies have shown an inverse relationship between vitamin A levels (or intake) and occurrence of cancer of various organs (13). The mechanisms whereby retinoids might exert this beneficial effect are still speculative. In addition to inactivating free radicals, vitamin A seems able to regulate cell proliferation (14) and to modulate the host immunologic defenses (15).

Low vitamin C consumption has been associated with a high incidence of cancer in general and of gastric and esophageal tumors in particular (16). Furthermore, animal studies have shown that vitamin C may prevent chemically induced carcinogenesis of the large bowel (17). Although these beneficial effects have not been confirmed by case-control studies (18), several possible mechanisms for the antitumoral effect of vitamin C can be considered (14). Finally, in a group of patients with adenomatosis coli, feeding of large doses of ascorbic acid after subtotal colectomy seems to reduce the recurrence rate of polyps in the residual rectum (19).

In some animal models inhibition of cancer has been observed after giving vitamin E (20, 21), but data in humans are scanty (14). As for the other protective vitamins, free radical scavenger activity has been shown and other mechanisms have been postulated (14).

Other antioxidants might be of clinical or experimental interest in cancer prevention. Glutathione is one of the major antioxidant and antimitogenic substances found in the soluble fraction of the cells (22). The administration of sulfur amino acids or analogues, such as acetylcysteine increase the concentration of glutathione and may reduce the oxidative toxicity of drugs like adriamycin and acetaminophen (23). The possible antineoplastic effects of these compounds need to be further evaluated.

The human colorectal mucosa is continuously exposed to substances derived from the incomplete absorption of foods and from bacterial metabolism. It is likely that in this situation several carcinogens (promoters) are formed that may affect epithelial cell kinetics in the colorectal mucosa and may lead to hyperproliferation, adenoma formation and, eventually, to cancer. It is not unreasonable to speculate that the administration of antioxidant vitamins in such situations might be effective in preventing the recurrence of polyps.

Dietary fiber remains one of the most interesting and intriguing substances in medicine and in cancer research. Although animal studies have shown that dietary fiber has a protective effect against colorectal cancer induced by chemical compounds (24), the results in humans are less clear and often controversial (25, 26). The beneficial effect of fiber might be due to several mechanisms including changes of large bowel transit time, dilution of the intestinal contents, chemical interaction with carcinogens or modifications of the bacterial flora. According to some authors, however, the weight of evidence tends to support the contention that fiber may protect against colorectal cancer (14). Fiber, therefore, can be considered as a potential preventer of polyp formation or recurrence.

Finally, recent studies suggest that oral calcium should be considered. Using an autoradiographic approach, Lipkin and Newmark showed that calcium feeding was associated with a significant reduction of the proliferative activity of the rectal mucosa in the relatives of patients with inherited tumors of the large bowel (27). It is possible that calcium interacts within the intestinal lumen with bile acids and ionized fatty acids, which may be converted to insoluble, less toxic compounds. The more quiescent, proliferative state of colonic mucosa after calcium feeding, therefore, could be a consequence of the reduced activity of potentially toxic substances. Since polyps may represent a dysproliferative disorder of the colorectal mucosa, it is important to determine whether calcium feeding can affect their recurrence rate.

PRELIMINARY RESULTS OF A RANDOMIZED CONTROLLED TRIAL IN THE PREVENTION OF THE RECURRENCE OF ADENOMATOUS POLYPS

On the basis of these considerations, a randomized controlled investigation was designed to assess the effect of lactulose and of antioxidant vitamins on the prevention of recurrence in patients who had undergone resection of large bowel polyps. The study, which started in May 1985, was designed to enroll 300 patients and to follow them for at least one year.

Patients were considered eligible for the study after a pancolonoscopic investigation during which one or more adenomatous polyps were removed and if they agreed to return semiannually for subsequent endoscopies. Eligible patients were informed about the purposes of the study and gave their oral consent. The patients were then randomized (using balanced blocks) into three groups.

By December 1986, 89 subjects had been entered into the study. Forty-seven patients had had follow-up colonoscopy after six to nine months of treatment.

Group A (lactulose)—patients received 20 to 40 g per day of pure lactulose (Epalfen®, Zambon Pharmaceuticals, Milan, Italy). The dosage was adjusted to stimulate two soft stools each day. If there were no changes in bowel activity, a lactulose syrup (65% g per dl) was given in doses of 30 to 60 ml per day. Twenty-seven patients have been randomized.

Group B (vitamins A, C, E)—patients received vitamins A, C and E at daily doses of 30,000 IU, 1 g and 70 mg, respectively. Thirty-one patients have been randomized.

Group C (control)—no therapy was administered. Thirty-one patients have been randomized.

All patients were asked to continue the scheduled treatment as outpatients without interruption to indicate any symptoms or adverse effects and to report the omission of therapy or withdrawal from the investigation.

The results in 47 patients who had had at least one follow-up endoscopic examination are shown in Table 1. Among the 16 patients who had received lactulose, 11 had normal endoscopy, two showed recurrent polyps, ie., the appearance of one or more new polyps, and three had nonspecific changes (i.e., nonspecific colitis and/or hyperplastic mucosa). Fifteen out of 18 patients treated with antioxidant vitamins had normal endoscopy, one showed a recurrence of polyps and two, nonspecific changes. Adenomatous polyps recurred in 4 of 13 untreated patients, whereas nonspecific changes were observed in one. Although the results are still insufficient for meaningful statistical evaluation, the recurrence rate of adenomatous polyps in the untreated group is significantly higher than that observed in patients who were given vitamins. A statistically nonsignificant trend in the same direction was noted in the patients who received lactulose.

TABLE 1. Endoscopic Findings Observed at the First Follow-up Examination after 6 to 12 Months of Treatment

	No. of patients	Normal endoscopy	Recurrence of adenomatous polyps	Nonspecific changes
Group A (lactulose)	16	11	2	3
Group B (vitamins A,C,E)	18	15	1	2
Group C (control)	13	8	4	1

SUMMARY

There is evidence in the literature which suggests that it is theoretically possible to prevent the occurrence and recurrence of adenomatous polyps of the large bowel. Although not all polyps become malignant, it is commonly believed that adenomas represent the natural precursor of colorectal cancer.

Thus, the prevention of their recurrence might represent a practical step in the control of this common neoplasm. At present, patients who have undergone endoscopic polypectomy are usually left without any specific therapy. Since the postulated therapies—lactulose and vitamins—are safe and well tolerated, it seems appropriate to undertake randomized controlled studies to evaluate the possibility of primary prevention of large bowel neoplasms.

The preliminary results of such a controlled investigation at our institutions are encouraging, suggesting a lower recurrence rate of polyps in patients given lactulose or antioxidant vitamins than in patients without therapy. Much more data and longer follow-up are needed, however, before any conclusions can be drawn.

REFERENCES

1. Feldman AR, Kessler L, Myers MH. The prevalence of cancer. N Engl J Med 1986; 315:1394-1397.

2. Lipkin M, Winawer SJ, Sherlock P. Early identification of individuals at increased risk for cancer of the large intestine. Part I: definition of high risk populations. Clin Bulletin 1981; 11:13-21.

3. Burt RW, Bishop DT, Cannon LA, et al. Dominant inheritance of adenomatous colonic polyps and colorectal cancer. N Engl J Med 1985; 312:1540-1544.

4. Wynder EL. The epidemiology of large bowel cancer. Cancer Res 1975;

35:3388-3391.

5. Hill MJ, Morson BC, Bussey HJR. Aetiology of adenoma-carcinoma sequence in large bowel. Lancet 1978; 1:245-247.

6. Bader JP. Screening of colorectal cancer. Dig Dis Sci 1986; 31:43S-56S.

7. Thornton JR. High colonic pH promotes colorectal cancer. Lancet 1981; 1:1081-1083.

8. Narisawa T, Magadia NE, Weisburger JH, et al. Promoting effect of bile acids on colon carcinogenesis after intrarectal instillation of N-Methyl-N'-nitro-N-nitrosoguanidine in rats. JNCI 1974; 53:1093-1097.

9. Macdonald IA, Webb GR, Mahony DE. Fecal hydroxysteroid activities in vegetarian seventh day adventists control subjects and large bowel cancer patients. Am J Clin Nutr 1978; 31:S233-S238.

10. Hennekens CH. Micronutrients and cancer prevention. N Engl J Med 1986; 315:1288-1289.

11. Kobayashi M, Kogata M, Yamamura M, et al. Inhibitory effect of dietary selenium on carcinogenesis in rat glandular stomach induced by N-Methyl-N'-nitro-N-nitrosoguanidine. Cancer Res 1986; 46:2266-2270.

12. Goodman DS. Vitamin A and retinoids in health and disease. N Engl J Med 1984; 310:1023-1031.

13. Kvale G, Bjelke E, Gart JJ. Dietary habits and lung cancer risk. Int J Cancer 1983; 31:397-405.

14. Willett WC, MacMahon B. Diet and cancer—an overview. N Engl J Med 1984; 310:633-638, 697-703.

15. Jurin M, Tannock IF. Influence of vitamin A on immunological response. Immunology 1972; 23:283-287.

16. Cameron E, Pauling L, Leibovitz B. Ascorbic acid and cancer: a review. Cancer Res 1979; 39:663-681.

17. Reddy BS, Hirota H. Effect of dietary ascorbic acid on 1-2, dimethylhydrazine-induced colon cancer in rats (Abstract). Fed Proc 1979; 38:714.

18. Jain M, Cook GM, Davis FG, et al. A case-control study of diet and colorectal cancer. Int J Cancer 1980; 26:757-768.

19. DeCosse JJ, Bussey HJR, Thomson JPS, et al. Ascorbic acid in polyposis coli. Colorectal Cancer: Prevention, Epidemiology, and Screening, 1980; 59-63.

20. Haber SL, Wissler RW. Effect of vitamin E on the carcinogenicity of methylcholanthrene. Proc Soc Exp Biol Med 1962; 111:774-775.

21. Cook MG, McNamara P. Effect of dietary vitamin E on dimethylhydrazine-induced colonic tumors in mice. Cancer Res 1980; 40:1329-1331.

22. Meister A. Selective modification of glutathione metabolism. Science 1983; 220:472-478.

23. Ames BN. Dietary carcinogens and anticarcinogens. Oxygen radicals and degenerative diseases. Science 1983; 221:1256-1264.

24. Reddy BS, Mori H, Nicolais M. Effect of dietary wheat bran and dehydrated citrus fiber on azoxymethane-induced intestinal carcinogenesis in Fischer 344 rats.

JNCI 1981; 66:553-557.

25. Manousos O, Day NE, Trichopoulos D, et al. Diet and colorectal cancer: a case-control study in Greece. Int J Cancer 1983; 32:1-5.

26. Dales LG, Friedman GD, Ury HK, et al. A case control study of the relationship of diet and other traits to colorectal cancer in American blacks. Am J Epidemiol 1978; 109:132-144.

27. Lipkin M, Newmark H. Effect of added dietary calcium on colonic epithelial-cell proliferation in subjects at high risk for familial colonic cancer. N Engl J Med 1985; 313:1381-1384.

25

HEPATIC ENCEPHALOPATHY IN THE 21ST CENTURY

DAME SHEILA SHERLOCK, M.D., HAROLD O. CONN, M.D.

It's difficult to make forecasts, especially about the future.
Samuel Goldwyn

Crystal ball reading is an ancient art form. The best practitioners of this art are neither charlatans nor frauds. However, they do not receive all their insights from the ball alone. Before rendering a reading they accumulate as much information as possible about the subject under analysis. They consider the purpose of the inquiry and, as best they can determine, the desires of the inquirers. Their predictions are based primarily on The Truth or on reasonable facsimiles thereof. They shrewdly incorporate all these diverse components. Thus, the finished product is not a series of guesses, but rather the thoughtful assimilation of educated guesstimates. The reading is presented in as an informative and entertaining manner as possible, ideally, one that comforts the inquirers and, if possible, a much wider audience. The presentation is by definition general rather than specific, although the incorporation of an occasional specific, sure longshot establishes credibility. Such seances are not empty exercises. Their purpose is to speculate publicly about specific aspects of the state of the art in order to stimulate new approaches. A good example is the speculation by Franz Ingelfinger that lactulose might play a role in the management of hepatic encephalopathy as mentioned in the preface to this volume.

THE DISORDER

Centuries have passed since Hippocrates described the patient with acute hepatic encephalopathy who barked like a dog and since Frerichs described coma in cirrhotic patients. The modern era started in the 1930s when Kirk in Norway and Van Caulaert in France observed disorders of consciousness when cirrhotic patients were given ammonium salts. Twenty years later McDermott and Adams noted intermittent stupor in a patient who had had a portacaval anastomosis in the course of a pancreatic resection.

The clinical syndromes of HE are relatively well established, and it is unlikely that any major changes in their presentation will take place. Changes in perception, however, will occur continually. The severity of HE will continue to be assessed by clinical-laboratory indices graded on crude, overlapping, but surprisingly useful, clinical I to IV grades. Many measurements will be shown to be more accurate yardsticks than are currently available in specific series of patients, but no one such measure will achieve a monopoly.

It is probable that unique neurologic presentations not recognized previously, such as cortical blindness (1) or conjugated deviation of gaze (2), will be reported, but these variants are fine points. The vague outlines of these syndromes will be perceived much as they are now, but with much greater insight.

It is likely that new precipitants of HE will be encountered, most likely by new pharmacologic agents with hitherto unrecognized metabolic intermediates. A prototype for such substances is valproate, the intermediate metabolic products of which are similar to cerebrotoxic substances seen in some variants of HE such as Jamaica vomiting sickness (3,4). It is probable that more accurate semiquantitative psychometric tests will be described for assessing HE earlier and more precisely. It is unlikely, however, that any will be simpler than the Number Connection Test (5).

The major clinical difference from the 20th century is that HE will be seen much less commonly by virtue of the elimination of HBV and nonA, nonB hepatitis by vaccination. Similarly, the eradication of schistosomiasis will reduce the frequency of portal hypertension and, therefore, to a certain extent the HE associated with it even though encephalopathy is an uncommon manifestation of schistosomial infestation. Continued use of the opiate of the masses, ethyl alcohol, will continue to be the basis for cirrhosis in the "civilized" world. As the underdeveloped countries become overdeveloped they too will assume this socially accepted hepatotoxin. This subtle pathogenetic transfer will compensate to some degree for the eradication of the infectious and infestational causes of cirrhosis. Eventually, educational programs akin to those which are now becoming effective for tobacco abuse may gradually become valuable in reducing alcohol abuse. In addition, we predict that substances, such as free radical scavengers that interfere with the injurious effects of alcohol when administered simultaneously with the beverage will be shown to reduce the hepatotoxicity of alcohol. Whether or not they will become widely accepted will depend on whether or not they affect adversely the flavor of the beverages or the euphoric effects of the alcohol.

Advances in genetic engineering will permit physicians to test for and abort fetuses with urea cycle enzyme deficiencies and related disorders that induce hepatic encephalopathy. Such developments may well precede the new century. Early in the century, gene replacement therapy (GRT) will allow corrected genetic sequences to be introduced into the fetal genome to reconstitute normal enzyme production.

Reye's syndrome will become even less common as the underlying viral disorders and the unidentified cofactors, whether genetic, environmental or pharmacologic, are identified and eliminated. On the other hand, the development of new pharmacologic agents will continue to induce variations of this variable syndrome.

Our understanding of the pathogenesis of hepatic encephalopathy will certainly improve. Future Nobel laureates still have the opportunity to discover the specific function or functions of the liver that permit optimal operation of the brain. Such advances, which are often recognized by identifying specific *dysfunctions*, may revolutionize the treatment of hepatic encephalopathy. Until that time, however, ammonia will continue to play the central role, although it will be recognized repeatedly that ammonia *per se* is not the toxic agent. Rather, combinations of ammonia with a variety of cofactors will be identified as precipitants that can induce a variety of related encephalopathic syndromes. Corrections of other coprecipitants of encephalopathy such as anemia and hypox-emia will decrease the prevalence of this disorder. Any search for a single, specific cause of all "hepatic" encephalopathy is doomed to failure, although these disorders may all be ultimately mediated via a single biochemical pathway.

The false neurotransmitter concept and the GABA hypothesis will have run their courses, having enlightened physicians about the nutritional and neurophysiologic mechanisms of hepatic encephalopathy. We doubt that either will give birth to specific, effective, therapeutic agents. Clearly, however, foods and nutritional supplements devoid of or with decreased amounts of comagenic content will be available. Other unpredictable, innovative, ingenious hypotheses supported by sound experimental data will appear periodically, run their courses, expand our horizons and disappear. Despite the introduction of more powerful investigative techniques and the accumulation of infinite amounts of important new data, the mechanisms of brain function and malfunction will remain complex and controversial and will never be fully elucidated.

THERAPY

It has been said that the efficacy of the treatment of any disorder is inversely proportional to the number of therapies used to treat it. HE, which is currently being treated a) by the restriction of dietary protein, b) by the lactulose-lactitol-lactose carbohydrate complex, c) by nonabsorbable antibiotics, d) by unnatural mixtures of amino acids and e) by a variety of other specific, unproved therapies, therefore, by definition, needs more effective treatment.

It is difficult to predict completely new therapeutic approaches. It is unquestionable that new therapies will be based rationally on the pathogenesis of these disorders. At present neomycin and metronidazole are standbys for treating acute coma. Unfortunately neither can be used on a long-term basis because of neuro- and ototoxicity. In the future, wide-spectrum, nontoxic, inexpensive antibiotics that specifically inhibit proteolytic, particularly comagenic, bacteria, but not fermentative organisms that activate lactulose, will be used. Such antibiotic agents may be used in combination with unabsorbed carbohydrates. Actually, fermentative bacteria rendered resistant to specific antibiotics may be administered as enteric-coated capsules to assure their presence in the large bowel.

In a similar approach lactase inhibitors that prevent the degradation of lactose in the upper intestinal tract and convert ingested lactose to a fermentable carbohydrate in the colon will be used as an adjunct to therapy.

Another pharmacologic approach to the same end point is the use of substances that inhibit the absorption of carbohydrate from the intestinal tract. The unabsorbed sugars will remain in the lumen to be degraded by bacteria. Such substances currently under development for the treatment of diabetes mellitus may well have a second application in the treatment of HE.

Hepatic encephalopathy rarely develops in patients with completely normal livers. True hepatoprotective drugs will be used to minimize the effects of environmental toxins much as exogenously administered prostaglandins can protect the liver against damage by carbon tetrachloride, galactosamine, acetaminophen or endotoxin (6).

For patients who develop recurrent encephalopathy secondary to dietary protein or to azotemia, immunization against bacterial urease, using an antigenically active, enzymatically-inactive analogue of urease will provide an effective form of prophylactic therapy. Such treatment would reduce the ambiant ammonia level and in effect raise the coma threshold. Similarly urease inhibitors like nicotinohydroxamate (7) that are nontoxic and well tolerated could function in a similar manner.

As outlined by Uribe (8), dietary management using vegetable proteins that are high in fiber content will be used, modified and extended. Indeed, the effects of dietary fiber on stool pH and bowel activity are similar to those of lactulose and lactitol (9). The application of known genetic principles to agriculture should permit the growth of vegetable proteins that contain a minimum of toxic amino acids, such as phenylalanine, tyrosine, tryptophan, methionine, etc., and an excess of noncomagenic and, perhaps, antitoxic amino acids, such as branched-chain amino acids (leucine, isoleucine and valine). Conceivably, some of the "amino" acids in these proteins will be synthesized as their keto analogues, which, by the incorporation of ammonia into the molecule, reduce the ammonia levels of tissue fluids. Keto analogues of amino acids are both malodorous and insoluble. These disadvantages will be corrected by complexing them with carriers which will facilitate their absorption and administered within microcapsules to protect the complexes until they are delivered to the target organs. Furthermore, the amount of insulin-stimulating amino acids will be kept sufficiently low to prevent over-stimulation of the beta-cells to produce insulin and, thereby, to minimize the prevalence of the insulinopenic diabetes of cirrhosis.

Furthermore, while the genetic engineers are creating new proteins they will have designed these crops to be easy to sow, rapid to ripen, economic to harvest and enjoyable to eat. To push the genetic therapeutic envelope for HE to its outermost limits, we predict that, in addition, they will have designed these proteins to have a high content of zinc and/or other substances that will have been shown to be beneficial in the treatment of HE.

Combinations of these various forms of prophylaxis and treatment may make HE a much more manageable and less distressing disorder.

The adverse effects of colonic carbohydrates will be little changed, but the employment of more predictably metabolized substances will reduce the prevalence of diarrhea. More effective hydrolysis of the carbohydrates, however, will permit the development of greater degrees of intestinal acidosis, which in turn may be associated with side effects such as rectal pruritus and burning. This will be treated by the use of alkaline, rectal ointments which will neutralize and soothe the acid-irritated rectal mucosa.

Hepatic transplantation, which has already been used to treat fulminant hepatic failure due to hepatitis viruses, drug hepatotoxicity, Wilson's disease and Budd-Chiari syndrome will have run its course. It will in the future be used for HE only when other measures have failed. When it is used, organ rejection will be controlled by the administration of substances derived from HIV that completely suppress the immunologic mechanisms of tissue rejection.

Fourth generation antagonists of benzodiazepine and related neuroinhibitory drug receptors will be used as non-specific "wake up" substances (10). These agents can convert encephalopathic patients at risk of aspiration and trauma to patients who are alert and responsive while the underlying cause of the encephalopathy is being eradicated.

In the 21st century the art of randomized clinical trials (RCTs) will have progressed in parallel with developments in biochemical and physiologic aspects of medicine. This progress will minimize the initiation and performance of RCTs with too few patients to achieve meaningful results. Indeed, as Orlandi et al. have lamented (11) in four-fifths of all the RCTs so far performed on lactulose the number of patients randomized has been less than 20. The greater acceptance of RCTs will result from the appreciation by the lay population of the necessity for and virtues of RCTs. Furthermore, teams of experienced RCTologists will be available to design and conduct such studies. In our brave new world of the 21st century, participation by patients in such studies will be covered by third party, medical insurance payers. The greater access to RCTs will permit physicians to determine which therapies are truly effective and which are ineffective or equivocal and should be discarded.

THIRD GENERATION LACTULOSES

The concept of disaccharides that are not absorbed in the upper GI tract but that are degraded by bacteria in the large bowel to create an intestinal, acid dialysis system is a fascinating one. We predict that other oligosaccharides that are metabolized more slowly than lactulose and lactitol and that have superior therapeutic properties will replace these agents. Crystalline lactulose will no longer be used since less expensive sugars that are simpler to manufacture will have made this pure preparation economically impractical. Some such substances like rhamnose are naturally occurring, and some are synthetic. These carbohydrates will be degraded more slowly than lactulose and lactitol resulting in the sustained release of acid that avoids peaks and valleys of pH which intermittently inhibit cathartic effects and induce bouts of diarrhea, respectively. Synthetic carbohydrates which are long, cellulose-like, digestible hydrocarbon molecules will be cheaper, have longer shelf-life and will be better tolerated than the substances in current use. In general the dosage of carbohydrates will be determined by the intracecal pH which will be noninvasively measured by ultrasonic inverse Doppler diffraction.

At present, lactulose is usually administered by mouth, but is sometimes given as an enema. In the future these bacteria-activated carbohydrates will be administered as carbohydrate suppositories that are rapidly broken down by bacterial action without the need to administer large enemas as are used at present. Furthermore, such carbohydrates need not necessarily be large, nonabsorbable, polysaccharide molecules to guarantee their delivery to the lower intestinal tract intact. Simpler, smaller, less expensive, more rapidly degradable sugars which can be brought into contact with the colonic flora directly by the rectal route will be used. After all, the intestinal bacteria are much less fastidious about the exact biochemical structure of the sugars and, more important, patients are less likely to complain about the sweetness or viscosity of sugars that are given *per rectum.*

Carbohydrate suppositories that incorporate bacteria which can degrade the carbohydrate in patients will be especially useful for patients who have been on antibiotic therapy which may have suppressed fermentative bacteria.

SUNDRY ASPECTS

Constipation will be one of the most common complaints of humans in the 21st century as it has been throughout recorded history. It can be confidently predicted that it will still be a common symptom in the 25th century and that Buck Rogers will probably complain of it.

Carbohydrate-induced acidification of the lower intestinal tract will be the most effective, the safest and the least expensive cathartic agents available. They will be universally used in adults, children and animals.

The lactulose-hydrogen breath test will still be the standard method for assessing intestinal transit time and carbohydrate malabsorption even though lactase deficiency will be easily managed by the oral administration of lactase early in the century and by gene replacement therapy later on.

Although lactulose had a brief trial use in the prevention of dental caries, later studies showed that topical antibiotic therapy is more effective in eradicating the cariogenic bacteria than the indirect method of creating a favorable gingival milieu for saprophytic organisms.

Perhaps, the most important indication for the administration of unabsorbable carbohydrates is the suppression of the growth of polyps of the colon and of the neoplasms that arise therein. The preliminary studies reported by Ponz de Leon in this volume showed that lactulose appeared to be effective (12). Later studies showed that sustained release "lactuloses" were even more effective. As might have been predicted (8), it was subsequently shown that vegetable diets supplemented by fiber are equally effective. Prophylaxis against colon cancer will evolve as dietary treatment as long as the pH of the colon lumen can be maintained below 5.5. If it cannot be maintained below this level, the diet must be supplemented by carbohydrates.

Finally, scientific advances in the fields of nutrition, agriculture and animal husbandry, stimulated by the search for less comagenic proteins, will have earthshaking ramifications. The ova of chickens will have disappeared almost completely from the diets of civilized humans. These experiments will produce a variety of semisynthetic meats, fish, cheeses and grains that are low in fat, sodium, cholesterol and carbohydrate, respectively. These new products of nutritional progress will be loudly proclaimed by nutritionists and by the Surgeon General of the United States for their neonutritional properties and for their lack of undesirable substances. These bland, unsatisfying foodstuffs will give rise to a new "la cuisine nouvelle." In a manner analogous to the lack of refrigeration in tropical countries for the past few centuries that resulted in the "hot" foods of Mexico, Thailand, India and China, these tasteless foods will also foster the use of spicy flavorings to make them more palatable. (It will be difficult for a sophisticated palate to differentiate Cajun cooking in Louisiana the late 20th century from continental cuisine in northern France at the end of the 21st century.)

Among the descendents of the 20th century, small, hardy bands of gourmets with long gustatory memories will survive and will worship the tasty, toxic foods of their youth, and will live their lives according to the culinary fashions of an earlier age. These pockets of people will also retain their appreciation of alcoholic beverages and will sometimes clone isolated cults in which cirrhosis and hepatic encephalopathy persist. No matter how effective and widespread anti-encephalopathic therapy becomes, we predict that some hepatic encephalopathy will always be with us.

REFERENCES

1. Naparstek Y, Shouval D, Auerbach E, et al. Transient cortical blindness in hepatic encephalopathy. Isr J Med Sci 1979; 15:854-856.

2. Sandyk P, Brennan MJW, Erdmann MWW. Conjugate deviation of gaze in hepatic encephalopathy (Correspondence). J Neurol Neurosurg Psychiatry 1982; 45:1168.

3. Tanaka K, Kean EA, Johnson B. Jamaican vomiting sickness: biochemical investigation of two cases. N Engl J Med 1976; 295:462-463.

4. Zimmerman HJ, Ishak KG. Valproate-induced hepatic injury: analyses of 23 fatal cases. Hepatology 1982; 2:591-597.

5. Conn HO. The trailmaking and number connection tests in assessing mental state in portal-systemic encephalopathy. Am J Dig Dis 1977; 22:541-550.

6. Abecassis M, Falk JA, Makowka L, et al. 16, 16 dimethyl prostaglandin E2 prevents the development of fulminant hepatitis and blocks the induction of monocyte macrophage procoagulant activity after murine hepatitis virus strain 3 infection. J Clin Invest 1987; 80:881.

7. Hirayama C, Ichida F, Takahashi Y, et al. A controlled clinical trial of nicotinohydroxamic acid and neomycin in advanced chronic liver disease. Digestion 1982; 25:115-123.

8. Uribe M. Dietary management of portal-systemic encephalopathy. In: Conn HO, Bircher J, eds. Hepatic Encephalopathy: Management with Lactulose and Related Carbohydrates. East Lansing, Michigan: Medi-Ed Press, 1988:95-112.

9. Weber F. Combination therapy with lactulose and antibiotics. In: Conn HO, Bircher J, eds. Hepatic Encephalopathy: Management with Lactulose and Related Carbohydrates. East Lansing, Michigan: Medi-Ed Press, 1988:207-218.

10. Mullen KD, Martin JV, Mendelson WB, et al. Could an endogenous benzodiazepine ligand contribute to hepatic encephalopathy? Lancet 1988; 1:457-458.

11. Orlandi F. Clinical trials of lactulose therapy in hepatic encephalopathy. In: Conn HO, Bircher J, eds. Hepatic Encephalopathy: Management with Lactulose and Related Carbohydrates. East Lansing, Michigan: Medi-Ed Press, 1988:191-198.

12. Ponz de Leon M. Lactulose in the prevention of the recurrence of adenomatous polyps. In: Conn HO, Bircher J, eds. Hepatic Encephalopathy: Management with Lactulose and Related Carbohydrates. East Lansing, Michigan: Medi-Ed Press, 1988:343-350.

INDEX

Alanine, 32-33, 36-38, 42, 44-49
Amino acids
branched-chain (*see also* Branched-chain amino acids)
hepatic uptake, 45
in treatment of HE, 129-139
insulin and, 46
nitrogen balance and, 137-138
urea cycle enzyme deficiencies, 319
false neurotransmitter theory, 20, 129
hepatic encephalopathy hypothesis, 89
hormonal control, 44-50
metabolism, 32, 41, 47-48
plasma patterns in chronic liver disease, 49, 100, 129
γ-aminobutyric acid, (*see* GABA)
Ammonia, (*see also* Blood ammonia)
and PSE, 3-12, 18, 20, 213-215
detoxication, 41-42, 47-49
diffusion, effect of pH, 91
from deamidation, 37
metabolism of, 31-38, 41-52
portal-arterial differences, 33-35
suppression
by antibiotics, 207-208
by lactitol, 249, 263
by lactose, 283-291
by lactulose, 108, 181-182, 306
by neomycin-lactulose, 213
toxicity 17-20
Ammonia tolerance test, 49
Analgesics, 4, 205
Antacids, effect on lactulose, 183, 205
Antibiotics
suppression of urease activity, 208
interaction with lactulose, 204
Antiendotoxin effect, 163-164
Apraxia, 16
Asterixis, 3, 6, 103
Astrocytes, 18-19, 22
Astroglial cells, 15, 17, 20, 26
Azotemia, 3-4, 12, 84, 202

Bacteria
in dental caries, effect of lactulose, 236-238
intracolonic, 96-97, 113-115, 120-122
lactitol vs lactulose, 263-264, 271-279
metabolism of lactulose, 153-158, 178-182
Bacterial flora, 32, 286
aerobic, 33, 264, 271-274
anaerobic, 33, 36, 180-181, 211, 264, 271-275
Barbiturate receptor sites, 62-63
BCAA (see Amino acids, branched chain;

Branched-chain amino acids)
Benzodiazepine receptors, 17, 21-22, 54, 56-59, 62-63
agonists, 66-75
antagonists, 22, 24, 54, 57-59, 63-75
binding activity, 64, 70, 74
Bicuculline, 66-70
Bile acids, effect of lactulose on, 160-163, 333-339
Blood ammonia (*see* Ammonia)
Blood-brain barrier, 19-22, 26
in FHF, 53
permeability to GABA, 71-73
Branched-chain amino acids (*see also* Amino acids, branched-chain)
in PSE and HE, 58, 129-139
Breath hydrogen, 114-116, 287, 318

Carbamyl phosphate synthetase, 6, 8, 320
Carbon dioxide narcosis, 3-4
Catharsis, effects of lactulose, 202, 303-311
Cathartics and lactulose, 202, 204, 303-311
Celiac disease, lactulose absorption, 150-153
Chloride channel blocker (IPPO), 66-67, 70
Chlortetracycline in acute HE, 31, 208
Cholesterol metabolism and lactulose, 160-163, 333-339
Colon
ecosystem, 283-284
pH, 85, 118-122, 155
transit time, 123-125
Constipants and lactulose, 204
Constipation, 4, 9, 303-304, 308-309

Dental caries and lactulose, 236-238
Diabetes
dietary fiber and, 105-106
lactitol as sugar substitute for, 240-241
Diarrhea (*see* Lactitol, side effects; Lactose, side effects; Lactulose, side effects)
Diazepam, 66-67
Dietary
compliance, 97
fiber, 96, 103, 105-109
management of PSE, 95-109
protein restriction (*see* Protein)
vitamin deficiency in PSE, 98

Eck fistula, 31, 100
EEG (Electroencephalography)
effect of lactitol vs lactulose, 249
effects of benzodiazepine receptor antagonist, 67-68, 71
effects of lactulose-neomycin, 213-215
effects of vegetable protein diet, 102-103
in PSE, 3-4, 7
Enema, treatment for encephalopathy
lactitol, 260, 296-298
lactose vs lactitol, 204, 260, 294-297
lactulose, 204

False neurotransmitter theory, 17, 20-21
Fiber, dietary, (*see* Dietary fiber)
Food efficiency of lactulose, 167
Formaldehyde, treatment of hyperammonemia, 87
Fulminant hepatic failure, 4, 9, 11-12, 16

GABA, 53-59, 61-75
concept, 15, 17, 21-26, 53-54
binding, 23, 62
from degradation of blood, 84
Galactosemia, effect of lactulose, 183, 204
Gas, intestinal (*see* Lactitol, side effects; Lactose, side effects; Lactulose, side effects)
Gastrointestinal bleeding, 11, 54, 84, 100
Glucagon
and nitrogen metabolism, 41, 45-48
effect on ammonia liberation, 49
Gluconeogenesis and insulin, 46
Glutamate, 17, 25, 87
Glutamate-aspartate neurotransmitter system, 24
Glutamic acid, biochemical conversion of ammonia, 31-33
Glutamine, 16-20, 31-32, 34, 36-38, 42, 44-49
Glutamine/alanine ratio, 36
Glycogen depletion, 49

Hepatic encephalopathies, 3-12
Hepatocytes, perivenous, 15-26, 47-48
Hormonal control of ammonia and amino acids, 41-50

Hyperammonemia
in chronic liver disease, 49
in inborn errors of metabolism, 320
in newborn, 320
in Reye's syndrome, 8-12, 320
in urea cycle enzyme deficiencies, 319-320
Hyperinsulinism, 46
Hypernatremia, side effect of lactulose, 201-202

Insulin and nitrogen metabolism, 41, 45-50

Jamaica vomiting sickness, 10

Lactase,
deficiency, 114, 201, 255
in treatment of PSE, 97, 284-286
Lactic acid, metabolite of lactulose, 120-121, 178, 202
Lactitol, 221-241, 245-265
absorption, distribution, and excretion, 232-233
analytical method for determining, 227
bacterial metabolism of lactitol vs lactulose, 264
biochemical aspects, 232-236
caloric value, 234
chemical properties, 225-227
chemical structure, 221
compliance, 194, 199
effect
on blood ammonia, 249, 263
on blood glucose, 227
on colonic flora, 246
on dental caries, 236-238
on intestinal flora, 271-277
on laxation, 234-235
on serum cholesterol in rats, 233
on stools, 250
enema, 260
enzymatic hydrolysis, 233
fermentability, 238, 271-273
metabolic energy, 233-234
nitrogen concentration, changes in, 272-277
pH, changes in, 272-277
preparation, 222
physical properties, 222-225
safety monitoring, 261-263
side effects, 234, 250-255
studies, 246-263
sugar substitute, 238-241
tooth-protective properties, 236-238
toxicology, 228-232
treatment
constipation, 234, 310
diabetic patients, 227, 238-241
dental caries, 236-238
vs lactulose, 263-264
Lactobacillus acidophilus, 97, 283
Lactobacillus bifidus, effect of lactulose, 113, 315
Lactose, 114, 200, 283-298
absorption and colonic digestion by fecal flora, 286
digestion in lactase deficiency, 285
effect on mental state, 288-289
blood ammonia, 283-289
NCT, 288-289
PSE Index (PSEI), 288-289
enemas, 260, 294-298
pharmacology, 284-285
plus antacids
plus neomycin, 292
effect on PSE Index, 293
side effects, 284-285, 289
treatment of chronic PSE, 288-289
treatment with, vs lactitol
in PSE, 290-292
constipation, 310
Lactulose
absorption, 145-150
acidification of intestinal lumen, 108, 306-307
bacterial metabolism, 120-122, 153-158, 180-182
cathartic properties, 303-311
chemical structure, 221
clinical trials, 111-195
compliance, 199
concomitant medications, 204-205
contaminating sugars in, 267, 269
crystalline form, 199, 267-269
degradation, 153-159, 305-306
gas production, 305

short-chain fatty acids and, 305-306
lactic acid, 153-155
effect on
ammonia metabolism, 181
bile acids, 160-163, 333-339
blood glucose, 147
cholesteral metabolism, 160-163, 333-339
fecal pH, 117, 179
intestinal absorption, 160
intestinal flora, 271-277
intestinal pH, 121-122, 155, 272-277
intestinal transit time, 307
mental state, 268
Number Connection Test, 268-269
enemas, 58, 181
excretion, 159
exsorption, 150
fermentability, 271-273
laxative, 182, 202, 303-311
luminal osmolality, 306
mechanism of action, 305-307
metabolism in colon, 113-126
nitrogen concentration, changes in, 272-277
pediatrics
constipation, 318-319
diagnostic purposes, 315-318
hyperammonemia, 319-324
disorders of urea cycle enzymes, 319-324
inborn errors of metabolism, 320-324
infantile PSE, 319-324
Reye's syndrome, 320-324
transient hyperammonemia of newborn, 320-324
protein restriction, 320
pharmacology, 145-171
clinical, 177-184
plus neomycin, effect on stool pH, 213-214
polyps, prevention of recurrence of, 343-347
side effects, 120, 126, 168-171, 179, 182-183, 194, 199-205, 268-269, 310.
teratogenic effects in mice, 168
toxicology, 165-171
treatment of PSE, vs lactitol, 263-264

Mental state (*see* Lactitol, side effects; Lactose, side effects; Lactulose, side effects)
consciousness, 5
disturbances of, 5, 15
effects of lactose, 287
effects of lactulose, 192
effects of lactulose-neomycin, 213
effects of vegetable protein diet, 102-103
in urea cycle abnormalities, 18
intellectual function, 5
Mercaptans, 3, 18, 20
Metabolic acidosis, 4, 202
Metabolic alkalosis, 4, 90
Methanethiol, 4, 84
Methenamine, 87-88

Neomycin
combined with lactulose, 207-215
treatment of HE, 31
Neurotransmitters
excitatory/inhibitory, 17
false (weak), 19, 130
false neurotransmitter theory, 17, 20-21, 129
theory, 21-26
Nicotinohydroxamate, 87-86
Nitrogen balance, 99,
with branched-chain amino acids, 130
Nitrogen metabolism in gut, 31-40
endocrine aspects, 41
Number Connection Test (NCT) (*see also* Lactitol, side effects; Lactose, side effects; Lactulose, side effects)
diagnosing HE, 16
effects of lactose, 290-291
effects of lactulose-neomycin, 214
effects of vegetable protein diet, 102-103

Ornithine transcarbamylase deficiency, 6, 10
in Reye's syndrome, 320

pH
    intestinal, 85, 118, 122
    stool,
        effect of lactulose and neomycin, 210-212
        effect of lactulose, 118
        effect of pH gradient, 91
Pneumatosis coli, 183, 202
Pneumatosis intestinalis, 183, 202-203
Polyps, colon, prevention of recurrence of, 343-347
Portacaval anastomosis, 5
Portal-arterial differences of amino acids and ammonia, 33-35
Portal-systemic encephalopathy (*see* PSE)
Portal-systemic Encephalopathy Index (PSEI) (*see* PSE Index)
Portal-systemic shunting 3, 5, 37, 49, 90
Protein,
    blood, 101
    dairy, 96, 101
    dietary, 99
        cause of PSE, 12, 95
        in pathogenesis of PSE, 84, 95
        metabolism, 44
        restriction in management of PSE, 58, 100-102
    meat, 101
    vegetable, in management of chronic PSE, 88, 101-106
PSE
    clinical picture, 3-5
    combination therapy with lactulose and antibiotics, 207-215
    diagnosis, differential, 4, 12, 16
    EEG in, 3-4
    induction
        by azotemia, 11
        by blood, 97
        by catabolism, 38
        by diuretics, 11
        by exercise, 97
        by methionine, 208
    therapy theory, 83-92
    treatment
        antibiotics, 207
        antibiotics plus lactulose, 209-215
        enema (*see* Enema)
        L-dopa, 20, 90
        lactose, 97, 283-298
        lactulose, 177-184
PSE Index (PSEI)
    components of, 194
    effects of lactitol vs lactulose, 252-253
    effects of lactose, 290-291
    effects of lactulose, 194
Pseudo-PSE, 10-11
Psyllium, 105-108, 161

Reitan Trailmaking Test (*see* Number Con nection Test)
Reticular activating substance, 17, 18
Reye's syndrome, 4, 8-12

Sedative/tranquilizers, 205
    GABA concept and, 21-22
    in PSE, 11
Short-chain fatty acids, 4
    absorption in colon, 179
    ammonia toxicity and, 18, 20
    from degradation of blood, 84
Small bowel transit time, with lactulose, 178
Stool pH
    effects of lactose, 290, 292
    effects of lactulose-neomycin, 210-212

Toxin concept, 17-20
Tranquilizers, 4, 205
Travasorb®, 58

Urea, 42
    degradation rate, 211
    production rate, 211
    source of ammonia, 85
    synthesis, 47-48
Urea cycle, 10, 320
Urea cycle enzyme disorders, 5-7, 319-320
Urea nitrogen excretion, 47

Vitamin deficiencies in liver disease, 98
Volatile fatty acids, 117-122, 178
Vomiting (*see* Lactitol, side effects; Lactose, side effects; Lactulose, side effects)
Visual evoked potentials, 16, 22, 54, 64

Zinc, 97, 99